# PSYCHOSOCIAL ASPECTS OF HEALTH CARE
## Second Edition

### Meredith E. Drench, PhD, PT

*Director*
*Adaptive Health Associates, Inc.*
*East Greenwich, RI*
*Adjunct Faculty*
*Department of Physical Therapy*
*Northeastern University, Boston, MA*

### Ann Cassidy Noonan, EdD, PT

*Associate Professor*
*Academic Coordinator of Clinical Education*
*Department of Physical Therapy*
*Northeastern University, Boston, MA*

### Nancy Sharby, MS, PT

*Associate Clinical Specialist*
*Department of Physical Therapy*
*Northeastern University, Boston, MA*

### Susan Hallenborg Ventura, PhD, MEd, PT

*Associate Clinical Specialist*
*Director of Clinical Education*
*Department of Physical Therapy,*
*Northeastern University, Boston, MA*

PEARSON
Prentice
Hall

Upper Saddle River, New Jersey 07458

**Library of Congress Cataloging-in-Publication Data**

Psychosocial aspects of health care / Meredith E. Drench . . .
[et al.].—2nd ed.
   p. ; cm.
Includes bibliographical references and index.
   ISBN 0-13-171674-3
   1. Clinical health psychology.   2. Medical personnel and
patient.   3. Social medicine.
   [DNLM: 1. Delivery of Health Care.   2. Psychology,
Social.   3. Adaptation, Psychological.   4. Attitude to Health.
5. Communication.   6. Professional-Patient Relations.
W 84.1 P9743 2007]   I. Drench, Meredith E.
   R726.7.P7953 2007
   616.001$$$'9—dc22
                                                2005027623

Notice: The authors and the publisher of this volume have taken care that the information and technical recommendations contained herein are based on research and expert consultation, and are accurate and compatible with the standards generally accepted at the time of publication. Nevertheless, as new information becomes available, changes in clinical and technical practices become necessary. The reader is advised to carefully consult manufacturers' instructions and information material for all supplies and equipment before use, and to consult with a healthcare professional as necessary. This advice is especially important when using new supplies or equipment for clinical purposes. The authors and publisher disclaim all responsibility for any liability, loss, injury, or damage incurred as a consequence, directly or indirectly, of the use and application of any of the contents of this volume.

The names contained in the journal entries found in this book are fictitious. Any connection to real people is unintended.

Publisher: *Julie Levin Alexander*
Publisher's Assistant: *Regina Bruno*
Senior Editor: *Mark Cohen*
Assistant Editor: *Melissa Kerian*
Editorial Assistant: *Karen DePodwin*
Marketing Manager: *Harper Coles*
Marketing Coordinator: *Michael Sirinides*
Marketing Assistant: *Patricia Linard*
Director of Production and Manufacturing:
   *Bruce Johnson*
Production Managing Editor: *Patrick Walsh*
Production Liaison: *Christina Zingone*

Production Editor: *Jan Pushand/Pine Tree Composition, Inc.*
Manufacturing Manager: *Ilene Sanford*
Manufacturing Buyer: *Pat Brown*
Design Director: *Maria Guglielmo Walsh*
Cover Photo: *Getty Images/Photographer Susan Strayer*
Cover Designer: *Amy Rosen*
Composition: *Pine Tree Composition*
Printing and Binding: *R.R. Donnelley & Sons, Harrisonburg, VA*
Cover Printing: *Coral Graphics*

Pearson Education Ltd., *London*
Pearson Education Australia Pty, Limited, *Sydney*
Pearson Education Singapore, Pte. Ltd.
Pearson Education North Asia Ltd., *Hong Kong*
Pearson Education Canada, Ltd., *Toronto*

Pearson Educación de Mexico, S.A. de C.V.
Pearson Education—Japan, *Tokyo*
Pearson Education Malaysia, Pte. Ltd.
Pearson Education, *Upper Saddle River, New Jersey*

10  9  8  7  6  5  4  3  2  1
ISBN 0-13-171674-3

# Dedication

*To our clients, for teaching us the art of healing and reinforcing the need to integrate psychosocial concerns into our therapeutic interventions*

*To our colleagues, for their collaboration, mutual teaching, and learning*

*To our families, for supporting, loving, and sharing us with this project*

*To our students, that they may understand that a key ingredient for clinical competence and professional excellence is based on compassion and understanding*

# Contents

## 4   Understanding Family Needs, Roles, and Responsibilities   81

## Part II Goal-Setting: Client–Professional Collaboration　105

## 5　Client Rights and Provider Responsibilities　107

## Part V  Responses to Illness and Disability That Complicate Care    293

## 15  Chronic Illness    295

# Preface

*Psychosocial Aspects of Health Care* addresses a variety of integrated psychosocial topics, involving clients, families, and other caregivers affected by pathology, impairment, functional limitation, and/or disability. This book is intended for students in the health care professions, such as nurses, physical and occupational therapists, speech-language pathologists, physicians and physician assistants, respiratory therapists, social workers, and students in medical laboratory sciences. While it targets students, the text may also serve as a reference for those already practicing in their respective disciplines.

As a textbook, it could fit well into various levels of the curriculum wherever a course specifically addresses or includes psychosocial aspects of illness and disability, such as courses in social psychology of disability and rehabilitation, chronic illness, and rehabilitation psychology. This textbook would also be useful in courses that include issues in communication, family relationships, client-professional relationships, characteristics of illness and disability, adaptation to impairment and disability, manifestations of client behavior, grieving and adjusting to loss, sources of stress and support, and attitudinal and cultural differences. Therefore, it can be thought of as multilevel, being incorporated into basic, intermediate, and advanced courses.

We had three compelling reasons to write such a text. The primary purpose is to help readers understand that a key ingredient for clinical competence and professional excellence is the human factor. Second, we strongly believe in the need for clinicians to understand psychosocial aspects of health care so that they may best help patients/clients optimize their therapeutic outcomes. This foundation area is often overlooked or devalued in favor of the "hard-core" components of health care. Last, as educators with collectively over 100 years of experience with clients and students, we are concerned with the reported and perceived lack of students' interest in textbooks, level of readership, and appreciation of the importance of this subject in their treatment armamentarium. We believe that the style and approach of this book will hold the readers' attention and enhance their understanding of the material.

The book is divided into five parts, each subdivided into chapters. Relevant clinical examples are interspersed throughout every chapter, punctuating topic points. Student journal entries introduce and are entwined throughout every chapter, reinforcing the subject and identifying biases and "too-quick" conclusions. The description and reflection of realistic clinical situations add to the fabric of the discussion, creating a real-life case study, an actual client problem. Reflective Questions and Case Studies with topical questions, new in the second edition, conclude each chapter, allowing for individual musings, classroom discussion, small group exercises, and student assignments. Additional Readings are suggested to engage readers in further personal accounts, histories, and insights. Readers will develop self-awareness as they learn more about the psychosocial issues of health care.

Part I, "Understanding Client-Professional Relationships," addresses components of recognizing your own beliefs and values as a health provider; communication; cultural aspects of therapeutic care; and understanding family needs, roles, and responsibilities. Part II, "Goal-Setting: Client-Professional Collaboration," explores quality of life, clients' rights and provider responsibilities, motivation and adherence, collaborative treatment planning, and the mind-body-spirit connection. Part III, "Changing Perspectives," discusses body image and self-concept, condition-specific characteristics, and sexuality. Part IV, "The Continuum of Loss, Grief, and Adjustment," delves into understanding loss, grief, and adjustment as related to disease, disability, and death. Finally, Part V, "Responses to Illness and Disability That Complicate Care," considers chronic illness, psychiatric disorders, and destructive behaviors.

Because readers of this text come from many health care disciplines, each with its own jargon, we have had to make editorial decisions for the sake of consistency. We have used "client" to name those with whom we work. "Caregiver" refers to personal caregivers and may be family, friends, or others with caregiving responsibilities. Variations of "health care professionals" and "health care providers" represent the readership, those who have chosen to make a career of providing care. Examples of clients and caregivers reflect both the diversity and lifespan issues inherent in today's health care environment. Similarly, the health professions and the students in the journal entries also depict our changing world.

This second edition includes updated information and references, where applicable, a change in sequencing of some of the chapters and parts, an integration of some topics with others, and an expansion and addition of some areas. The pedagogical alterations, including the addition of Case Studies with topical questions at the end of each chapter, are based on our own experience and the feedback of other faculty and students who have used this text in learning about psychosocial aspects of health care.

# Acknowledgments

A work of this nature is not created in a vacuum. We express our thanks and gratitude to all those who have helped us in our journey toward the publication of this book. Throughout our lives, many have nurtured us, taught us how to nurture others, and provided lessons in the costs and rewards of caregiving.

Special thanks to our families and friends, who supported us throughout this project. They have forgiven our occasional absences from social events and family meals, as well as late hours spent at the computer, rather than in front of the fire.

We also thank the many educators who have facilitated our development, including George Goldin, Ruthie Hall, Ruth Purtilo, Shirley Stockmeyer, Fran Tappan, and Marie Winston. They helped shape our ability to provide skilled and compassionate care that is based on a strong moral and ethical foundation.

We are grateful for the review and critique of selected material by David Karp, PhD, Professor, Department of Sociology at Boston College, for his encouragement; David Borrelli, MD, Psychiatrist, Massachusetts General Hospital, for his time, wisdom, and clarification of the psychiatric concepts described in Part V; and Ronnie Leavitt, PhD, PT, Professor, Department of Physical Therapy at the University of Connecticut, whose expertise in multicultural settings was invaluable in the preparation of Chapter 3. We appreciate the insights of the people at the Manic Depressive-Depressive Association, McLean Hospital Chapter, whose struggles and successes of living with mental illness remind us of the resilience of the human spirit.

We also acknowledge the members of our professional communities, who challenge and guide us. Northeastern University, in particular, facilitated this endeavor by providing a climate conducive to intellectual pursuits. Special thanks to our work-study students for the hours spent "in the stacks" and to Meredith Harris, EdD, PT, for her administrative support.

Finally, we recognize Mark Cohen, Executive Editor and Melissa Kerian, Associate Editor at Prentice Hall, for their belief in this project and its valuable contribution to health care.

# Reviewers

## Reviewers of the Second Edition

**Debbie Amini**
Occupational Therapy Assistant Program
Cape Fear Community College
Wilmington, North Carolina

**Kimberly K. Cleary, PhD, PT**
Associate Professor of Physical Therapy
Idaho State University
Pocatello, Idaho

**Yolanda Griffiths, OTD, OTR/L, FAOTA**
Department of Occupational Therapy
Creighton University Medical Center
Omaha, Nebraska

**Larry Chinnock, PT, EdD, MBA**
Department of Physical Therapy
Loma Linda University
Loma Linda, California

**Harriet Lewis, PT, MS**
Academic Coordinator of Clinical Education
Physical Therapy Program
Angelo State University
San Angelo, Texas

**Cathy Hinton, PhD, PT**
Associate Professor
School of Physical Therapy
Belmont University
Nashville, Tennesse

## Reviewers of the First Edition

**Denise Abrams, PT, MASS**
Physical Therapist Assistant Program
Broome Community College
Binghamton, New York

**Sherry Borcherding, MA, OTR/L**
Associate Professor
Department of Occupational Therapy
University of Missouri
Columbia, Missouri

**Donna Calvert, PhD, PT**
Professor
Physical Therapy Education Department
Rockhurst University
Kansas City, Missouri

**Peggy DeCelle Newman, PT, MHR**
Program Director and Professor
Physical Therapist Assistant Program
Oklahoma City Community College
Oklahoma City, Oklahoma

**Elaine Eckel, PT, MA**
Department Chair
Physical Therapist Assistant Program
Fayetteville Technical Community College
Fayetteville, North Carolina

**Joan E. Edelstein, MA, PT, FISPO**
Special Lecturer
Program in Physical Therapy
Columbia University
New York, New York

# Part I

# *Understanding Client-Professional Relationships*

Extensive knowledge about health care practices is obtained in the classroom. We are taught anatomy, physiology, and how to examine and assess clients' abilities and develop a plan of care. In addition, in order to efficiently treat clients, we must effectively communicate with them and develop a sense of rapport.

Part I focuses on the skills required to develop effective client-professional relationships. As individuals, we develop personal beliefs and attitudes at a very early age. Our values are usually influenced by what our parents taught us, as well as our cultural context. These may expand and change as we mature and meet new people. As we enter a health profession, we are also expected to embrace professional values. People tend to feel more comfortable with those who are like themselves. In Chapter 1, readers learn to recognize their own beliefs and values and identify ways these affect attitudes and behaviors toward others. The concepts of overt and covert stigma, prejudice, and discrimination in health care delivery are explored. Tolerance, mutual respect, appreciation, and teamwork are also explained.

Chapter 2 discusses the importance of communication, including using "people-first" language and being mindful, or present, in the moment. Components of communication, such as vocabulary, paralanguage, active listening, and nonverbal communication, are presented. Barriers to effective communication and strategies for overcoming them are identified.

Conflict is also examined. Despite negative connotations of conflict, it has both positive and negative elements. Managed effectively, conflict can lead to beneficial changes and help clinicians develop problem-solving strategies that may result in improved client care. Personal, interpersonal, and intragroup conflicts are explored and components and sources of conflict defined. Readers will learn about the advantages and disadvantages of different strategies to manage conflict. Methods for conflict negotiation and mediation are also presented.

Health care providers interact on a regular basis with clients, families, colleagues, insurance providers, and others. Appreciating diversity and respecting human differences are necessary components of health care delivery, particularly when we encounter individuals from a culture that differs from our own or when values and priorities are in conflict with ours.

The United States is a nation that is rich in diversity, made up of people from different races, ethnic groups, cultures, and lifestyles. To provide effective health care services, we need to put aside some of our own values, attitudes, and behaviors to accommodate the enormous variations presented by clients and families with whom we work. It may be difficult to embrace health practices that seem to be based more on history or tradition than on science or to accept the belief that an imbalance between mind, body, and spirit may cause disease. However, we must learn to understand and respect the beliefs and practices of people from other cultures in order to develop collaborative relationships that meet the diverse needs of our clients.

In Chapter 3, we present information on race, cultures, and ethnicity and examine how they affect our relationships with clients. A client's worldview may be quite different from our own, and failure to appreciate these differences can present barriers to effective cross-cultural interaction. Understanding basic differences in worldview can help us reframe our attitudes and offer more culturally congruent therapeutic recommendations. The culture of medicine is also explored in this chapter. Strategies for bridging the gap between traditional Western medical care and the care that clients from other cultures may desire or expect are described.

In today's health care environment, the need for interdependence and teamwork is evident. Health providers need to be aware of their own biases and prejudices and accept the value systems of others if they are going to provide culturally sensitive health care.

Chapter 4 helps readers understand that when people develop an illness or disability, their life-roles change, either temporarily or permanently. As a result, the roles of family members and friends may also be altered. Health care professionals need to understand individual family members' responsibilities when caring for a child, spouse, parent, or sibling. The concept of caregiver burden and ways to minimize it are introduced.

Developing an open and trusting relationship with a client enhances your effectiveness as a caregiver. This process requires patience, understanding, and active listening.

# 1

# *Recognizing Beliefs and Values*

I was sitting in the conference room today, waiting for our team meeting to begin. I couldn't believe the discussion that was going on. Mrs. Garjulo had been admitted last night with a left hip fracture, secondary to falling out of bed. Apparently, she was well known to the staff, with a long history of obesity, diabetes, coronary artery disease, and arthritis. She was now scheduled to undergo surgery. I couldn't believe what the staff members were saying. One of them actually said it was her own fault, and she deserved what she got.

Angie, the nutritionist, stated, "I've worked with her over and over again. I've explained the importance of a balanced diet to her, but she just doesn't listen. She always loses weight while she's in the hospital, but as soon as she's home, she's back to her old habits of eating candy, ice cream, and cookies. The pounds go right back on. I've warned her that it's affecting her health, but she doesn't seem to care."

Pam, the physical therapist, said, "I'm glad I'm rotating to the outpatient department tomorrow. I would hate to be the one to have to get her out of bed and walking. She's so big! She only fits into one of the wheelchairs in the hospital. Every time she's admitted, I end up wasting time trying to find it."

At that point, the charge nurse arrived, and the conference began. All day long, I kept thinking about poor Mrs. Garjulo. Imagine how she would feel if she knew what the staff thought about her. I've always been a few pounds overweight myself, but I've never thought too much of it. Now, I began to wonder if others talked about me behind my back.

—*From the journal of Donald Spencer, occupational therapy student*

As health care professionals, we are presumed to treat all individuals with respect and dignity. Codes of ethics provide us with a list of professional values and describe ethical responsibilities we are expected to uphold. It is important to recognize, however, that as we enter into therapeutic relationships, we, as well as our clients, do so having developed our own personality, temperament, natural abilities, and talents. Lessons we learned in life shape the way we view the world and define us as the unique individuals we are. Understanding ourselves and our clients with all of our strengths and limitations is an important personal and professional lesson. We begin to develop personal values at a very early age. Parents, extended families, society, schools, and culture all serve to mold and shape personal values. People tend to be more comfortable when they are with individuals who are similar to themselves. While hesitant to admit it, we all have personal biases. We may be aware of some, but others exist in our subconscious minds. Both overt and covert prejudices can affect our interactions with clients and colleagues. When we are aware of our biases, we are less likely to make inappropriate or incorrect judgments about others.

This chapter discusses the importance of recognizing our own beliefs and values and identifying the ways in which they affect our attitudes and behaviors. Developing awareness helps us avoid discrimination. The importance of valuing interdisciplinary viewpoints and working together as teams is emphasized. Recommendations to promote cultural awareness and team-building among health care professionals are included.

# Understanding Values

"The less a person understands his own feelings, the more he will fall prey to them. The less a person understands the feelings, the responses, and the behavior of others, the more likely he will interact inappropriately with them" (Gardner, 1993, p. 254). To develop a sense of self, every individual needs to develop both intrapersonal and interpersonal intelligence. Intrapersonal intelligence involves developing an understanding of one's own feelings and emotions. Interpersonal intelligence includes understanding the feelings, behaviors, and motivations of those around you (Gardner, 1993). It is by developing a sense of self that someone is able to grow, mature, and interact intelligently and appropriately in society. In order to do this, a person must also begin to understand his or her own value system.

Values are strong beliefs and attitudes about the worth of a thought, idea, object, or course of action (Purtilo & Haddad, 1996). These beliefs and attitudes develop during our formative years, as parents teach us their values, and we learn what is important to them. These values may include religious beliefs, honesty, the importance of a good education, a strong work ethic, and/or taking care of family. Socioeconomic status and culture influence our value systems. What is valued in one culture may not be universal. Personal values vary between individuals. It is important to note that values change or evolve over time. As children mature and meet new people, they encounter outside influences. Family values are examined and questioned as young adults begin to make their own decisions about what is important. Understanding your personal value system increases self-awareness and promotes personal growth (Schoenly, 1994).

When an individual enters a health profession, he or she is expected to embrace professional values. Formulated over many years, professional values express ideals that members of the organization believe are important, such as punctuality, competency, and courtesy. They are also reflected in professional ethics and are typically presented in the form of a code of ethics. Principles, such as autonomy, beneficence, justice, nonmaleficence, and equal distribution of resources are codified and interpreted (Kasar & Clark, 2000; Nosse, Friberg, & Kovacek, 1999). See Chapter 5 to explore this further.

In determining how to most effectively treat individual clients, health care providers recognize that they will not be able to serve all of these principles equally at all times. When there is a short supply of resources and high demand, decisions need to be made to determine who receives the limited assets. Priorities and decisions that achieve a balance of these principles and serve the best interest of the clients are made in conjunction with clients, families, and other health care providers.

Sometimes, the values of a health professional are in conflict with those of clients or colleagues. It is the provider's responsibility to respect clients' and colleagues' values, while maintaining his or her own personal values (Seroka, 1994). For example, consider Mrs. Mahoney, who has been receiving treatments for several months for cancer. She calls the clinic and indicates that she has decided to terminate conventional therapy and substitute herbal treatments. You may believe that this will be detrimental to her health and explain why she should continue treatments. However, she insists on her new course of action. While you may disagree with her decision and rationale, you need to respect her right to make her own decisions regarding her health care.

# Attitudes and Behavior

Values, socioeconomic and cultural background, and attitudes of health care professionals affect interactions with clients and colleagues. These attitudes are favorable or unfavorable emotions or sentiments toward people that strongly predict behavior toward those individuals (Greenwald & Banaji, 1995). Although we may believe that we are unbiased and treat all individuals fairly, hidden or covert biases may emerge.

People within a particular group tend to share common values, habits, and customs, which they may not share with those from outside the group (Erlen, 1998). Individuals often feel more comfortable with people who they perceive are similar to themselves and favor members of their own social group (Brewer, 1979; Sumner, 1906). Favoritism for like individuals is so well-imbedded in people's value systems that pronouns such as "us" are more favorably valued than those such as "them" (Perdue, Dovidio, Gurtman, & Tyler, 1990). Social behavior often operates in an unconscious manner, and people may not realize that past experiences affect future judgments. This supports the findings that people who adamantly disavow prejudice have been shown to discriminate against others (Bargh, 1994; Greenwald & Banaji, 1995).

Are we unknowingly prejudiced? How do we determine who we will help and who we will avoid? Weiner (1980) found that individuals are more inclined to help others when they perceive that people seeking help have no control over their situation. In a series of experiments, individuals approached and helped someone who had fallen when that person was carrying a cane and appeared to have a disability. In contrast, they avoided a person in the same situation who appeared intoxicated. Human nature may foster feelings of helping for a person who appears to be "innocently" ill but not for someone who may be responsible for his or her condition. Do you have less empathy for a client diagnosed with liver failure if there is a history of alcohol abuse? Conversely, do you care more for an individual dying from lung cancer if you know that person never smoked?

# Stigma and Prejudice in Health Care Delivery

The term stigma has a negative connotation and refers to someone or something that is not highly valued. Goffman (1963) identified three classes of stigmatization: physical deformities, character deficits, and "tribal" stigma, related to race, national origin, or religion. People frequently stereotype stigmatized individuals or groups. As a result, erroneous assumptions are made. Stereotyping can lead to avoidance and lack of respect for those who are stigmatized. Studies show that health care professionals frequently stigmatize and discriminate against individuals or groups who have certain diagnoses or come from different cultures (Brink, 1994; Crisp, Gelder, Rix, Meltzer, & Rowlands, 2000; Davies, 2000; Erlen, 1998; Kaminski & Harty, 1999; Minkoff, 1997; Ritson, 1999). Recognizing personal bias, understanding cultural differences, and avoiding stigmatization and discrimination are important components of providing effective health care. This section describes many common personal biases. Developing awareness of biases can help reduce stereotyping and discrimination and increase appreciation for diversity and respect for all clients and colleagues.

## Blaming the Clients

As a result of advances in health care, risk factors for many illnesses have been identified. Some are within a person's control, such as cigarette smoking, substance abuse, obesity, sedentary lifestyle, multiple sex partners, and failure to wear seat belts (Gunderman, 2000). Consequently, some health care providers "blame" clients for their illnesses or conditions because they failed to take responsibility for their personal well-being. However, other factors are involved: Socioeconomic, cultural, educational, and geographical influences all affect behaviors. We may lose patience and blame those who overreact to illness or who fail to recognize they are sick and wait until it is too late to seek help. When unable to "cure" a client, it is sometimes easier to say the client "failed to respond to treatment," when in truth we may have failed to find a cure. Are we uncomfortable or avoid clients with chronic illnesses? Often the answer is a resounding "yes."

Do we try to separate ourselves from our clients, forming an "us" and "them" mentality? Many practitioners prefer clients who are in better health (Hall, Epstein, DeCiantis, & Mc-Neil, 1993). Therefore, "sicker" clients may receive less time and attention from their health care providers, resulting in a detrimental effect on health outcomes. Individuals with chronic illnesses typically report that although they have a thorough knowledge of their symptoms, conditions, and needs, health care providers often ignore their input. Clients with diabetes, who have been monitoring their own insulin intake at home for many years, have serious conflicts with health care professionals regarding their insulin dosages while they are hospitalized. Others state that health professionals "ridiculed" them when they presented their own theories about what exacerbated their symptoms. Clients with long-term problems were often labeled as "complainers." Health care providers maintained a distance, attending to clients' medical concerns but avoiding their psychosocial needs. Perhaps this behavior is the result of frustration experienced by health care professionals because they cannot "cure" clients with chronic illnesses (Minkoff, 1997; Thorne, Nyhlin, & Paterson, 2000).

The role of health care professionals is not to blame but to assist clients with their illnesses or disabilities. While it is appropriate to inform clients as to how their habits may be jeopardizing their health, "blaming the victim can inhibit care-seeking, erode hope, and undermine the therapeutic alliance between clients and health professionals" (Gunderman, 2000, p. 10).

## Cultural Bias

Culture includes the values, language, beliefs, and customs shared by a group of people (Dennis, 1997). As individuals grow and develop, cultural values, beliefs, and customs are incorporated into their lives. This enculturation influences behaviors and attitudes (Erlen, 1998). Sumner (1906) first introduced the term ethnocentrism to describe the phenomenon in which people of one culture see themselves as part of the "us" or "we" group and those of another culture as part of the "them" or "out" group. As discussed earlier, there is a normal tendency for people to view members of their own group more favorably than members of the "out" group. Ethnocentrism is a normal part of development, and children as young as 6 years old have been shown to be ethnocentric (Nyatanga, 1998). As a result of ethnocentrism, health professionals may be knowingly or unknowingly biased toward individuals from other cultures, a situation that could create prejudicial health care practices.

It is important to recognize that within every large culture, there are a number of smaller subcultures. Members of each subculture have their own value systems that may differ from those of another subculture (Erlen, 1998). Within the United States, there are distinct subcultures based on gender, age, race, religion, ethnicity, and sexual orientation. Individuals may belong to more than one subculture. Members of one subculture may have difficulty relating to those of another, even though they both belong to the same larger culture. To provide culturally competent care, health care professionals need to develop an understanding and respect for these differences. However, this does not always occur.

Following interviews with nurses caring for culturally diverse clients, Kirkham (1998) discovered that nurses' attitudes and behaviors toward their clients ranged from being resistant to caring for clients to being impassioned about their work. Resistant nurses considered cultural differences as an inconvenience or problem. Their knowledge regarding other cultures was limited and based on negative stereotyping. They ignored requests based on cultural values and practiced both overt and covert racism. The nurses were frequently overheard complaining about clients.

Further along the continuum were nurses who provided what Kirkham (1998) termed "generalist" care. They gave respectful and individualized care to all clients. While their knowledge of other cultures was also based on generalizations and stereotyping, their attitudes were positive. Although they admitted seeing discrimination practiced by their colleagues, they chose to accept it rather than address it.

The nurses who provided culturally diverse clients with "impassioned" care went beyond accommodation to an appreciation of diversity. They did not stereotype patients but saw each as an individual with varying needs. Having knowledge about or working with people from other cultures seemed to promote what these nurses called an "awakening" to the need for culturally sensitive care. The researcher concluded that, although the nursing profession pays great attention to issues related to cultural diversity, the goal of culturally sensitive care remains in the distant future (Kirkham, 1998). Understanding cultural differences and respecting diversity is further explored in Chapter 3.

## Gender Bias

The Society for the Advancement of Women's Health Research was founded in 1990 to bring national attention to the problem of gender bias in health care research and to promote a women's health research agenda (Greenberger, 1999). Until that time, women's health issues were largely ignored. Most medical research focused on a white male population, and findings could not be generalized to a larger, diverse, clinical population, including women (Marrocco & Stewart, 2001). Although more women are entering the field of medicine today, generations of gender inequities in health care have not yet been eliminated (Cohen, 1999).

In the past, the major focus on women's health issues was reproduction. Today, there is an emphasis on providing comprehensive care for women, including both physical and mental health. However, in reviews of the literature regarding health care, a number of deficiencies related to women's health were found regarding both topic and content. Few studies made reference to the gender of clients. Most were based on standards related to manifestations of diseases in men. Therefore, it was difficult to determine whether the results could be generalized to a female population. Erroneous assumptions could be made that men's health status is the "norm," and women's health status is a "deviation from the norm." When a topic was covered, important implications specific to women's health issues were not addressed. For example, in describing rheumatoid arthritis, key information was often missing about how the use of oral contraceptives, hormone replacement therapy, or pregnancy might affect the disease process (Nicolette & Jacobs, 2000).

As a result of these findings, several problems were identified. It is important for all health care professionals to recognize that men and women respond differently to disease processes and present varying symptoms. In addition, since women's complaints often differ from men's, systemic problems might be overlooked. Gender-specific, evidence-based information needs to be made available to women and their physicians. Researchers have become aware of the importance of including women in medical studies, but they frequently fail to analyze the data according to gender.

Failure to distinguish the differences between men's and women's symptoms perpetuates gender bias in health care (Marrocco & Stewart, 2001; Nicolette & Jacobs, 2000). Consider heart disease, which has traditionally been regarded as primarily affecting men. Today, we know this is not true. The incidence of cardiovascular disease among women is now recognized as a major challenge and is the leading cause of death among older women. However, symptoms of angina and myocardial infarction in women do not conform to the classic symptoms described by men. Women are more likely to present with nausea or pain in the back, jaw, or neck. Because these are not the chief symptoms emphasized in the media, women may misinterpret their symptoms and not seek health care. Health care providers may also mistake these atypical symptoms as being noncardiac related. This could prevent early intervention and result in treatment delay (Goodman & Kirwan, 2001; Wenger, 1999).

Existing gender bias in the diagnosis and referral rates for coronary artery disease in women results in the perception that women have less exertional angina than men. This is not true (Goodman & Kirwan, 2001). In addition, women with symptoms similar to those of men are less likely to be referred for cardiac catheterization than are men (Nicolette & Jacobs, 2000; Schulman et al., 1999; Weitzman et al., 1997). Men are also counseled more frequently about the importance of exercise, diet, and weight control in avoiding heart disease. If women are unaware of the fact that they are at risk, they may be less likely to take preventive measures (Wenger, 1999).

It is also interesting to note that a study of internists at a health maintenance organization found that male physicians liked male clients better than female clients (Hall et al., 1993). Why might this be true? In comparing men and women, Gilligan (1982) stated that women use a language of "caring and relationships," while men use one of "justice and rights." It has also been suggested that male physicians might have difficulty interpreting their female clients' complaints. Women are more likely to include affective comments in describing their symptoms. This communication gap may foster gender bias (Hatala & Case, 2000). In an attempt to eliminate attitudinal bias among male physicians, many medical schools now include women's health curricula, which presents physical, behavioral, and psychological effects related to gender. It has been shown that these types of programs do improve students' ability to appropriately assess women's health status (Hatala & Case, 2000).

As discussed in Chapter 5, health care has moved from a medical model based on paternalism to one based on client autonomy. In this system, communication and collaboration between clients and health care professionals is critical. Clients need to be informed and included in decision making. Studies show that female physicians spend more time with their clients and facilitate partnerships with them more often than male physicians. They are also less verbally dominant during interactions. While the researchers do not suggest that all female physicians communicate better than their male counterparts, they note the findings are statistically significant and should send a message to all health care providers (Roter & Hall, 1998). Whether men or women, we must ensure that we take the time to listen to all clients. We also need to guard against dismissing women's complaints just because they do not fit into predetermined categories. Despite recent gains in identifying women's health issues, societal stereotyping and gender bias still exist.

## Ageism

Hattie Williams worked part time as a fashion designer, right up until her stroke 3½ weeks ago. I'm totally amazed at how sharp she is! She has a quick wit and is the "youngest" 84-year-old person I've ever met.

Yesterday, I commented on the new bathrobe she was wearing. She wrinkled her nose and said, "My daughter-in-law bought it for me. She's very sweet and means well, but this is for an old lady. It's too frumpy! I'd have picked one that is stylish."

I see her improve everyday, and she's able to do more independently. We've been discussing where she might go after discharge. Although her son wants to bring her into his home, the doctor thinks she should go to a nursing home

> "because she's 84 and has had a stroke." Hattie, however, wants to go to her own house. I hope they don't make this decision based on age alone.
> —*From the journal of Diane Patel, social work student*

In a society that emphasizes youth and beauty, the tendency to view aging in a negative light is common. There are fewer positive images in the media of older people, especially older women. As a result, some older individuals fear declining health and the potential lack of independence. Yet, many older adults maintain health and independence well into their 90s and beyond. Chronological age is not necessarily a reflection of biological age (Shortt, 2001). However, health care professionals, perhaps because of their frequent exposure to older clients who are "ill," have been shown to be particularly susceptible to ageism, and caring for the elderly is often an unpopular career choice (Kearney, Miller, Paul, & Smith, 2000).

Unfortunately, "a client's age is often inappropriately used as a factor to choose treatment options" (Madan, Aliabadi-Wahle, & Beech, 2001, p. 282). Chronological age has been used as one criterion for discontinuing life support. Underrepresentation of older clients in research studies has been shown to lead to health care decisions based on assumptions, observations, past experiences, and bias rather than on evidence-based practice (Kearney et al., 2000).

Older clients are sometimes not offered the same medical treatments as younger clients (Madan et al., 2001). While biological factors and comorbidities may limit the use of certain procedures, ageism may also influence the options offered to older clients. In one study, researchers found that when treating clients diagnosed with breast cancer, second-year medical students did not offer the same options regarding breast reconstruction to clients over age 59 as they did to those under age 31. However, they would choose the option they suggested to younger clients if they or their family members were placed in a similar situation (Madan et al., 2001). Health professionals must guard against such stereotyping. Decisions need to be made using evidence-based criteria, not the health care provider's attitudes and beliefs. Regardless of client age, all available options need to be presented to clients, and they should be included in determining which treatment option is the best one for them (Shortt, 2001).

As discussed in Chapter 4, older adults represent the fastest growing population in the United States, and their needs for health care services are expanding. Many older adults complain that in today's managed care system, doctor–client communication suffers due to productivity demands and time constraints. Older clients tend to have more complex medical problems and may require more time and attention. However, as we have discussed, some practitioners prefer healthier clients to their sick counterparts (Hall et al., 1993). These factors can cultivate bias against older clients. As a result of subtle or not so subtle ageism, older adults may find themselves at risk for passive relationships with their health care providers (Roter, 2000). In fact, gerontologists concur that prejudice against older people in the United States is a major problem (Palmore, 1999).

A review of the literature regarding younger adults' attitudes toward older adults confirms that, in general, some negative stereotypes do exist. However, studies show that older adults are viewed as multidimensional people with both positive and negative attributes (Slotterback & Saarnio, 1996). Feldman (1999) found that although most of the older women he contacted had good relationships with their health care providers, they also experienced subtle biases by some health professionals. Study participants offered the following suggestions for improvement:

- Encourage health care providers to view elderly clients as individuals.
- Avoid stereotyping and patronizing comments.
- Take time to listen to each person's concerns.
- Respond to clients' complex medical and psychosocial needs in a language they can understand.

In addition, avoid using negative terms to describe older people, such as "deteriorating." It is more appropriate to use neutral or positive terms, such as "senior," "elder," "retired person," or "veteran" (Palmore, 2000).

## Ethnic Bias

While the population in the United States continues to grow increasingly diverse, "segregation, disparate treatment, and racism continue to contribute to the epidemiologic gap between minorities and whites. The significant underrepresentation of minorities in the health professions and in the health care industry is one reason behind the disparity" (Gonzales, Gooden, & Porter, 2000, p. 56).

Ethnicity also affects the course of illness, treatment availability, and medical outcomes. It is important to study the impact of ethnicity on health care for several reasons. Ethnic background influences health and susceptibility to various diseases. Medical treatments, including drug therapy, may be more or less effective depending upon the client's ethnic background. Ethnicity also affects communication: What is said may not always be what is heard (Dimsdale, 2000).

While it is expected that health professionals examine and evaluate all clients objectively, a review of the literature indicates that this does not always exist. Due to time constraints, work overload, and ethnocentrism, stereotyping of clients does occur. As a result, clients may be treated differently depending upon their race and socioeconomic status. In a survey of client–doctor encounters, doctors rated black clients as being of lower intelligence and at higher risk for noncompliance with rehabilitation than white clients. In addition, the doctors perceived black clients to be less rational and pleasant than white clients. The researchers conclude that it may be unrealistic to assume that practitioners can completely avoid stereotyping. However, they stress the need for interventions to reduce stereotyping and offer recommendations. More training is needed to make health care providers more conscious of the effects of stereotyping. In addition, organizational changes can help reduce stress to allow time to elicit and absorb individual client information and incorporate it into treatment plans (van Ryn & Burke, 2000).

While ethnicity influences client–practitioner communication, it also influences decisions regarding diagnostic tests and interventions. In a study comparing clients with identical medical histories, women of color were less likely to be perceived as having coronary artery disease and referred for cardiac catheterization than any other clients (Dimsdale, 2000; Schulman et al., 1999).

There are many erroneous assumptions about the effect of ethnicity on pain tolerance. In a study of 250 clients who had undergone open reduction and fixation of an extremity fracture, white clients received significantly more narcotics than did Hispanic or black clients. To receive medication, clients had to first request it, and a nurse had to respond and agree that medication was warranted. The researchers wondered what, if anything, was influencing these ethnic variations. In an attempt to answer this question, they conducted a second study in which clients self-administered medication through a bedside pump. Hispanic and Asian clients received less pain medication than either black or white clients. Differences among both groups of clients were not attributed to injury, severity, or social class. However, it was determined that the doctors had preprogrammed the pumps differently, so that the Hispanic and Asian clients received less medication than black or white clients. It appeared that the doctors had predetermined the client's need for pain medication based on ethnicity rather than illness. The physicians were not even aware of their behavior (Dimsdale, 2000).

Covert bias can affect future health care professionals as well as clients. Physical therapy students are required to complete clinical education experiences as part of their educational programs. Faculty rely on physical therapy practitioners to evaluate student competencies. In one study, students were videotaped reciting identical scripts about one client's status. A group of physical therapists was then asked to rate the students' abilities on several measurement criteria. The black student consistently received lower ratings than the white, Hispanic, or Asian students (Haskins, Rose-St. Prix, & Elbaum, 1997). It would appear that ethnic bias influenced the opinions of the physical therapy practitioners involved in the study.

Race-associated differences in health outcomes are routinely documented in this country but are poorly explained. Jones (2000) attributes these differences to racism, which can exist on three levels: institutional, personal, and internalized. Institutionalized racism is defined as differential access to opportunities, goods, and services. As a result of institutionalized racism, members of one race may have inadequate access to education, employment, and medical facilities. They would receive poorer quality medical care, if they received care at all.

Personally mediated racism is defined as prejudice and discrimination toward others based on their race. This can be intentional or unintentional and includes both acts of commission and omission. As a result of personally mediated racism, one may show lack of respect toward another. This, too, could negatively affect one's ability to administer or receive adequate health care.

Internalized racism is acceptance of the perception by members of one race that they are not as good as people of another race. As a result of internalized racism, someone may have a lower level of self-esteem, perhaps evidenced by dropping out of school or engaging in risky health practices. While we must address racism at every level, it is most important to eliminate institutionalized racism. If that can be eliminated, the other forms of racism will, hopefully, disappear over time (Jones, 2000).

People who have experienced discrimination in the past are more likely to blame current hardships on those events. This can lead to high stress levels that negatively affect health outcomes (Clark, Anderson, Clark, & Williams, 1999). In today's global economy, there is a great need for health care professionals to develop an understanding and respect for clients of all cultures. It is important to emphasize diversity training with both developing therapists and students. By the year 2040, it is estimated that over half of the population of the United States will be made up of ethnic minorities (Brooks, 2001). To support culturally sensitive health care, we need to recruit individuals from a variety of ethnic groups into the health care professions. In addition, health care providers can be encouraged to learn a second language to better prepare for communication with their clients. In locations where it is feasible, students may want to volunteer their services assisting individuals from other cultures. This would allow them the opportunity to immerse themselves in the culture and give them time to begin to know the people and their customs.

## HIV and AIDS Bias

People living with human immunodeficiency virus (HIV) and acquired immune deficiency syndrome (AIDS) are subjected to discrimination within the health care system. Attitudes toward clients with HIV and AIDS may be influenced by race, socioeconomic status, gender, sexual orientation, and their positive-HIV status (Bunting, 1996). In one study, many women who were HIV-positive tried to hide their diagnosis from others in an attempt to protect themselves and their family members from being stigmatized. They hid their medications so that no one knew they were sick. When symptoms were apparent, they endeavored to cover them up, suggesting they had diseases they did not have rather than admitting to being infected with HIV. They also avoided participating in support groups because of a fear of being discovered. While some of the clients indicated that their health providers were supportive, provided them with information, and addressed their concerns, others complained of a lack of acceptance by health professionals. The women indicated that their health care providers commonly avoided looking at or touching them. These behaviors caused the clients to feel further stigmatized (Ingram & Hutchinson, 1999).

> Touching becomes very important to me, being able to hold people and be caring. This has been unique for me. I've been a psychiatric nurse for a long time, and touching is not a normal part of what I do with patients. Touching the client is a big difference in working with people with HIV (Drench, 1998, p. 165).

In the early 1990s, many professionals considered leaving health care because of perceived risks of HIV infection (Jemmott, Jemmott, & Crus-Collins, 1992). Although they face transmission risks from hepatitis, tuberculosis, and HIV, it is frequently the perception of risk more than the actual risk that results in fear and avoidance (Drench, 1996). Although knowledge regarding the transmission of HIV has improved, fear of contagion remains a major concern among health care workers. This is a strong predictor of unwillingness to provide care to clients with AIDS, regardless of health care providers' educational background. It seems that only increasing cognitive knowledge about AIDS and infection control may not always influence fears of contagion or reluctance to treat clients with AIDS (Kemppainen, Dubbert, & McWilliams, 1996). Clarification of values and attitudes, as well as knowledge and skills, is also beneficial in improving emotional responses to HIV/AIDS.

Improvements are being made, albeit slowly. In a recent study of nurse practitioners, certified nurse midwives, and physician assistants, more than 80 percent of the respondents indicated they would provide care to clients infected with HIV (Martin & Bedimo, 2000). Respondents who indicated they would refer clients to other practitioners indicated they would do so primarily because of their lack of experience and the availability of more experienced providers rather than because they chose not to treat clients who were HIV-positive.

As with other stigmatized conditions, self-awareness of potential bias is important. When health professionals ask clients how they became infected, the clinicians need to know why they are asking. Is it out of curiosity about the client's lifestyle, or is it to enable them to provide more effective client education? Will a health provider's attitude toward a client change if the client was infected as the result of a blood transfusion rather than as the result of using a tainted needle or participating in unprotected sex (Bormann & Kelly, 1999)? Inviting clients who are infected with HIV/AIDS to interact with health care students has been shown to help students separate the person from the illness, reducing the risk of future stereotyping (Campbell, Maki, Willenbring, & Henry, 1991).

AIDS was originally known as GRID, gay-related immune deficiency, but that acronym was a misnomer. We now know that this disease affects people with heterosexual as well as homosexual orientations, children and adults, whites and people of color, and those who are affluent and poor. The virus depresses immune system functions so that the people who are HIV-positive cannot fight off certain bacteria, viruses, fungi, yeast, and protozoa. AIDS is a far more accurate name. Because HIV/AIDS had initially been strongly associated with gay men, homophobia escalated, along with fear of contagion with a virus that is, as yet, not curable. As with all people, those with a homosexual orientation fear rejection, discrimination, and violence. Consequently, many spend considerable time monitoring their behavior so that they are not "found out." This stigmatization may also result in chronic stress that can affect health (Meyer, 1995). Practitioners need to assess their attitudes and behaviors toward their clients to ensure that they treat all clients with respect and dignity.

> That is one of the shocking things about a hospital: its leveling of you to your body's weakest link. The PhD in Comp. Lit., the years in Paris, the wall of books—you do not wear these badges on your johnny gown. No wonder I was forever giving our résumés to doctors and nurses, as if to beg them to see us for real, see what happy lives we had left at the border, which waited still like a dog on the front stoop (Monette, 1988, p. 74).

## Mental Illness Bias

Members of our society have historically stigmatized people diagnosed with mental illness (Davies, 2000; Fraser, 1994; Kaminski & Harty, 1999; Socall & Holtgraves, 1992). Medical and mental health providers are influenced by this stigma and bias, and many health professionals choose not to work with clients with mental illness, describing the work as unrewarding and lacking in prestige (Minkoff, 1997; Shera & Delva-Tauiliili, 1996). Among those who do choose to work with this population, negative attitudes and biases may affect treatment outcomes.

Clients diagnosed with mental illness are frequently perceived as being dangerous, unpredictable, and difficult. They are often blamed for their own disability. It has been suggested that they have a high rate of noncompliance and frequently drop out of treatment programs (Crisp et al., 2000; Hayward & Bright, 1997; Wahl, 1992). Employers often consider people with psychiatric illnesses as liabilities. As a result, many of these individuals remain unemployed (Davies, 2000).

Clients who have been diagnosed with a mental illness often perceive themselves as different, and they may be ashamed of their illness. Their quality of life is often adversely affected. Many are neglected by family, friends, and health care providers. Their self-confidence is unfavorably affected by their own perceptions, attitudes, and practices, as well as those of others (Gallo, 1994). Although few clients with mental illness behave in ways that are dangerous to society, public opinion is too often generalized to include all clients with psychiatric diagnoses (Crisp et al., 2000). The stigma associated with mental illness is mirrored in our language and society. Some people still refer to those with mental illness as being "mad" or "loony" (Kaminski & Harty, 1999). Casual use of disparaging labels such as "crazy" perpetuates the negative bias toward clients who have mental illness.

Efforts to change public and professional attitudes toward clients with mental illness are needed (Byrne, 1999). Research has indicated that such efforts can be successful. One training program promoted individual values clarification and self-awareness. Participants were made aware of language they used and accepted from others, referring to clients diagnosed with mental illness. Through this educational program, an attempt was made to close the gap between the "them" and "us" mentality. As a result of the training sessions, participants recognized their covert biases and raised their awareness of the stigma associated with mental illness (Kaminski & Harty, 1999).

Research also suggests that having personal contact with people who have psychiatric disorders improves a person's acceptance of members of this group (Kolodziej & Johnson, 1996; Lyons & Hayes, 1992; Shera & Delva-Tauiliili, 1996). Attitudes can be changed. Positive attitudes are required if we are to effectively treat members of this client population.

---

When I walked into class yesterday, there was a nicely dressed older man standing with the instructor. He was the guest speaker and told us that he had been depressed since he was 2 years old. However, at the age of 43, he was finally diagnosed with clinical depression. If he had come to my clinic for treatment of diabetes, asthma, or something else, I never would have guessed he had a mental illness.

Over the years, he's been hospitalized several times, including once after a suicide attempt. I don't think I'll ever stereotype patients with mental illness again.
—*From the journal of Tran Nguyen, medical laboratory science student*

---

## Obesity Bias

In the United States, people who are obese face discrimination by the media, the clothing industry, public transportation systems, and health care providers. Cultural assumptions suggest that obesity is equated with being lazy, stupid, and overindulgent. The resulting psychological trauma can be devastating and often leads to poor self-esteem (Brink, 1994; Goodman, 1995). Many people believe that obesity and other eating disorders are self-inflicted, perpetuating stereotypes and stigma. Little empathy exists for people who are obese (Crisp et al., 2000).

Medical assessment of the significance of a client's body weight is often arbitrary in nature and not based on empirical evidence. In one study, doctors were more likely to discriminate against women who were overweight than their male counterparts. Male doctors tended to withdraw treatment from the women, sending them home to lose weight, prior to performing a scheduled operation. This was not true for the men. Surgeons, anesthetists, and nurses sometimes made unnecessary, rude, and derogatory comments about women who were overweight. These remarks occurred in the operating room or at the nurses' stations. While most nurses admitted feeling uncomfortable hearing these comments, they also believed they were unable to refute or challenge such attitudes (Wright, 1998).

Obesity is a chronic disease affected by genetic, environmental, and behavioral factors. There are no easy remedies. Although dieting may result in short-term success, most weight is later regained (Wadden, 1993). If you are overweight, would you feel comfortable discussing the dangers of obesity with your clients? As health professionals, we need to understand our own lifestyle choices and the effect they may have on our ability to relate to clients.

By avoiding the subject, we do a disservice to our clients. In addition, most studies of weight loss have been conducted using participants who are white and have a high socioeconomic level, making the findings invalid to generalize to other populations (Wilson, 1994).

The health care professionals discussing Mrs. Garjulo, in the journal entry at the beginning of this chapter, seemed to believe that she was undisciplined and self-indulgent. With such an attitude, would they be able to develop an honest rapport with her and provide effective treatment?

## Substance Abuse Bias

While health care professionals should treat all clients equitably and fairly, this does not always happen. Many clinicians avoid treating clients who have drug and/or alcohol addictions (George & Martin, 1992). Practitioners who do care for those who use alcohol and/or illegal drugs describe the experience as extremely challenging (McLaughlin & Long, 1996). Stigma may also contribute to the difficulties some clients with drug or alcohol problems have seeking help (Ritson, 1999).

Some health professionals think they lack the necessary training and support to treat clients with these problems. Others prefer not to work with them. Clients may be perceived as out-of-control, self-indulgent, and having self-inflicted problems. Practitioners may fear that clients are unpredictable and dangerous, and they expect clients to relapse. This leads to feelings of frustration, pessimism, and anger. Derogatory comments made by health professionals may contribute to clients' hiding their problems. Clients may also internalize detrimental comments, resulting in depression, self-criticism, and possibly a return to drugs or alcohol in an attempt to escape these negative feelings (Howard & Chung, 2000).

Treatment is available for substance abuse problems, and some clients do recover. It is encouraging to note that studies confirm that recent graduates have more positive, optimistic attitudes toward clients with alcohol or drug problems than earlier graduates (Howard & Chung, 2000).

## Disability Bias

"Stereotypical assumptions about disabled people are based on superstition, myths, and beliefs from earlier, less enlightened times" (Barnes, 1994, p. 36). Filmmakers and both classical and popular authors of stories and fairy tales frequently depict people with disabilities as being villains or other evil characters. These negative images promote discrimination and exclusion. Little has been done to counteract this view (Barnes, 1994; Roush, 1986; Shakespeare, 1994).

Our socialization, professional education, and health profession specialization all influence and shape our perceptions of disability (French, 1994b). Perceptions are further affected by the media, which often portrays people with disabilities as being either helpless, in need of protection, or exceptional, thus minimizing their "real" problems. Many health providers have a distorted perception of disability. Although health professionals frequently view disability as a result of functional limitations, clients often view their disability as a result of society's neglect to care for people's social and physical environmental needs. These differing perceptions may interfere with a health professional's ability to advocate effectively for people with disabilities (Oliver, 1990).

As a result of well-intentioned fundraising campaigns, people with disabilities may be stereotyped as having suffered great misfortunes. They may be looked upon as individuals whose lives have been damaged forever. When pursuing their interests and strengths, they may be perceived as compensating for their disabilities. Yet, when they hold back from engaging in certain activities because they recognize their limitations, they may be viewed as inferior to others (Wright, 1983). People are often amazed when they see a person with a disability who is happy and leading a successful life. It is not expected. Some members of our society believe that having a disability must be intolerable and that people with disabilities must spend their entire lives wishing they were "normal" (Morris, 1994).

As a result of this stigmatization and stereotyping, people may try to hide their disabilities (French, 1994a). A person who has limited sight may pretend to be lost. An individual diagnosed with multiple sclerosis may pretend to be clumsy. The time and energy spent "hiding" the disability results in high stress levels for them, which may affect their overall health. However, some people would prefer to hide their disabilities rather than face the pity they fear from their peers who are not disabled.

People often stare at individuals who have disabilities. Some ask questions about the disability or personal life that cross standard social boundaries (Morris, 1994; Roush, 1986). While overt negative comments may be infrequent, people who do not have disabilities often express benevolent, patronizing attitudes toward those with disabilities. As we have seen, these adverse comments can become internalized, resulting in diminished self-esteem (Morris, 1994).

Typical reactions toward individuals with disabilities include feeling uncomfortable, guilty, or fearful. Susan Roush, a physical therapist with a disability, states that health care professionals may be more sensitive than the general public when in a structured, "clinical" situation, but outside of that setting, they are no different from the general population. She describes situations in which people followed her around stores asking her numerous questions about her disability. There is a need for people to see the person rather than only seeing the disability. Using "people-first" language, as described in Chapter 2, and stressing the need to increase public awareness of disabilities to decrease attitudinal barriers can promote inclusivity and debunk stereotypes (Roush, 1986).

People project their uneasiness and fears about their own limitations and mortality onto individuals who have disabilities (Shakespeare, 1994). As health care professionals, it is our duty to nurture equality for all. Do we treat individuals with disabilities one way in the clinic and another way in the grocery store? While society has improved access for individuals with disabilities, we still have a long way to go. In 1986, Susan Roush wrote, "the true challenge for rehabilitation in the 1980s is not the development of new technology and miracle drugs but to overcome attitudinal barriers to interaction and relationships through understanding and acceptance" (p. 1551). It would appear that challenge is still with us today.

# Becoming Competent, Unbiased Health Care Practitioners

Most health care curricula focus on providing students with evidence-based scientific knowledge. While this is important, it must be balanced with information that helps us understand ourselves and our clients (Seroka, 1994; Swick, 1998). It is imperative that we not only recognize that cultural and other biases exist, we also need to understand and respect differences and attempt to eliminate our own biases (Erlen, 1998). Clients cannot be expected to "fit into" our way of doing things, but rather health care practices must be developed that "fit into" the clients' world (Markakis, Beckman, Suchman, & Frankel, 2000; Rowley, Baldwin, Bay, & Cannula, 2000; Schoenly, 1994; Shelton, 1999; St. Clair & McKenry, 1999).

Shedding our biases requires discussing values, beliefs, and attitudes. This involves taking risks, and people must feel safe and accepted before they become involved in these dialogues. Exposure to culturally diverse clients in clinical settings helps health care professionals develop a true understanding of the needs, beliefs, and values of individuals from different cultures and provides a context for these discussions.

While knowledge and attitudes have been shown to improve following educational programs (Rowley et al., 2000), the long-term effects on changes in practice are not known. It is clear that it takes longer to change attitudes than it does to improve knowledge. Continued interaction with individuals who differ from us, attending continuing education programs and seminars, and receiving institutional support all help to reduce bias and positively motivate practice in the health care environment (Howell, Butler, Vincent, Watt-Watson, & Stearns, 2000).

# Cross-Professional Values and Biases

Technological advances, a focus on health promotion, changes in reimbursement policies, and a movement away from acute care to outpatient and home-based services have all affected the role of health professionals. Years ago, the emphasis was on clinical skills, but today's health care professional is in a leadership or managerial role, with an emphasis on delegation, education, and supervision (Mawn & Reece, 2000). In this new system, no one works alone. To be effective, health providers must learn to work as members of a health care team. Members of a team need to understand each other's roles and contributions and be clear about how they are going to work together (Martin, 2000). This is not always as easy as it might seem. Our personal beliefs and values, as well as our professional socialization, may be in conflict with those of our colleagues. When this happens, we must communicate with each other to overcome obstacles and work cohesively.

The health care system is another example of a culture. Within that culture exist many subcultures, such as nurses, doctors, physical therapists, occupational therapists, speech and language pathologists, dieticians, and social workers. Professional ethnocentrism, based upon the "in" and "out" group model described earlier, may pose a barrier to effective communication. Members of each "in" group share a specialized educational experience, culminating in a specific degree and/or license. Each group has an umbrella organization that affords its members greater professional identity and separateness. To work together effectively, members of each group must first acknowledge the existence of professional ethnocentrism, recognize each others' strengths, and then work together for the common goal of promoting optimal health care for all (Nyatanga, 1998).

Success in today's health care system demands a balance between quality client care and cost-effectiveness. Information from all involved disciplines must be obtained, consolidated, updated, and shared continuously to ensure quality care. Communication among team members is vital. Team meetings can help to facilitate this exchange. Each team member needs to develop an understanding of his or her dependence on coworkers to provide appropriate information to the team. Respect for the members of each discipline involved in client care is critical. Achievement of the team and the quality of client care is based upon the success of each (Miceli, 1999).

In order for a team to be effective, three conditions must be present. First, there must be trust among all members. Second, there needs to be a sense of group identity. Members must all feel that they belong to a unique and worthwhile team. Finally, there must be a sense of group efficacy. Members need to believe that they can be more effective working together, rather than as individuals, and that each person on the team can perform competently. While a team may function when one or more of these conditions are missing, it will not be as effective (Druskat & Wolff, 2001).

The foundation for building a team is based upon human emotions. Individuals need to understand and be able to control their emotions, be sensitive to others, and compel the emotions of their team members. When individuals accurately listen and assess each other's feelings and concerns, they are more willing to cooperate with each other, improving morale. If one team member is being disruptive, other members of the team must be willing to confront the individual. This can be accomplished in a positive way that conveys the message that his or her contributions to the group are valued. However, it must be clear that disruptive behavior will not be tolerated. Similarly, if an individual appears upset, members need to acknowledge that person's feelings and convey a caring attitude. If emotions are not addressed early, disruptive behaviors can escalate and erode any sense of trust in the team.

Taking time to build team spirit and allowing members to vent frustrations help develop effectiveness. Emotionally intelligent groups make better decisions, develop creative strategies for problem solving, and are more productive than others. Health care professionals can foster emotional intelligence by comprehending their own personal and professional identity, as well as gaining a clear awareness of their colleagues' strengths and skills. As a by-product, quality of care improves, and everyone benefits (Campion-Smith, 2001).

## SUMMARY

This chapter addressed the importance of understanding personal and professional values. The significance of identifying attitudes and recognizing how they affect behaviors was explored. We described how both overt and covert personal biases can result in stigmatization, generalization, and stereotyping of individuals who are different from "us." The need for group cohesiveness when working in interdisciplinary teams was explained. Competent health care interactions require knowledge, experience, mutual respect, and tolerance.

## REFLECTIVE QUESTIONS

1. a. List ten values that are personally important to you such as faith, appearance, power, and success.
   b. Once you have completed your list, prioritize your values in order of importance to you.
   c. Discuss how your values affect your behavior.
   d. How do you feel about people whose behavior conflicts with your values?
2. Imagine you have a colleague who makes offensive comments about people.
   a. How would you feel?
   b. What would your opinion be about this person?
   c. What would you do?

3. Although we may consider ourselves fair and unbiased, it is likely that we harbor stereo-types or negative images toward some individuals or groups, to varying degrees. Consider your feelings and beliefs carefully and honestly.
   a. Do you hold negative stereotypes about any racial or ethnic groups, older people, those with mental retardation or mental illness, people with HIV/AIDS, or others? If so, describe what they are.
   b. Biases and stereotypes can interfere with our ability to be nonjudgmental, build relationships, and work effectively with clients. What can you do to move beyond your current beliefs, attitudes, and feelings?
4. People with disabilities often complain that health care providers have lower expectations and goals for them than they themselves do. What rights do you think people with disorders or disabilities have to be fully integrated into daily life?
5. a. What might your response be to clients with disabilities who you consider to have unrealistic goals or expectations for their rehabilitation?
   b. How might you support them in achieving goals?

## CASE STUDY

As part of the service learning component of her nursing curriculum, Dawn has been assigned to volunteer in a shelter for homeless women, located in the inner city. Having grown up in an affluent suburban neighborhood, she is very uncomfortable taking the bus into the city and is somewhat afraid of the clients. Although she is unaware of their medical status, several appear to her to have some form of mental illness, while others appear to be drug- or alcohol-dependent. Many do not speak English.

Dawn is expected to spend 3 hours each week assisting the nursing staff and serving the clients. Her role includes monitoring vital signs, preparing and serving meals, discussing the importance of diet and exercise and other healthy behaviors, and spending time talking with the women.

1. Discuss Dawn's possible preconceived biases and how she may have internalized these values.
2. What can Dawn do to modify her beliefs and values to reduce her biases?
3. Stigma is a large obstacle for people perceived to be out of the mainstream, such as the women in this shelter. Identify how stereotypes and biases can create barriers to care.
4. What can health care providers do to eliminate barriers to care for stigmatized populations?

## REFERENCES

Bargh, J. A. (1994). The four horsemen of automaticity: Awareness, intention, efficiency, and control in social cognition. In R. S. Wyer, Jr., & T. K. Srull (Eds.), *Handbook of social cognition* (2nd ed., Vol. 1, pp. 1–40). Hillsdale, NJ: Erlbaum.

Barnes, C. (1994). Images of disability. In S. French (Ed.), *On equal terms: Working with disabled people* (pp. 35–46). Oxford, UK: Butterworth-Heinemann.

Bormann, J., & Kelly, A. (1999). HIV and AIDS: Are you biased? *American Journal of Nursing, 99*(9), 38–39.

Brewer, M. (1979). In-group bias in the minimal intergroup situation: A cognitive motivational analysis. *Psychological Bulletin, 86,* 307–324.

Brink, P. J. (1994). Stigma and obesity. *Clinical Nursing Research, 3*(4), 291–293.

Brooks, A. M. (2001). Cultural diversity: Getting to a viewing point. *Journal of Professional Nursing, 17*(1), 4.

Bunting, S. (1996). Sources of stigma associated with women with HIV. *Advances in Nursing Science, 19*(2), 64–73.

Byrne, P. (1999). Stigma of mental illness: Changing minds, changing behavior. *British Journal of Psychiatry, 174,* 1–2.

Campbell, S., Maki, M., Willenbring, K., & Henry, K. (1991). AIDS-related knowledge, attitudes, and behaviors among 629 registered nurses at a Minnesota hospital: A descriptive study. *Journal of the Association of Nurses in AIDS Care, 2*(1), 15–23.

Campion-Smith, C. (2001). Putting patients first will help interprofessional education. *British Medical Journal, 322*(7287), 676.

Clark, R., Anderson, N. B., Clark, V. R., & Williams, D. R. (1999). Racism as a stressor for African-Americans: A biopsychosocial model. *American Psychologist, 54*(10), 805–816.

Cohen, J. J. (1999). Still seeking gender equity in health care. *Academic Medicine, 74*(11), 1226.

Crisp, A. H., Gelder, M. G., Rix, S., Meltzer, H. I., & Rowlands, O. J. (2000). Stigmatization of people with mental illnesses. *British Journal of Psychiatry, 177,* 4–7.

Davies, M. R. B. (2000). The stigma of anxiety disorders. *International Journal of Clinical Practice, 54*(1), 44–47.

Dennis, B. P. (1997). Bridging cultures: African-Americans and nursing. In J. C. McCloskey & H. K. Grace (Eds.), *Current issues in nursing* (5th ed., pp. 595–602). St. Louis, MO: Mosby.

Dimsdale, J. E. (2000). Stalked by the past: The influence of ethnicity on health. *Psychosomatic Medicine, 62,* 161–170.

Drench, M. E. (1996). Lowering the risk: Fears and facts of HIV transmission to health care professionals. In M. L. Galantino (Ed.), *Issues in HIV rehabilitation* (pp. 9–28). Alexandria, VA: American Physical Therapy Association, Oncology Section.

Drench, M. E. (1998). *Red ribbons are not enough: Health caregivers' stories about AIDS.* Wilsonville, OR: BookPartners.

Druskat, V. U., & Wolff, S. B. (2001). Building the emotional intelligence of groups. *Harvard Business Review, 79*(3), 81–90.

Erlen, J. A. (1998). Culture, ethics, and respect: The bottom line is understanding. *Orthopaedic Nursing, 17*(6), 79–82.

Feldman, S. (1999). Please don't call me "dear": Older women's narratives of health care. *Nursing Inquiry, 6,* 269–276.

Fraser, M. E. (1994). Educating the public about mental illness: What will it take to get the job done? *Innovations and Research, 3*(3), 29–31.

French, S. (1994a). Dimensions of disability and impairment. In S. French (Ed.), *On equal terms: Working with disabled people* (pp. 17–34). Oxford, UK: Butterworth-Heinemann.

French, S. (1994b). What is disability? In S. French (Ed.), *On equal terms: Working with disabled people* (pp. 3–16). Oxford, UK: Butterworth-Heinemann.

Gallo, K. (1994). First person account: Self-stigmatization. *Schizophrenia Bulletin, 20,* 407–410.

Gardner, H. (1993). *Frames of mind: The theory of multiple intelligences.* New York: Basic Books.

George, M., & Martin, E. (1992). General practitioners' attitudes toward drug users. *British Journal of General Practice, 42*(360), 302.

Gilligan, C. (1982). *In a different voice: Psychological theory and women's development.* Cambridge, MA: Harvard University Press.

Goffman, E. (1963). *Stigma.* New York: Simon & Schuster.

Gonzalez, R. I., Gooden, M. B., & Porter, C. P. (2000). Eliminating racial and ethnic disparities in health care. *American Journal of Nursing, 100*(3), 56–58.

Goodman, J., & Kirwan, L. (2001). Exercise-induced myocardial ischemia in women: Factors affecting prevalence. *Sports Medicine, 31*(4), 235–247.

Goodman, W. C. (1995). *The invisible woman: Confronting weight prejudice in America*. Carlsbad, CA: Gurze Books.

Greenberger, P. (1999). The women's health research coalition: A new advocacy network. *Journal of Women's Health and Gender-Based Medicine, 8*(4), 441–442.

Greenwald, A. G., & Banaji, M. R. (1995). Implicit social cognition: Attitudes, self-esteem and stereo-types. *Psychological Review, 102*(1), 4–27.

Gunderman, R. (2000). Illness as failure: Blaming patients. *Hastings Center Report, 30*(4), 7–11.

Hall, J. A., Epstein, A. M., DeCiantis, M. L., & McNeil, B. J. (1993). Physicians' liking for their patients: More evidence for the role of affect in medical care. *Health Psychology, 12*(2), 140–146.

Haskins, A. R., Rose-St. Prix, C., & Elbaum, L. (1997). Covert bias in evaluation of physical therapist students' clinical performance. *Physical Therapy, 77*(2), 155–168.

Hatala, R., & Case, S. M. (2000). Examining the influence of gender on medical students' decision-making. *Journal of Women's Health and Gender-Based Medicine, 9*(6), 617–623.

Hayward, P., & Bright, J. A. (1997). Stigma and mental illness: A review and critique. *Journal of Mental Health, 6,* 345–354.

Howard, M. O., & Chung, S. S. (2000). Nurses' attitudes toward substance misusers. I. Surveys. *Substance Use and Misuse, 35*(3), 347–365.

Howell, D., Butler, L., Vincent, L., Watt-Watson, J., & Stearns, N. (2000). Influencing nurses' knowledge, attitudes, and practice in cancer pain management. *Cancer Nursing, 23*(1), 55–63.

Ingram, D., & Hutchinson, S. A., (1999). HIV-positive mothers and stigma. *Health Care for Women International, 20,* 93–103.

Jemmott, L., Jemmott, J., & Crus-Collins, M. (1992). Predicting AIDS patient care intentions among nursing students. *Nursing Research, 41,* 172–177.

Jones, C. P. (2000). Levels of racism: A theoretic framework and a gardener's tale. *American Journal of Public Health, 90*(8), 1212–1215.

Kaminski, P., & Harty, C. (1999). From stigma to strategy. *Nursing Strategy, 13*(38), 36–40.

Kasar, J., & Clark, E. N. (2000). *Developing professional behaviors*. Thorofare, NJ: Slack.

Kearney, N., Miller, M., Paul, J., & Smith, K. (2000). Oncology healthcare professionals' attitudes toward elderly people. *Annals of Oncology, 11,* 599–601.

Kemppainen, J. K., Dubbert, P. M., & McWilliams, P. (1996). Effects of group discussion and guided patient care experience on nurses' attitudes towards care of patients with AIDS. *Journal of Advanced Nursing, 24,* 296–302.

Kirkham, S. R. (1998). Nurses' descriptions of caring for culturally diverse clients. *Clinical Nursing Research, 7*(2), 125–146.

Kolodziej, M. E., & Johnson, B. T. (1996). Interpersonal contact and acceptance of persons with psychiatric disorders: A research synthesis. *Journal of Consulting and Clinical Psychology, 64*(6), 1387–1396.

Lyons, M., & Hayes, R. (1992). Students' perceptions of persons with psychiatric and other disorders. *American Journal of Occupational Therapy, 47*(6), 541–548.

Madan, A. K., Aliabadi-Wahle, S., & Beech, D. J. (2001). Ageism in medical students' treatment recommendations: The example of breast-conserving procedures. *Academic Medicine, 76*(3), 282–284.

Markakis, K. M., Beckman, H. B., Suchman, A. L., & Frankel, R. M. (2000). The path to professionalism: Cultivating humanistic values and attitudes in residency training. *Academic Medicine, 75*(2), 141–150.

Marrocco, A., & Stewart, D. E. (2001). We've come a long way, maybe: Recruitment of women and analysis of results by sex in clinical research. *Journal of Women's Health and Gender-Based Medicine, 10*(2), 175–179.

Martin, J. E., & Bedimo, A. L. (2000). Nurse practitioner, nurse midwife and physician assistant attitudes and care practices related to persons with HIV/AIDS. *Journal of the American Academy of Nurse Practitioners, 12*(2), 35–41.

Martin, V. (2000). Developing team effectiveness. *Nursing Management, 7*(2), 26–29.

Mawn, B., & Reece, S. M. (2000). Reconfiguring a curriculum for the new millennium: The process of change. *Journal of Nursing Education, 39*(3), 101–108.

McLaughlin, D., & Long, A. (1996). An extended literature review of health professionals' perceptions of illicit drugs and their clients who use them. *Journal of Psychiatric Mental Health Nursing, 3,* 283–288.

Meyer, I. H. (1995). Minority stress and mental health in gay men. *Journal of Health and Social Behavior, 36,* 38–56.

Miceli, C. (1999). Building staff communication. *Provider, 25*(8), 59–61.

Minkoff, K. (1997). Resistance of mental health professionals to working with people with serious mental illness. In L. Spaniol, C. Gagne, & M. Koehler (Eds.), *Psychological and social aspects of psychiatric disability* (pp. 334–347). Boston: Center for Psychiatric Rehabilitation, Sargent College of Allied Health Professions.

Monette, P. (1988). *Borrowed time: An AIDS memoir.* New York: Harcourt Brace Jovanovich.

Morris, J. (1994). Prejudice. In S. French (Ed.), *On equal terms: Working with disabled people* (pp. 61–67). Oxford, UK: Butterworth-Heinemann.

Nicolette, J., & Jacobs, M. B. (2000). Integration of women's health into an internal medicine core curriculum for medical students. *Academic Medicine, 75*(11), 1061–1065.

Nyatanga, L. (1998). Professional ethnocentrism and shared learning. *Nurse Education Today, 18,* 175–177.

Oliver, M. (1990). *The politics of disablement.* London: Macmillan.

Palmore, E. (1999). *Ageism: Negative and positive.* New York: Springer.

Palmore, E. (2000). Guest editorial: Ageism in gerontological language. *The Gerontologist, 40*(6), 645.

Perdue, C. W., Dovidio, J. F., Gurtman, M. B., & Tyler, B. B. (1990). Us and them: Social categorization and the process of intergroup bias. *Journal of Personality and Social Psychology, 59,* 475–486.

Purtilo, R., & Haddad, A. (1996). Health professional and patient interaction (5th ed.). Philadelphia: W. B. Saunders.

Ritson, E. B. (1999). Alcohol, drugs, and stigma. *International Journal of Clinical Practice, 53*(7), 549–551.

Roter, D. L. (2000). The outpatient medical encounter and elderly patients. *Clinics in Geriatric Medicine, 16*(1), 95–107.

Roter, D. L., & Hall, J. A. (1998). Choices: Biomedical ethics and women's health. Why physician gender matters in shaping the physician–patient relationship. *Journal of Women's Health, 7*(9), 1093–1097.

Roush, S. E. (1986). Health professionals as contributors to attitudes toward persons with disabilities. *Physical Therapy, 66*(10), 1551–1554.

Rowley, B. D., Baldwin, D. C., Bay, R. C., & Cannula, M. (2000). Can professional values be taught? A look at residency training. *Clinical Orthopaedics and Related Research, 378,* 110–114.

Schoenly, L. (1994). Teaching in the affective domain. *Journal of Continuing Education in Nursing, 25*(5), 209–212.

Schulman, K. A., Berlin, J., Harless, W., Kerner, J., Sistrunk, S., Gersh, B., Dube, R., Taleghani, C., Burke, J., Williams, S., Eisenberg, J., & Escarce, J. (1999). The effect of race and sex on physicians' recommendations for cardiac catheterization. *New England Journal of Medicine, 340,* 618–626.

Seroka, A. M. (1994). Values clarification and ethical decision-making. *Seminars for Nurse Managers, 2*(1), 8–15.

Shakespeare, T. (1994). Cultural representation of disabled people: Dustbins for disavowal? *Disability and Society, 9*(3), 283–298.

Shelton, W. (1999). Can virtue be taught? *Academic Medicine, 74*(6), 671–674.

Shera, W., & Delva-Tauiliili, J. (1996). Changing MSW students' attitudes towards the severely mentally ill. *Community Mental Health Journal, 32*(2), 159–169.

Shortt, S. (2001). Venerable or vulnerable? Ageism in health care. *Journal of Health Services Research Policy, 6*(1), 1–2.

Slotterback, C. S., & Saarnio, D. A. (1996). Attitudes toward older adults reported by young adults: Variation based on attitudinal task and attribute categories. *Psychology and Aging, 11*(4), 563–571.

Socall, D. W., & Holtgraves, T. (1992). Attitudes toward the mentally ill: The effects of label and beliefs. *The Sociological Quarterly, 33,* 435–445.

St. Clair, A., & McKenry, L. (1999). Preparing culturally competent practitioners. *Journal of Nursing Education, 38*(5), 228–234.

Sumner, W. G. (1906). *Folkways.* Boston: Ginn.

Swick, H. M. (1998). Academic medicine must deal with the clash of business and professional values. *Academic Medicine, 73*(7), 751–755.

Thorne, S. E., Nyhlin, K. T., & Paterson, B. L. (2000). Attitudes toward patient expertise in chronic illness. *International Journal of Nursing Studies, 37,* 303–311.

van Ryn, M., & Burke, J. (2000). The effect of patient race and socioeconomic status on physicians' perceptions of patients. *Social Science and Medicine, 50,* 813–828.

Wadden, T. A. (1993). Treatment of obesity by moderate and severe caloric restrictions: Results of clinical research trials. *Annals of Internal Medicine, 119,* 688–693.

Wahl, O. F. (1992). Mass media images of mental illness: A review of the literature. *Journal of Community Psychology, 20,* 343–351.

Weiner, B. (1980). A cognitive (attribution)–emotion–action model of motivated behavior: An analysis of judgments of help-giving. *Journal of Personality and Social Psychology, 39*(2), 186–200.

Weitzman, S., Cooper, L., Chambless, L., Rosamond, W., Clegg, L., Marcucci, G., Romm, F., & White, A., (1997). Gender, racial and geographic differences in the performance of cardiac diagnostic and therapeutic procedures for hospitalized acute myocardial infarction in four states. *American Journal of Cardiology, 79,* 722–726.

Wenger, N. K. (1999). Should women have a different risk assessment from men for primary prevention of coronary heart disease? *Journal of Women's Health and Gender-Based Medicine, 8*(4), 465–467.

Wilson, G. T. (1994). Behavioral treatments of obesity: Thirty years and counting. *Advances in Behavior Research and Therapy, 16,* 31–75.

Wright, B. (1983). *Physical disability: A psychosocial approach* (2nd ed). New York: HarperCollins.

Wright, J. (1998). Female nurses' perceptions of acceptable female body size: An exploratory study. *Journal of Clinical Nursing, 7,* 307–315.

# 2

# *Communication*

Patrick was late again! In frustration, I asked the nurse why he was never down in physical therapy (PT) for his scheduled appointments. She said he was "the most impossible amputee" she'd "ever worked with. Come with me, and you'll understand." As we approached his room, she shouted, "Patrick, get out of bed!" and threw up the shade. Depressed and angry, Patrick shouted obscenities at the nurse and pulled the covers over his head.

I was absolutely appalled at her lack of sensitivity and compassion. No wonder he refused to have PT that day. I determined another strategy was in order. The following morning, I entered Patrick's room, smiled, and said, "Patrick, it's time to get up for PT. Your appointment is in 30 minutes. Will that work for you?" He nodded, and I left. One half hour later, on the dot, Patrick wheeled his chair into the clinic.

—*From the journal of Lindsay Cushing, physical therapist student*

Health care providers are required to communicate on a daily basis with clients, clients' families and friends, third-party payers, equipment vendors, and other health care professionals. First and foremost, it is the means by which we establish a therapeutic relationship. Unless we are able to do this, we will be ineffective, regardless of our clinical skills. Second, we determine the clients' needs and understand their medical history and current problems, concerns, and goals. Third, we provide the clients with information. We may supply them with verbal or written facts about their diagnosis and/or refer them to other resources. Plans of care and protocols are also discussed in this mode. Finally, we interact with them to develop and achieve appropriate collaborative goals (French, 1994; Purtilo & Haddad, 1996; Swain, 1997).

Good communication skills allow health care providers to accurately exchange information between the clients and themselves, determine a problem list, and formulate therapeutic management.

In practice, however, it is not uncommon for a health care professional to ask a question, such as "What brings you here today?" and not wait for a response. In addition, health care workers might not fully listen to what the client replies or interrupt the client after a brief time has elapsed. More than two decades have passed since research showed that patients were interrupted on the average of 18 seconds after beginning to explain their problems, and less than 2 percent were able to complete their explanations (Beckman & Frankel, 1984). How much has changed since then? Contemporary managed care, with its high productivity demands, continues to impose time constraints that restrict the interchange between clients and providers. Diagnosis, prognosis, management strategies, and client/family education must be accomplished within a compressed period.

For professionals to fully understand clients' needs and for clients to understand their problems and what they need to do, clear communication needs to occur within that time. It is important to begin by introducing yourself and identifying your discipline. The onus falls on the health care provider to intently listen to clients' stories, understand their needs within the context of their lives, create an appropriate plan of care, and collaborate with and teach clients and their families (Vanderhoff, 2005).

In a study on expert practice, listening was found to be an essential evaluation tool (Jensen, Gwyer, Shepard, & Hack, 2000). Expert clinicians maintain a focused interaction with clients. They allow the clients time to tell their stories, rather than relying on structured questionnaires, and then pose additional questions based on earlier responses.

Health care professionals agree that they must possess effective communication skills to motivate clients, promote compliance with treatment protocols, and ensure appropriate, cost-efficient outcomes (Pettrey, 2003; Vanderhoff, 2005). Henkin, Dee, and Beatus (2000) suggest "the need for more formal communication training that is professionally relevant, efficient, and designed to strengthen desired communication competencies" (p. 32). They and others (Ang, 2002) stress the importance of including communication and other professional behaviors in health care curricula to supplement other rigorous program requirements. Learning to value clients' self-knowledge and actively listening to them are essential for all health care practice.

Studies show that poor communication often results in many negative consequences. For example, if information is not relayed adequately, inaccurate diagnoses can result (Sutcliffe, Lewton, & Rosenthal, 2004). In addition, stress levels may increase in all parties. Practitioners can become frustrated and develop symptoms of burnout. Clients may grow dissatisfied with health care providers and become nonadherent with treatment plans or even seek alternative care, resulting in higher medical costs (Davis & Fallowfield, 1991).

As health care practitioners, we need to recognize that while we may believe we are clearly conveying a message to someone, the receiver may not always hear the message we thought we sent. In the opening journal entry, we recognize that there was a lack of communication between Patrick and the nurse. In this chapter, we discuss the components of effective communication.

# Elements of Effective Communication

"Communication is one of those terms which have an intuitive and obvious meaning but are hard, if not impossible, to define precisely" (Swain, 1997, p. 247). It involves the sending and receiving of information, emotions, messages, and thoughts through visual, auditory, and kinesthetic channels (Barringer & Glod, 1998).

Communication begins when the sender expresses an idea, either verbally or nonverbally. Verbal messages are influenced by paralanguage cues, such as tone of voice, pitch, volume, and speed. Nonverbal messages may be sent intentionally or unintentionally. They include facial expression, touch, proxemics, and behavior. The receiver interprets the message, which is mediated by these influencing factors. The receiver's understanding of the meaning of the message is further affected by what he or she sees, hears, understands, and feels. People's perceptions may vary depending on social role, cultural background, personal needs, age, and prior life experiences. Finally, the physical context in which the discussion takes place, the time of day, the individual's mental status, and other factors occurring in one or more of the participants' lives may influence the communication process (Adler & Rodman, 1994; Barringer & Glod, 1998; French, 1994; Swain, 1997).

Communication between health care providers and clients differs from day-to-day social interactions with friends or family members. Individuals choose their friends, but not necessarily their clients. Social relationships are often based on fun and mutual satisfaction, while professional affiliations exist for the benefit of the client. A health professional may elect to end a friendship based on another individual's unacceptable social demeanor but may be forced to continue treating a client who behaves similarly. During social interactions, individuals equally share problems and experiences, whereas in therapeutic situations, the focus is on the client's concerns. In social surroundings, people often speak without thinking beforehand about what they are going to say or how it will influence others. In health care settings, communication strategies should be planned in advance, whenever possible, to facilitate accurate communication (Barringer & Glod, 1998).

To ensure that messages are being correctly interpreted by both sender and receiver, health care professionals need to continuously observe and analyze their interactions with others, rather than take them for granted, as they might do in their personal communication (Vanderhoff, 2005). Providing feedback and paraphrasing messages may help ensure clarification (Davis, 1998; French, 1994; Purtilo & Haddad, 1996).

## Levels of Communication

Communication occurs at four levels. It starts at the *intrapersonal level,* as we absorb information from our environment and begin to develop and formulate our thoughts and ideas. Once we decide to send a message to another person, we start to communicate at the *interpersonal level.* Here, the opportunity for misinterpretation begins. A higher level of communication takes place when we participate in a *small group discussion* with more than one other individual. This frequently occurs at team and family meetings. People enter with differing goals, objectives, and backgrounds, and the chances of misinterpretation and/or conflict increase. Finally, organizational communication takes place when *several groups* within a facility meet to discuss problems or establish policies. Egos, personal agendas, and professional differences may all interfere with the exchange. Everyone needs to strive to keep the channels of communication open and effective (Adler & Rodman, 1994; Barringer & Glod, 1998).

# Developing Practitioner–Client Rapport

As health care professionals, we are sometimes so busy that we neglect to think about the culture shock that clients experience when they encounter the health care setting. Clients enter with their own concerns, anxieties, and value systems. They have their personal routine and may be accustomed to privacy. In an inpatient setting, they suddenly "get" an unknown and unwanted roommate, which the system (us) provides. We socialize them into *our* world. We often require them to wear particular attire and eat at preset times. They select what they are eating from limited menus. In addition to coping with their illness, disease, or disability, we expect them to value our expertise and follow our instructions. Is it any wonder why clients may begin to feel dependent, vulnerable, and afraid?

In Patrick's case, the nurse probably thought she was clearly communicating to Patrick that it was time for him to get ready for physical therapy. She was undoubtedly quite busy and had many other client responsibilities. Her assessment was that Patrick was being unreasonable and difficult. Listening to her message, we, and probably Patrick, detect impatience, frustration, and lack of respect.

In a busy health care setting, we are frequently under stress. It may be easy to fall into the habit of concentrating on the illness, disease, or injury rather than on the client as a person. While this may be an appropriate response in the emergency room, it is not appropriate in most other cases. Before we can effectively "treat" a client, we must develop a relationship or rapport with him or her (Adler & Rodman, 1994; Davis, 1998; French, 1994; Northouse & Northouse, 1998; Purtilo & Haddad, 1996; Schneider, Kaplan, Greenfield, Li, & Wilson, 2004).

Prior to entering a client's room or greeting a client in the clinic or home setting, try to clear your mind of other thoughts and focus on the person you are about to meet. It is said that a picture is worth a thousand words. Your face and posture may be the first "picture" or impression the client receives, depending on his or her learning style, cultural context, and other factors. Smile and take a moment to introduce yourself. Tell the client who you are and why you are there. If the client is in bed, pull a chair next to the bed and sit down so that you are at eye level with one another. In the clinic or home setting, try to find a comfortable area where you can both sit to communicate. Take time to get to know the client. It is unwise to make judgments based on first impressions.

Ask clients about their health practices. Do they eat a balanced diet? Do they exercise regularly? Do they use seatbelts? Do they consume drugs or alcohol? As they talk, take the time to listen to what they have to say. Lean forward in your chair so that they know you are listening. Nod appropriately and ask questions to clarify issues. While some clients find touch comforting, others do not. If you feel comfortable, and believe the client is comfortable with you, it may be appropriate to touch the client's arm or shoulder to show that you care. If the client withdraws or appears uncomfortable, remove your hand and avoid unnecessary touch in the future.

Before you begin to examine or treat clients, let them know what you are going to do. Once you have developed a sense of mutual trust and respect, you are ready to begin your treatment. The few extra minutes it takes to develop this sense of rapport will be worth the effort as your treatment program progresses.

Although the nurse in Lindsay's journal entry expected Patrick to rise and shine and be ready for treatment, how many of you jump out of bed early in the morning, ready to face the day? As health care professionals, we need to be aware of and reflect on our own attitudes, styles, and approaches to clients. Rather than assume that a client is "difficult," we should question our own attitudes and develop more effective strategies.

From this journal entry, we are unaware of Patrick's history. Following his amputation, he may be questioning his ability to return to work or family life. He may be depressed. When Lindsay approached Patrick in a caring manner and allowed him time to prepare for treatment, he was cooperative and willing to participate. Payton and Nelson (1995) believe that involving clients in decision making and allowing them to assume responsibility for their care promotes adherence and ensures optimal benefit from their treatments. This is especially important in a health care environment in which clients are quickly discharged. The health care provider must play the roles of educator and facilitator, helping clients become independent in their own care (Vanderhoff, 2005).

## Client-Sensitive Language

As Martin (1999) notes, "language shapes thought" (p. 44). Thinking about clients as their disabilities reinforces emotional detachment. For some, the person *becomes* the disability, which frames how we connect with him or her. Focusing on people first enables us to see their abilities, needs, desires, and goals rather than their impairments. For example, the common expression of "confined to a wheelchair" promotes a negative connotation of being limited, even imprisoned. The wheelchair, in fact, is just the opposite. It is liberating, providing a means of mobility, of accessing the world. Refer to Table 2–1 for other examples of diminishing and empowering language.

In addition to empowering clients, we show respect by using "people-first" language. The terminology we use reflects how we think about clients (Martin, 1999). Consider how the nurse in Lindsay's journal referred to Patrick as "the most impossible amputee." Patrick is not the amputation. He is a person who has undergone a surgical amputation of his lower limb. We often hear health care workers using terminology such as "that CVA," "the shoulder," or "the arthritic client." Those people are not their impairments, functional limitations, or disabilities, but rather the person with a stroke, the woman with a shoulder problem, the client with arthritis. Acknowledging their individuality and totality is part of a therapeutic outcome. We need to be aware of this and encourage other health care providers to avoid referring to clients by their diagnoses or body parts.

Similarly, choice of words, tone, and volume can communicate certain messages, even when they are unintended. For example, by referring to clients as "honey" or "dear," health providers may inadvertently transmit messages of "dependence, incompetence, and control" to older adults by infantilizing them, using what has become known as elderspeak (Williams, Kemper, & Hummert, 2004, p. 17).

TABLE 2–1    Communicating with People with Disabilities

| Diminishing Terminology | Empowering Terminology |
| --- | --- |
| • stroke victim | • person who has had a stroke |
| • stricken with polio | • person who has polio |
| • afflicted with cerebral palsy | • person with cerebral palsy, diagnosed with cerebral palsy |
| • suffers from Parkinson's disease | • person who has Parkinson's disease |
| • mute, dumb | • person who is unable to speak |
| • confined to a wheelchair | • uses a wheelchair |
| • the handicapped, impaired, disabled, crippled, deformed | • person with a disability or impairment |
| • normal (as though a person with a disability is not normal) | • person without a disability |
| • the blind | • person who is visually impaired, person who is blind |
| • the deaf | • person who is hard of hearing, person who is deaf |
| • epileptic | • person with epilepsy, person with a seizure disorder |
| • schizophrenic | • person with schizophrenia |
| • alcoholic | • person with alcoholism |
| • victim of domestic violence | • survivor of domestic violence |
| • fits | • seizures |
| • victim | • survivor |
| • suffering from | • diagnosed with |

# Mindfulness: Being Present in the Moment

Today, I had an experience that made me very sad. I've been on my rotation at the hospital for three months, and my supervisor seems very pleased with my skills. I have a lot of independence and am responsible for my own caseload. A therapist was out sick with the flu today, and I was asked to pick up two of her clients on top of my own. Boy, was I overwhelmed! I only had time to skim the charts and then rush in and do the best treatment I could with very little information.

Unfortunately, I also had an examination to do on Ms. Jones, a newly admitted client. She's a 23-year-old woman who was in a car accident two months ago that caused a fracture-dislocation of L4-L5 in her back. At this time, she has total paraplegia, with no sensation in her lower extremities. I was feeling so rushed that I just barged into her room and quickly introduced myself before I started bombarding her with questions about her past medical history and current status. Then I began running through the items on the evaluation form as quickly as I could.

She started crying and then shouted, "You're just like all the others! I'm a person." I felt so terrible. I realized I was not treating her as a client, but as an object. I quickly apologized and fled the room. I know I could have done a better job, but I'm not sure what I should have done.

*—From the journal of Mark Smart, occupational therapy student*

Today, high productivity is a significant demand in the health care industry. The ability to simultaneously perform multiple tasks is expected. While running from client to client, it is easy to forget that each person is a unique human being. What messages do you think this behavior conveys? When we work with one client but are preoccupied with our next or previous task, we risk giving the client the impression that he or she is "in the way" and "unimportant." To avoid this, we should practice mindfulness. This requires that we fully attend to each task (Kabat-Zinn, 1994; Mentgen, 2001).

How do we become mindful in the midst of a chaotic health care environment? We must first become self-aware, clearing our minds of mental clutter, so that we are able to focus on the present moment (Kabat-Zinn, 1994; Mentgen, 2001). It only takes a minute to focus and give complete attention to the client. This small intervention can greatly enhance the effectiveness of the treatment. Clients are aware of the state of mind we bring to the interaction. Had Mark, the occupational therapy student, been able to eliminate the distractions and fully attend to Ms. Jones, he might have developed a rapport with her and been more successful in eliciting information. She might have become a partner in her care and been spared feeling like a "victim" of *his* distress.

# Verbal Communication

## Vocabulary

As stated earlier, communication involves sending a message to a receiver, in effect, an audience. When sending a message, keep in mind who that audience is and what its needs are. First, consider the importance of vocabulary. When talking to another health care professional who shares our common language, we should use medical terminology. However, when speaking with a client, we need to use words that the client understands. We would not use the same language with an adult who had a heart transplant as we would with a child with a developmental delay. Sometimes clients nod and smile, apparently signaling that they understand, although they actually might not. Checking with clients to determine what they have heard helps avoid misunderstanding. We can ask them to repeat the information or ask questions to determine clarity of understanding.

Routine terminology used by medical staff members may frighten clients. A nurse might suggest that a client go to a short-term care facility for rehabilitation following surgery. This message may be routine to the nurse. However, the client may hear, "I am being sent to a nursing home. I will never go home again." The distress that may ensue can leave the client unable to absorb and interpret any further information or instructions the nurse might provide (Adler & Rodman, 1994; Northouse & Northouse, 1998).

To avoid such miscommunication, observe clients' nonverbal responses. If they appear upset by something you said, ask questions to clarify any misconceptions or concerns, prior to moving on to new topics or activities. Whatever vocabulary we choose, it is essential to speak with clients at their level of understanding and not patronize them by "talking down" to them in a condescending manner (Vanderhoff, 2005). Words are building blocks, but they are only a part of verbal communication.

## Paralanguage

Paralanguage, including pitch, tone, speed, volume, emotional quality, stress, and accent of our formal language, is an important component of verbal communication (Adler & Rodman, 1994; Purtilo & Haddad, 1996; Swain, 1997). The phrase, "It's not what you say but how you say it that counts," illustrates the idea that what we say can be interpreted many different ways. Sometimes, especially when we are stressed, busy, or impatient, what we planned to say comes out sounding all wrong.

When we are in a hurry, we tend to talk faster. When we are excited or angry, we talk louder or "yell." If we are nervous, the listener may detect a higher pitch or tone in our voice. When communicating with clients, it is important to appear calm, concerned, and in control. Try to maintain an appropriate tone and volume in your voice so that you convey a sense of trust and interest. Take time to emphasize key words so that the listener "hears" them and recognizes their importance. Your volume should vary depending upon the size of the room and your audience's hearing capabilities. If you are next to a client, there is no need to "yell." If the room is large or noisy or if the person has impaired hearing, you can adjust accordingly.

## Active Listening

It is common for clients to feel nervous or afraid in a health care environment. This can lead to miscommunication. Consider this scenario: A busy phlebotomist enters a client's room to draw blood and discovers the speech language pathologist in the midst of treatment. Knowing how many clients he still needs to see, he yells, "You'll have to stop for a minute. I need to draw blood immediately. I'm in a hurry." The phlebotomist is responding emotionally. Although the therapist may have the urge to shout back, anger will not resolve the situation and may even inflame it. It is far more effective for the therapist to employ active listening techniques.

In discussing active listening, Davis (1998) includes a three-step framework: restatement, reflection, and clarification. Through this process, you let the speaker know that you heard what he or she said. You describe how you think the person feels and give him or her an opportunity to clarify those feelings. Finally, you summarize the situation. Active listening is a challenging skill to develop and requires practice. When used effectively, it can diffuse angry situations and lead to effective solutions.

Applying this process to the above scenario, the therapist might reply to the phlebotomist, "I understand that you're in a hurry and want to see this client immediately. It sounds like you're having a busy day and are upset." The speech-language pathologist could stop treatment for a moment or two to allow the phlebotomist to proceed. If not, she might indicate how long she expects to be and ask the phlebotomist to come back later. Either response would reduce conflict and allow both health care providers to proceed with client care. We must keep in mind that the client should come first. What are the medical priorities? What would most benefit the client at this time?

It is not always easy to be "therapeutic" in your approach, especially when you are the target of disappointment, frustration, and blame. Expert clinicians do not judge or categorize clients as difficult or noncompliant. Instead, they evaluate the challenge and take responsibility to develop alternate communication solutions (Jensen et al., 2000). Consider Joyce, a woman with multiple sclerosis, who bellowed at the occupational therapist, "When I came here, they told me that I would be able to dress myself within a week. Well, I can't. It's all your fault! If I had a better therapist, I would be home by now." Although you might reflexively respond defensively, it is therapeutically beneficial to take a different approach. In this case, the occupational therapist could say, "I understand that when you first came to this hospital you thought you'd be able to take care of yourself. You now see that this will take more time and be more involved than you anticipated. You sound frustrated. Unfortunately, there are no quick solutions. We have to work on your balance and strength so that you're able to be more independent." Keep this in mind when you are with clients. How will you react the next time you are confronted by an angry client or colleague? How will you respond to others when *you* are angry?

We know that when we are under stress, we are often tempted to respond inappropriately. We must be aware of this. When we are emotionally upset, we should state how we feel. In that way, we are taking responsibility for our own emotions and are not blaming others. It is particularly important for clinicians to develop active listening skills. These include maintaining eye contact, sustaining focus on the interaction, and positioning ourselves on the same level as the client, i.e., if a client is seated in a wheelchair, it helps if you sit, as well. Active listening skills also include restating what the clilent is saying to ensure your understanding and asking questions based on what the client is telling you (Jensen et al., 2000).

Not all situations will work out the way we would like, even for expert clinicians. People are emotional; they may become angry and frustrated and verbally "strike out" when they feel they cannot control the situation. We must do our best to maintain a level head, control our own emotions, and respond appropriately to clients, family members, and other health care professionals. If, however, you say something inappropriate, a well-timed apology is in order. These strategies not only improve our communication capabilities but also allow us to provide more effective client care.

At times, clients may bring up issues we do not know how to handle. For example, they may mention that they are having suicidal thoughts or report that they are being abused at home. A student should immediately inform his or her supervisor if this occurs. As a licensed professional, the supervisor can speak with the client to further explore the issue and perhaps determine if he or she needs to be referred to another health care provider for additional assistance. It is the wise professional who knows the scope of his or her practice and ability and refers clients to mental health professionals, such as psychiatrists, psychologists, rehabilitation counselors, and social workers.

## Nonverbal Communication

While verbal communication is important, we must recognize that people convey messages without saying a word. It is imperative to "tune in" to the nonverbal cues we give and receive. Nonverbal communication is open to ambiguous interpretation, is not always easy to understand, and strongly influences the meaning of messages received (Adler & Rodman, 1994; Davis, 1998; Northouse & Northouse, 1998; Purtilo & Haddad, 1996; Swain, 1997).

You enter a client's room and find him in tears. Do you immediately assume that he is depressed about his condition? Do you avoid interacting, or do you open a dialogue? You may be surprised to find out that he is shedding tears of joy over news of a grandchild. This information may motivate him to achieve the goal of returning home. It is important to verify assumptions and not accept seemingly pat conclusions.

## Facial Expressions

Facial expressions are important because they convey emotions. Following a biopsy, a frightened client is alert to the expression on the doctor's face as she walks into the room to announce the diagnosis. Is the news good or bad? Afraid and lacking information, we attempt to learn what we can by watching people. What do your facial expressions convey to clients? What do clients' expressions convey to you?

When treating a client, it is important to be aware of the expression on the person's face. Consider the adage, "The eyes are the mirror of the soul." Is the person in pain? Does he or she wince when moved from the bed to the chair? While some clients report when they feel pain, others are stoic and silent. Observing facial expressions and nonverbal language assists us in understanding what clients may be thinking and feeling. As we stated earlier, it is essential to verify our assumptions.

## Touch

Touch is another form of nonverbal communication. In health care settings, we touch clients to examine, evaluate, treat, and comfort them. In fact, as health care professionals, we often have intimate contact with clients that otherwise would be restricted to their significant others.

There are several forms of touch. Procedural or instrumental touch occurs when our hands come in contact with clients as we carry out interventions, such as moving a client into bed, performing range-of-motion exercises, or drawing blood. Expressive or caring touch involves contact that is meant to convey emotional support. This may include resting a hand on a client's arm or shoulder (Barringer & Glod, 1998; McCann & McKenna, 1993; Routasalo, 1999). Although expressive or caring touch may be "therapeutic," there is a complementary/alternative approach known as "therapeutic touch." This a technique in which a health care practitioner combines mindfulness, intent, and hand movements to promote healing by balancing energy fields. Hands may be placed directly on the skin, over clothing, or several inches above the client's body (Hayes & Cox, 1999; Herdtner, 2000; Krieger, 1979; Umbreit, 2000).

Health professionals' touching style is influenced by their cultural backgrounds, previous experience, and education (Estabrooks & Morse, 1992). While many studies show that touch does have a calming and comforting effect on clients, individual responses to touch vary, depending on age, gender, parts of the body being touched, physical environment, cultural heritage, prior experience, and personal interpretation of the meaning of the touch (McCann & McKenna, 1993; Routasalo, 1999).

Like verbal communication, the true meaning of a touch may be misinterpreted by either a client or health care provider. Touch, intended to be comforting, may be perceived as controlling or as a sexual advance (McCann & McKenna, 1993). Therefore, it is important to inform clients about what you are going to do and the reason for it. Touch should be firm enough to let the client feel safe and secure but should not be so firm as to cause unnecessary discomfort. We constantly need to assess how clients are responding to our touch. Do they withdraw? Do they appear physically or emotionally uncomfortable? If so, we may want to clarify the response with them. Keep the lines of communication open.

## Spatial Distances/Proxemics

Spatial distances also convey nonverbal information. Sitting down to speak with someone seated in a wheelchair puts you at the same level as the client and conveys respect. Standing over clients and talking down to them conveys a message of superiority. Standing in a doorway and listening or shouting to clients may imply that you are too busy to interact with them or that you do not really care what they have to say. Moving closer to clients sends a positive message that you are interested.

The concept of proxemics represents another aspect of spatial distances. Proxemics identifies the distances we maintain while communicating with others (Hall, 1966). As we will discuss in Chapter 3, these distances are culturally determined. What is important to note here is that every culture defines intimate and personal zones, typically entered only for physical intimacy, aggression, and comforting. However, when we provide health care interventions, we frequently enter these more private zones. We must do so sensitively. For example, you could say, "I need to take your blood pressure. May I please hold your arm?"

## Distracting Behaviors

Constantly checking your watch while you are with clients conveys a message that you are really too busy to be with them and have other things to do. Clients may become uncomfortable and feel unimportant. They may fail to relay valuable information because they do not want to "hold you up" or think you do not care.

It is important to remember that clients and families do not always share the perspective or priorities of health care providers (Woltersdorf, 1998). While providers are usually goal-centered, clients and family members tend to be emotionally centered. Through listening, observing, and avoiding distracting behaviors before we speak, we can learn about clients' emotional needs and discover how best to help them.

# Written Communication

Written communication is extremely important in the health care setting (French, 1994; Purtilo & Haddad, 1996). For example, letters are written to doctors to describe client progress, to third-party payers to justify treatments and request equipment, and to other health care professionals who are collaborating with us to provide client care. In addition, information is recorded in the medical record. Finally, we write client instructions and care plans to assist them in following through with recommended suggestions.

One advantage of written over verbal communication is that the printed material is more permanent (Vanderhoff, 2005). Providers can refer to notes to review client progress. Clients can refer to the written word to remind them, for example, what medications to take and how often. They can reread it at their own pace, as often as necessary. However, it is critical to keep your target readers uppermost in your mind. Many studies have identified incongruencies between the reading levels of written health care materials and the literacy skills of the intended audience (McCray, 2004).

When preparing written documentation, keep in mind the rules for verbal communication: Write to your audience; use appropriate terminology; and ensure that the information is accurate, clear, concise, and legible.

### Electronic Communication

The media is a significant shaper of values and attitudes. It is becoming increasingly common for health care professionals to take their message to the airwaves, such as television and radio broadcasts and Internet websites, as well as print media, like newspapers, magazines, and bulletins. They are also communicating their positive messages at wellness fairs and public forums.

Media and electronic communication systems are transforming the way health care professionals and clients gather information and interact. Clinical decision-making software and online sources of medical information that clients explore are two such examples. Rapid Internet access and inexpensive web cameras have made videoconferencing possible, and that same technology allows a professional to assess a situation, such as the status of a wound, without an additional clinic visit (Jadad & Delamothe, 2004).

Electronic transmissions can have a broader audience, thereby making confidentiality issues a paramount concern. In addition, clients may seek information on websites that provide inaccurate data, but health care professionals can guide clients to preferred reliable sites. Although there is no opportunity to read nonverbal cues through email, many clients favor communicating with their practitioners electronically, a trend that is anticipated to become more prevalent in the future (Kummervold, Trondsen, Andreassen, Gammon, & Hjortdahl, 2004).

Electronic communication can be a detriment or boon for people with disabilities and those who are aging. Not everyone is computer literate or has access. Conversely, large print, talking computers, and various modes of operation provide flexibility of communication and improved access to information.

# Grasping the True Meaning of What the Client Is Saying

Despite our best efforts to pay attention to verbal and nonverbal language, we may fail to understand the true meaning of what the client is saying (Vanderhoff, 2005). We often work with very distressed people. The resulting emotional strain can affect their ability to communicate. Our attempts to deal with difficult situations can also affect our own ability to communicate and be compassionate.

In our efforts to be compassionate, we should never offer false reassurances. Refrain from using the statement, "I know how you feel"—we do not know how they feel. Instead, you might say, "This must be difficult for you," "Tell me how this is affecting you," or "How are you feeling?" Similarly, we may not be able to tell them that "everything will be all right." Clients have a right, and often a need, to express their emotions regarding their illness or disability. Our role is to listen.

In addition, we need to avoid judgmental responses that indicate approval or disapproval. In the opening journal entry, Lindsay believed that Patrick would benefit from getting out of bed and attending therapy. She didn't yell at him, "Patrick, you're acting like a 2-year-old. Get out of bed!" Instead, she reframed the situation, giving him the opportunity to take control and "save face." By choosing the high ground, Lindsay was far more successful in motivating him. As a health professional, your role is to provide clients with factual information that helps them formulate their own decisions, not to offer value judgments. Grasping the meaning of what the client is truly saying is a key element in promoting optimal care.

# Using Humor to Communicate

There are many strategies to assist us in developing relationships with clients. When used appropriately, humor can be one of them. It may open the lines of communication, decrease stress, and establish a sense of camaraderie. Although humor does not *solve* problems, it can diminish their impact.

With all of the books, audio- and videotapes, and compact discs devoted to the subject, a newcomer to our world might think that humor was a new phenomenon. Corporations are hiring humor consultants, and anything billed as "humor" is almost a guaranteed drawing card to sessions at conferences. Is "Laughter the Best Medicine,®" as the popular column in *Reader's Digest* has been telling us for decades? Is there a role for humor in health care? Can injury or disease be appropriately funny? Think of all the humorous get-well cards and the jokes circulating about today's health care.

Humor in medicine as a concept may appear new, but it has been around longer than you might think. The Bible reminds us in Proverbs 17:22 that "a merry heart doeth good like medicine, but a broken spirit drieth the bone." In Moody's (1978) retrospective search on the healing power of humor, he highlighted three people. In the early 1900s, James Sully noted the positive effects that laughter has on respiratory, circulatory, and nervous systems. During the eighteenth century, German philosopher Immanuel Kant discussed the physiological benefits of laughter. Parson and scholar Robert Burton, who penned *Anatomy of Melancholy* in the 1600s, incorporated the work of many scholars to support his premise of laughter being a therapeutic measure.

Today, we know that laughter involves every major system in the body (Black, 1984; Hassed, 2001; Leiber, 1986; Robinson, 1983). When you laugh, you enjoy yourself, blissfully not thinking about the release of catecholamine, which will boost your alertness and enhance your ability to problem solve. You probably are not focusing on your dilated blood vessels, increased heart rate, and circulation spreading a high density lipoprotein, which may lower your risk of heart disease. Your lungs expand more, bringing in more oxygen and expelling more carbon dioxide than you did before you laughed. Your muscular tension is released, as you exercise your diaphragm, facial, upper extremity, thoracic, and abdominal muscles. Stress hormones are lowered. Chemical chain reactions occur (Black, 1984; Leiber, 1986; Robinson, 1983). Cortisol, a derivative of the hormone cortisone, is secreted from the adrenal glands and has an anti-inflammatory effect, improving immune system function. Increases of immunoglobulin help fight viral infections, particularly those of the upper respiratory tract. Endorphins are released (Siegel, 1986). Those natural pain relievers probably played a role in Norman Cousins's self-prescribed pain control regimen to battle his ankylosing spondylitis. This former editor of the *Saturday Review* would watch hours of funny movies and shows. His belly laughs, of even 10 minutes, could reduce or eliminate his pain for 2 hours (Cousins, 1979).

Humor has other health benefits: It decreases feelings of anxiety, apprehension, helplessness, anger, and hostility; it can be a tonic against staff fatigue and burnout; it can improve communication and interactions between clients and their health care providers (Robinson, 1991; Siegel, 1986).

Schmitt's (1990) research indicates that clients welcome laughter. The majority of clients in her survey strongly agreed that "Laughing helps me get through difficult times," "Sometimes, laughing works as well as a pain pill," "When I laugh, I feel better," "I appreciate an opportunity to laugh when I feel sad," and "Rehabilitation hospitals should encourage laughter to help clients feel better about their stay" (p. 145). Clients perceive that nurses who laugh with them are being therapeutic.

For example, consider Mr. Elliott, whose use of a postsurgical ventilator precluded him from speaking. He was using pantomime to communicate with the staff in the intensive care unit. One day, no matter how hard he tried, he could not make the staff understand what he was trying to tell them. He finally reached for the nearby clipboard and scribbled, "I thought actions speak louder than words!" That small action alleviated a lot of anxiety and frustration for the staff and Mr. Elliott. They were able to "take a step back" and try again. Humor is appropriate when it improves social relations and dispels harmful emotions (Harvey, 1998). When clients feel overwhelmed, humor may be therapeutic, alleviating stress and helping them cope.

Appropriate use of humor may help lighten the mood and facilitate adjustment. For example, Mrs. Williams had undergone a transtibial amputation of her right lower extremity, secondary to complications from diabetes. Recently back at work, she found herself embroiled in a conflict with a coworker. Realizing that there was no way she was going to convince this man of the validity of *her* point of view, she retorted, "I'd continue arguing, but I can see that I don't have a leg to stand on." At first flabbergasted, the man softened after she burst out in laughter.

When used inappropriately, however, humor may interfere with communication or offend others. At its extreme, it may even cause psychological harm. Struggling to maintain his sitting balance, a 25-year-old man with a traumatic brain injury wildly threw a ball, which landed far from the desired target. The recreation therapist responded, "Well, we won't be picking *you* to pitch on the Center's team." Although she was trying to lighten his mood, the client, a former semi-professional baseball player, took this message to heart and became quite depressed. He refused to "try again," thus setting back his progress.

When stress levels are high and people feel anxious, humor may be perceived as caustic and damaging. Mr. Carlin thoroughly researched all of his medical care and confronted the team's wisdom at every turn. He was well known to say, "That's not what I read in the book." One day, the team leader, at her wit's end, shared a remark attributed to Mark Twain: "Be careful about reading health books. You may die of a misprint." The medical staff all laughed, relieving their tension. The client, however, was very offended, feeling as though they were laughing at his expense.

Inappropriate humor may antagonize and alienate people. Once this has occurred, it can be difficult or impossible to reestablish a therapeutic relationship. Make sure you know and understand your client prior to injecting humor into your conversation. If a client appears offended by something you said, apologize to the client, assure him or her that you meant no disrespect, and be sure to avoid such topics in the future. Attempt to reestablish a sense of rapport and mutual respect with the client. If, over time, you believe that is impossible, suggest to your supervisor that the client may benefit if care is transferred to someone else.

Think about the potential impact of humor. Try to put yourself in the position of the client, friend, or family member. Does the humor have the same effect on you as it did before? Clients are in a vulnerable position when they come to you. Although humor can be an excellent communication tool when used in a therapeutic manner, it can also have undesirable effects. You may be unaware of where sensitive areas lie. Avoid jokes related to gender, politics, religion, culture, or sexual orientation. It is wise to proceed with caution.

# Barriers to Effective Communication

### Role Uncertainty

Communication can be negatively affected by a number of factors, such as role uncertainty. Clients may not know what we expect of them and not know what to expect of us. Many older clients are accustomed to a paternalistic health care system in which no one questioned the doctor. Health professionals held all of the power and had the responsibility of making clients "better."

In today's health care environment, practitioners expect to include clients in treatment-planning. This may be uncomfortable to older clients, who may be reluctant to ask questions. They may appear passive to a younger generation of clinicians. It is important to encourage them to assume a more active role in their communication. In an inpatient setting, it is common for clients to have contact with many different professionals during the course of a day. Team members may have different expectations for them, further contributing to their role uncertainty. Another complicating factor is that everyone is in a hurry, which may confuse the patient, who may hesitate to ask questions or discuss physical or psychosocial concerns (Northouse & Northouse, 1998).

Florence Nightingale is reported to have said, "We must not talk to them [clients] or at them but with them" (Attewell, 1998). Active listening shows clients that you are fully present in the moment, grasping the meaning of what they are saying. One difference noted between "expert" and "novice" physical therapists (Jensen et al., 2000) relates to the importance of listening. Skilled clinicians claim that they "got much more information from listening than from structuring questions" and that "if you go in and listen to the clients, they will tell you" (p. 33). It is very powerful for the client to feel your complete presence.

### Sensory Overload

Sensory overload may adversely affect both receptive and expressive communication (Purtilo & Haddad, 1996). People process information at varying rates. Instructions to a client may seem abundantly clear to us, but they may not be easy for others to fathom. Health care professionals need to be aware of the cognition, intelligence, and educational level of clients and use plain terminology, to avoid overloading them with information they do not comprehend. It also helps diminish sensory overload if we speak at a rate of speed that is easy to follow.

Are directions understandable, amidst a frightening environment of intravenous poles and buzzing machines? Institutional smells, distracting visual stimuli, and unfamiliar touch can also bombard clients' senses. As a result, clients may become unable to organize their thoughts to effectively communicate.

## Physical Appearance

There is an adage that says, "First impressions are lasting." We often judge others based on their appearance, which may include height, weight, hairstyle, clothing, skin color, accessories, and physical attractiveness (French, 1994; Swain, 1997). As discussed in Chapter 1, we tend to gravitate to individuals who are similar to ourselves and may have overt or covert biases against those who differ from us. As health care professionals, we need to be aware of our biases and refrain from making judgments about clients based on their physical appearance. How do you perceive clients who appear "rich," "poor," "well-dressed," or "slovenly"?

Sometimes, we may misinterpret apparent physical limitations. One study of people who are blind or have low vision identified barriers to receiving effective health care (O'Day, Killeen, & Iezzoni, 2004). As a result of physical appearance and assumed disability, health providers and office staff perceive that their clients cannot fully participate in their own care.

Clients may also judge us using these same criteria. In addition, uniforms, stethoscopes, and other tools of our trade convey messages. While a professional appearance may help inspire trust and confidence in clients and allay a measure of anxiety, it may create a barrier for others.

Customizing communication, listening actively, and being open-minded and avoiding assumptions all show respect and facilitate client-centered care. For example, in the O'Day et al. study noted above (2004), clients had difficulty communicating with health providers and office staff. Although written materials were provided, they were in a format that could not be used by the clients who were blind or had low vision, i.e., not written in Braille or in large print and not available on audiotape.

## Voice and Word Choice

We must be sure to give clear, simple instructions in a tone and volume that are easy to hear and comprehend. Whenever possible, provide the client with written instructions, including pictures if this enhances understanding. You may ask the client to repeat the directions or demonstrate a task. If the instructions are for home use, you might ask, "Can you picture yourself doing this on your own at home?" If the client says no, you have time to ask why not. You are creating an opportunity to promote understanding and allow the client to voice questions or concerns in a safe environment. It is wise to give instructions in a quiet room to minimize distractions. Whenever possible, give the client a period of time to think about the instructions. Review them at the next session and see if the person still understands or has any questions.

## Language Barriers

In today's multicultural environment, we may find that language barriers affect our ability to communicate effectively. If a client speaks a language different from our own, it is important to provide an interpreter to assist with the communication process. Family members may or may not be the most appropriate resource. Clients do not always want to discuss their situation in front of family. In certain cultures, for example, men do not reveal their problems in front of their wives or children. Well-intentioned family members may edit or misinterpret messages being translated. We must be sensitive to these issues. We explore cross-cultural communication in greater depth in Chapter 3.

Not only may we speak different languages, we may misinterpret values, beliefs, emotions, and nonverbal language. While people from some cultures are encouraged to cry when they feel pain, individuals from other cultures are discouraged from doing so, and in fact may hide their pain (Trill & Holland, 1993). This could certainly affect our treatment intervention.

Ideally, administrators should recruit and hire health professionals who share a common language and culture with the people who live in the communities being served. However, this may not be feasible. It is advisable to learn as much about the culture and language of the community as possible. This can assist you in understanding and communicating with clients. If possible, consider taking a language course so that you can understand and speak with clients. In all settings, clear, written instructions, complete with pictures and/or videotapes, available in various languages, greatly enhances communication with clients whose primary language is not your own.

According to Houts, Bachrach, and Witmer (1998), using pictures and audiovisual aids to explain medical procedures and treatment protocols may be an effective method of interacting with and teaching clients who are illiterate or who have poor comprehension skills. Using pictures along with written material significantly improves short-term memory recall of medical instructions. Simplify language and use these tools whenever possible.

Other language barriers may also exist. For example, a traumatic brain injury or cerebral vascular accident (stroke) may result in expressive and/or receptive difficulties. Stuttering can render speech unintelligible. Not understanding the client, health care providers may feel angry, frustrated, or embarrassed. They may even avoid the client. Even though you may feel uncomfortable, it is important to take the time to listen closely (Pore, 1995). If the client perceives that you are uncomfortable, he or she may become anxious, making speech even more difficult to comprehend. If you do not understand, let the client know. Do not allow him or her to keep talking before you gently interrupt. Consider using the following strategies:

- Provide cues, such as nodding, when you do understand.
- Ask questions for clarification.
- Do not pretend to understand.
- Maintain eye contact.
- Speak slowly and directly to the person, not to a surrogate, unless the client has directed you to do so.
- Modulate your tone and volume of voice, based on the situation.
- Enunciate clearly.
- Schedule treatments in a quiet room when possible.

Sometimes we can understand the client's speech but are unwilling to listen. We do not want to hear what he or she has to say. We may believe that a client is a "complainer" and is wasting our time. Clients may state that no one has the time or wants to listen to them. In a busy health care environment, time is limited, and it becomes even more important to spend that time wisely. Therefore, we must learn to direct the client's conversation so that we hear the information we need. There may be times when we have to inform a client that we do not have time to "chat" today. We need to keep the conversation focused. However, there will be other times when we may have a few extra minutes to look at family photographs. Sometimes, this is just what the client needs to become refocused.

Selective listening and incorrect perceptions are other obstacles to effective listening (Conine, 1976). As health care providers, we hear many similar stories from clients. As a result, we may have preconceived ideas of how the client is going to answer our questions. In selective listening, health professionals anticipate what they expect to hear and focus on that information. As a result, they may fail to absorb information relative to the individual client's needs. Health providers may also assume that they understood the message, but that may not be an accurate perception. It is important to seek clarification by asking probing questions, such as "Do you mean . . .?", "Have I understood this correctly . . .?", "This is what I hear you saying. . . ." Focused, active listening ensures that the listener receives the messages the speaker intended to transmit. However, this is not always enough to make us successful.

# Conflict

Health care providers interact daily with clients, families, colleagues, insurance providers, and others. Everyone brings his or her background, culture, beliefs, and goals into the workplace, and viewpoints vary. Even when people share similar goals, they may have different perspectives and priorities to reach those goals. Conflict becomes inevitable (Xu & Davidhizar, 2004). Although some people seem to thrive on conflict, many are uncomfortable with it and try to avoid it or handle it poorly. To manage conflict effectively, we need to change our own behavior or alter the situation.

Despite the negative connotations of conflict, it has both positive and negative elements. Managed appropriately, conflict can lead to positive changes, such as decreased stress levels, improved staff cohesiveness, job satisfaction, and creative problem solving, resulting in improved client care. Ignored, avoided, or poorly managed conflict negatively affects all people involved. It can permeate an organization, group, or relationship, decreasing everyone's ability to work effectively (Dove, 1998; Henrikson, 1998; Lipcamon & Mainwaring, 2004; Marcus, Dorn, Kritek, Miller, & Wyatt, 1995; Northouse & Northouse, 1998). Sometimes, people are able to adequately resolve their issues independently. At other times, the assistance of managers, supervisors, or neutral third parties is needed.

Conflict involves tension or disagreement between two or more opposing forces. It is "a process in which one party perceives that its interests are being opposed or negatively affected by another party" (Wall & Callister, 1995, p. 517). Once that occurs, people need to decide how to deal with the situation, even if their choice is to do nothing. They respond emotionally, and actions lead to reactions. Conflict is underway.

In the health care system, individuals work both independently and interdependently. Opinions about the most appropriate form of care may differ. In one study of clinical decision making in intensive care units, physicians and nurses identified conflict during patient management discussions (Coombs, 2003). Other research supports this. With more than 200 patients in intensive care, doctors and nurses documented 248 conflicts concerning vital matters of patient care, as well as disputes between teams and families, team members, and among family members (Studdert et al., 2003). In addition, time constraints and limited resources influence decision making. As health professionals work together to provide client-centered care, roles may overlap and lines of authority for ultimate decision making may blur. Conflict is often a by-product.

Although it may be unsettling, conflict is neither "good" nor "bad." Rather, it is how well we deal with conflict that is important. Our behavior and ability can affect client outcomes, interpersonal relationships, and sometimes our own health (Lipcamon & Mainwaring, 2004; Miller, 1998; Northouse & Northouse, 1998; Strutton & Knouse, 1997).

---

**M**y supervisor reprimanded me this morning in front of a client and his daughter. I was so embarrassed! I became so nervous that my hands were shaking as I tried to continue with the treatment. I knew Mr. Chen had lost all confidence in my abilities. He looked as if he feared I was going to hurt him. His daughter asked me if I was sure I knew what I was doing. Finally, my supervisor suggested I leave and finish up some paperwork while he completed the treatment. I left the room and ran to the ladies room in tears, to hide and compose myself. Later in the day, my supervisor acted as if nothing had happened. We continued to treat other patients. I was anxious and afraid I would make another mistake, but I didn't say anything to him.

Tonight, I talked with my roommate. She told me that I should confront my supervisor first thing in the morning and discuss the situation. I know she's right. I can accept constructive criticism, but I think he handled it inappropriately. He could have directed me to correct my error and then talked to me later in the staff room, away from the client and his daughter. The client's safety wasn't at risk. As much as I hate confrontation and would like to pretend this never happened, I know my roommate is right. If I don't say something, I'll always be afraid that he'll do this to me again, and my ability to learn will be in jeopardy. He probably doesn't even know how he made me feel.

*—From the journal of Shannon Sullivan, nursing student*

---

While Shannon would prefer to ignore this conflict, she realizes that this strategy will not solve her problem and may negatively affect her educational experience and her ability to treat clients effectively. If she is able to discuss her feelings and situation with her supervisor, she may be able to develop a better working relationship with him. Together, they could develop learning objectives and discuss appropriate feedback mechanisms. Shannon might be more at ease treating clients in the presence of her supervisor, and she could learn how to improve her nursing skills from him.

## Levels of Conflict

### PERSONAL CONFLICT

Conflict can occur at personal, interpersonal, intragroup, or intergroup levels (Dove, 1998; Wall & Callister, 1995). At the personal level, conflict occurs within an individual. He or she may receive pressure from colleagues to do something that is not in accordance with his or her personal value system. For example, a supervisor may suggest that an occupational therapist delegate portions of a client's treatment to an occupational therapy assistant in order to increase productivity. The occupational therapist may believe that the client requires the attention and skills of a therapist and that it is inappropriate to delegate this part of the care. As a result, the occupational therapist may feel internal personal conflict and have to decide whether to adhere to the supervisor's suggestion or confront the supervisor to discuss the situation. The ultimate decision will be influenced by how strongly the occupational therapist feels about the level of care needed, the experience of both the occupational therapist and the assistant, and the conflict-management style the occupational therapist uses in this situation.

An individual may also experience interrole conflicts at a personal level. Consider Tim Gallagher, a nurse in the intensive care unit in a large urban hospital. Toward the end of his shift, Tim hurries to complete paperwork, ignoring the patients' call buttons buzzing around him. Other nurses leave their documentation to respond to the patients' needs. While Tim always leaves on time, the other nurses work overtime to complete their duties. Although they do not confront Tim, they ventilate their anger among themselves. When one of the nurses finally tells him how much the others resent his behavior, he reminds her that he is a single parent, caring for two preschool-age children. If he does not pick the children up at the day-care center at the appointed time, he is charged a penalty for each minute he is late. He cannot afford to be late. Torn between his parental role of needing to get his children on time and his professional role of being a team player and attending to client care and documentation, Tim may be experiencing personal conflict of an interrole nature. This conflict is causing internal stress for him and creating an interpersonal conflict between Tim and the other nurses.

### INTERPERSONAL CONFLICT

Conflict develops at the interpersonal level when two or more individuals exhibit conflicting values or beliefs (Dove, 1998; Wall & Callister, 1995). For example, interpersonal conflicts frequently occur between nursing home staff members and residents' family members (Nelson & Cox, 2003; Pillemer, Hegeman, Albright, & Henderson, 1998). Nursing homes are structured organizations with rules and regulations. Sometimes they promote impersonal client care. Family members, however, may provide more personal, albeit infrequent, care. Discrepancies about what is best for the client may arise.

While staff members focus on the technical aspects of care, families may perceive that the emotional components are lacking and that their experiences are undervalued. Similarly, staff members might feel unappreciated by families. Because many nursing home residents, especially those with cognitive impairments, are unable to provide accurate information about their experiences, well-intentioned families may misinterpret what they see. Interpersonal conflict may ensue. If time restrictions further limit communication between staff and families, minor interpersonal conflicts can escalate into larger problems (Pillemer et al., 1998).

## INTRAGROUP CONFLICT

Intragroup conflict exists when members within a group disagree with each other as to what course of action should be taken (Dove, 1998; Wall & Callister, 1995). Consider the Minelli family. For more than 10 years, Mr. Minelli has been caring for his wife at home. As her Alzheimer's disease progresses, she has started to wander and is becoming combative. Mr. Minelli is seeking advice from his children. Of the six adult children in the family, three of them work in health care. Only the youngest daughter lives nearby.

The local daughter is the mother of five young children and has a husband who frequently travels for business. Experiencing interrole conflict between her roles as a mother, wife, and daughter, she cares for her nuclear family, while cleaning her parents' house and doing their laundry and shopping. Exhausted and frustrated, she suggested to her father that he consider placing her mother in a nursing home. The oldest son, who is a pediatrician, disagrees and has offered to pay for daytime respite care. The oldest daughter, who is a nurse, agrees with her younger sister. She believes her mother would receive excellent care in a long-term facility and that her father would be relieved of the burden. The youngest son, who is a pharmacist, thinks that everyone should "chip in" to build an apartment for the parents attached to his sister's house, making it easier for her to assist them. Her husband does not support this idea. Other family members are divided as to how their father should handle the situation.

This family is experiencing intragroup conflict. The situation and the intragroup conflict that the family is experiencing is tearing them apart. Mr. Minelli wants to do whatever is best for his wife, but he does not know what that is. He loves his children and does not want to hurt their feelings, yet he is unable to make a decision. Siblings have heated arguments over the telephone and by email correspondence. Alliances and counteralliances have developed. If the conflict remains unresolved, the family may be further torn apart. The Minelli family may need a neutral party, such as a social worker, to mediate the situation.

## INTERGROUP CONFLICT

Intergroup conflict arises between two or more groups of people, departments, or organizations that have conflicting beliefs or needs (Dove, 1998; Wall & Callister, 1995). Consider Carmen Garcia, a 94-year-old woman recovering from a motor vehicle accident in which she sustained multiple fractures and internal injuries. She was in both the intensive care and regular units for several weeks and is now ready to be discharged from the acute care hospital. The health care team recommended that she go to a transitional care unit, where she will receive nursing care and therapy to increase her strength and endurance. In contrast, Mrs. Garcia and her family want her to go home. Her children and grandchildren believe that their cultural values oblige them to care for her at home, out of respect for her position in the family and their love.

Members of the health care team are quite concerned about the family's ability to care for Mrs. Garcia at home because she is weak and cannot bear weight on her casted right leg. She also has a fracture of her left humerus. Hospital staff members fear that either she will be further injured at home or that a family member will get hurt trying to help her.

The meeting between the two groups was confrontational. Even though a social worker attempted to mediate the situation, members of both groups refused to change their positions. Christmas was fast approaching, and both Mrs. Garcia and her family believed that this would be her last one at home. They wanted to spend it together in a family environment, not in the cafeteria of a health facility. The family ultimately brought Mrs. Garcia home, discharged against medical advice.

## Sources of Conflict

Conflicts include content, psychological, and procedural components (Moore, 1996). Content issues are related to specific factors, such as time and money. In today's managed health care environment, a primary care physician may be in conflict with an insurance provider over how long a client may be able to stay in an acute care hospital following surgery. A physical therapist and a parent may be in conflict over the appropriate care of a child.

> I visited my client and her family today. It was time to discuss the possibility of ordering a wheelchair for Brenda. Her mother became extremely insistent that Brenda's stroller was just fine for getting her around and that the use of a wheelchair would make her appear much more disabled. By using some support blocks I had available, I was able to demonstrate that a more supported sitting posture would actually make Brenda significantly more functional and, therefore, appear less disabled.
> —*From the journal of Ron Johansen, physical therapist student*

By reframing the above situation, Ron was able to suggest an alternate perspective. The wheelchair became a symbol of independence rather than disability.

The psychological elements of conflict include aspects such as trust, respect, and the desire for inclusion (Moore, 1996). Involving clients, families, and appropriate care providers in decision making, introducing change slowly, and encouraging feedback can help reduce conflict (Davidhizar, Giger, & Poole, 1997). Using active listening techniques, described earlier, can improve communication and diminish conflict. Listening to concerns and ideas attentively, eliminating unnecessary interruptions, and ensuring confidentiality will help develop a sense of trust. Providing adequate information and showing respect for everyone increases the probability that all involved will be able to manage conflict without the need for outside interventions (Davidhizar, 1994; Marcus et al., 1995).

Procedural components of conflict involve issues, such as policies, the chain of command, and decision-making responsibility. When policies are unclear, individuals may interpret them differently, resulting in conflicting views as to the appropriate course of action. Because content, psychological, and procedural components are interrelated, a conflict cannot be completely resolved until all three elements in this "satisfaction triangle" have been addressed (Moore, 1996).

Conflict can emanate from many sources. As discussed earlier, differing personal beliefs, goals, interests, and values may lead to conflict (Seroka, 1994; Wall & Callister, 1995). Possible incompatibilities, based on temperaments, race, religion, culture, or other biases, may also result in conflict (Greenwald & Banaji, 1995). Members of different cultures view conflict in different ways, a factor that must be taken into consideration when dealing with both clients and colleagues (Xu & Davidhizar, 2004; Nibler & Harris, 2003) (see Chapter 3).

In the health care arena, there is much ambiguity. Individuals interpret available information in different ways, depending upon their backgrounds and life experiences. There may be uncertainty about options and potential outcomes. Decisions are complex, as many individuals are involved at different levels, and there is competition for power, prestige, and status.

Lack of communication and unclear expectations are also sources of conflict. For example, in health care settings, clients may receive conflicting information from different staff members. Consider Nancy, a new mother who is having difficulty breastfeeding. Nurses on each of three successive shifts have offered her different and conflicting strategies. She is frustrated, confused, and anxious.

In today's health care environment, clients are sometimes encouraged to discuss questions or problems with their health care providers via the Internet. However, email messages lack both the verbal and nonverbal cues of face-to-face communication, leaving room for misinterpretation. In addition, people tend to respond instantaneously to email messages, not always taking the time to consider what they are going to say. To prevent unnecessary conflict, it is important to follow up on email messages with regular phone calls and face-to-face meetings to clarify questions or concerns (Umiker, 1997; Zweibel & Goldstein, 2001).

Life circumstances may also result in conflict (Northouse & Northouse, 1998). For example, in contemporary society, family members often live long distances from each other, creating a form of structural barrier when adult children attempt to assist parents with medical problems. Older adults sometimes fail to ask pertinent questions of their health care providers, and, therefore, clients may not receive the necessary services to which they are entitled. Consider Ramona, a medical assistant working in southern California. Her elderly parents are both ill and live on the east coast, without relatives living in their area. Ramona's mother has heart problems and goes for dialysis treatments twice a week. Her father has difficulty walking, following total hip arthroplasties. In addition, he has a long history of smoking and emphysema.

Ramona has attempted to contact her parents' primary care physician but has had difficulty connecting with him. Frustrated, she believed that the physician was not doing everything he could to help her parents and accompanied them to an appointment during an infrequent visit home. She described how much difficulty her parents were having and suggested that the physician request a homemaker to assist with routine housecleaning, as well as Meals on Wheels, so that her parents could receive at least one well-balanced, hot meal each day. The doctor did not know they were having such difficulties in the home setting because they had never mentioned their problems or concerns. Appropriate resources were immediately put into place. While phone calls and emails may reduce some structural barriers, these issues remain a concern for clients, families, and health care providers.

Lack of advance directive from a legally incompetent client may be another source of conflict. There are many questions about what is the "right" or "best" thing to do. Health care providers and a client's medical care surrogate, such as a family member, may have conflicting opinions regarding the most appropriate care for a client who is unable to express his or her own wishes. Alpers and Lo (1999) describe a case in which a client who no longer had decision-making capabilities had not left a clear advance directive as to his future care. The client and his family believed in the sanctity of life. Despite no hope for recovery, family members wanted the health care providers to prolong his life as long as possible. The health care professionals thought that the client was enduring unnecessary pain and suffering while life support systems kept him alive. Although his wife agreed with the health care team in principle, she would not go against the wishes of her children. This illustrates the stress and need for support that family surrogates experience and presents an issue of conflicting values. Providing accurate, understandable medical information, and allowing a surrogate time to understand the circumstances and express personal concerns, fosters communication and reduces conflict.

# Strategies to Manage Conflict

Four elements affect the outcome of conflict: the issues at hand, cooperation among involved parties, the power bases of the participants, and the effectiveness of their communication skills (Miller, 1998). When conflict concerns relatively minor issues, cooperation and resolution may be fast and easy. At other times, conflict is related to substantive issues where individuals or groups interpret facts differently, have opposing goals, or disagree on acceptable methods. When conflicting parties disagree on principles, cooperation may be nonexistent and resolution will be more difficult to achieve.

While many health care professionals consider clinical skills as being most important for competent practice, they sometimes fail to recognize that communication and the ability to manage conflict successfully are of primary importance in assuring effective health care outcomes (Pettrey, 2003). This is especially true in today's health care environment where there is an emphasis on interdisciplinary care. There is a tendency for individuals to "band together" in the "us" against "them" mentality described in Chapter 1. This can result in intragroup and intergroup conflict. It has been shown that teams that work together to openly discuss differences and solve problems are much more effective than those that set up competitive goals (Alper, Tjosvold, & Law, 1998).

The ability to communicate effectively greatly assists people and groups to resolve conflicts. It is imperative to focus on the pertinent issues and avoid blaming and name-calling. When participants lose focus, the number of issues involved tends to expand, and the emphasis shifts toward winning rather than compromising. People begin to attack each other rather than the issues. Power tactics, including coercion and deception, are often employed. Asking open-ended questions that encourage people to reveal their true concerns helps us focus on the important issues and allows us to resolve conflict in its early stages (Rakley, 1999).

A good communicator expresses his or her own viewpoints, listens carefully to opponents' opinions, and works collaboratively with others to develop cooperative problem-solving strategies that lead to solutions acceptable to all parties (Marcus et al., 1995; Miller, 1998; Umiker, 1997).

Thomas and Kilmann (1974) identified five styles of managing conflict: *avoidance, accommodation, competition, compromise,* and *collaboration*. These styles continue to be studied today (Lipcamon & Mainwaring, 2004). Most authors agree that no one single strategy is best. Rather, each situation needs to be evaluated to determine which strategy would be the most effective (Eason & Brown, 1999; Henrikson, 1998; Marcus et al., 1995; Milstead, 1996; Northouse & Northouse, 1998; Spickerman & Brown, 1991; Umiker, 1997; Wall & Callister, 1995). While we have the ability to utilize each of the strategies in a given situation, each of us has our own preferred style of managing conflict. Understanding the strengths and weaknesses of each strategy and learning to identify our own, as well as our colleagues' and clients' preferred styles, will help us become better communicators and more effective health care providers. The following section describes the strengths and liabilities of each of these styles of managing conflict.

## Avoidance

Avoidance is an unassertive and uncooperative conflict management strategy in which individuals simply ignore or evade the fact that a conflict exists (Eason & Brown, 1999; Henrikson, 1998; Marcus et al., 1995; Milstead, 1996; Northouse & Northouse, 1998; Spickerman & Brown, 1991; Umiker, 1997; Wall & Callister, 1995). People who are passive and uncomfortable addressing conflict frequently use this style. Avoidance can be counterproductive, often prolonging rather than resolving issues and increasing stress levels. Consider a staff therapist who works in a large medical center. As clients are referred to the department, their names are posted on the bulletin board, and therapists select them. While most of the staff members add clients to their caseloads as the names become available, one therapist purposely avoids "difficult" patients, leaving colleagues to care for the more complicated clients.

However, there are times when avoidance is a positive and/or necessary strategy. If individuals are angry, avoidance can allow for a cooling-off period. It provides people with time to gain composure and gather additional information prior to addressing the issues. If a problem is perceived to be trivial, people may prefer to ignore it rather than deal with it. In addition, some problems resolve themselves over time. In those cases, they may not be worth the time and energy needed to confront them. When a problem is not yours, or there is nothing you can do about it, you may want to avoid becoming involved. In health care, people may need to overlook minor personality conflicts to ensure effective client care.

## Accommodation

Accommodation is an unassertive but cooperative approach to conflict management. A person neglects his or her own needs to meet the needs of others. Those who seek constant approval frequently use this strategy (Eason & Brown, 1999; Henrikson, 1998; Marcus et al., 1995; Milstead, 1996; Northouse & Northouse, 1998; Spickerman & Brown, 1991; Umiker, 1997; Wall & Callister, 1995). While this approach may appear to promote harmony and solve conflicts quickly, it may also be superficial and temporary. People who accommodate may feel angry and frustrated because they failed to seize the opportunity to express their own thoughts, opinions, and feelings. For example, Shelley, a respiratory therapist, initially volunteered to work on major holidays so that her colleagues, whose extended families lived out of state, could have the time off. What began as "team player behavior" became expected by the staff. Now harboring feelings of frustration, she would like to have a holiday off but continues to accommodate colleagues' expectations. A better resolution may have been discovered if the group had taken the time to consider everyone's ideas.

Accommodation is an appropriate strategy to use when one realizes that the other party is right or when there is little chance of "winning." It can also be used when one has little interest in the situation or when the outcome does not particularly affect you. In health care settings, accommodation may sometimes be useful to promote harmony and maintain good interpersonal relationships among staff members within a department or interdisciplinary team.

## Competition

Competition is an aggressive, uncompromising approach to managing conflict. It is power-driven and frequently used by assertive individuals interested in pursuing their own goals, even at the expense of others (Eason & Brown, 1999; Henrikson, 1998; Marcus et al., 1995; Milstead, 1996; Northouse & Northouse, 1998; Spickerman & Brown, 1991; Umiker, 1997; Wall & Callister, 1995). Think of a situation in which a student clinician proposes an alternative evidence-based treatment approach. The supervisor refuses to consider the plan or listen to the rationale, insisting that it be done her way. This style may result in quick, short-term agreements. However, the results are based upon an "I win, you lose" strategy, which may be counterproductive over time. When competition levels are high, communication may become hostile and potentially damaging to relationships.

In contrast, healthy competition among health care providers may result in improved services for clients. It is also appropriate in an emergency situation when someone needs to make a quick decision to save a client's life or preserve the person's safety. It may also be appropriate when legal and ethical violations need to be addressed.

## Compromise

Compromise is a strategy midway between competition and accommodation. It includes an element of assertiveness, as well as a component of cooperation (Eason & Brown, 1999; Henrikson, 1998; Marcus et al., 1995; Milstead, 1996; Northouse & Northouse, 1998; Spickerman & Brown, 1991; Umiker, 1997; Wall & Callister, 1995). People who compromise use a "give-and-take" strategy. They are concerned with their own needs, as well as the needs and concerns of others, and realize that neither side can win completely. While both parties agree to the final outcome, neither side is perfectly satisfied with the results. Whereas this method may result in faster resolution of problems, more innovative and satisfying results may be achieved if the parties continue to negotiate.

Compromise can be an effective means of settling conflict. Consider Melissa, a 15-year-old girl with juvenile rheumatoid arthritis. Her medication made her drowsy and impaired her ability to think clearly, affecting her schoolwork. Her physician compromised and prescribed another medication that was not as effective but had fewer side effects.

## Collaboration

Collaboration involves both assertiveness and cooperation. It is a problem-solving approach in which all parties want to fully address the concerns of everyone. It is designed to promote a "win–win" solution, with everyone committed to the final outcome. Participants believe that the achievement of mutual goals is more important than individual objectives (Eason & Brown, 1999; Henrikson, 1998; Marcus et al., 1995; Milstead, 1996; Northouse & Northouse, 1998; Spickerman & Brown, 1991; Umiker, 1997; Wall & Callister, 1995). Imagine a situation in which a manager enlists the input from the entire staff to address how they might change the hours and staffing patterns of their operation. While most authors agree that this is the preferred approach to managing conflict, it is the most difficult and often the most time-consuming to achieve and, therefore, may not be practiced in all situations.

People need to explore differences, identify commonalities, and work together to develop problem-solving strategies and initiate solutions acceptable to all involved. This requires everyone's dedication and hard work. As a result of the time and energy expended, innovative, cost-effective solutions usually result. Because both sides "win," everyone tends to feel satisfied. This helps build stronger relationships, promotes trust, and sets the stage for more positive conflict resolution in the future.

It is important to note that these five styles of managing conflict may be used to varying degrees or in combination with one another, depending upon the circumstances in each situation.

## Mediation

Sometimes, individuals or groups may be unable to resolve conflict, and it escalates. Members of each side may try to convert otherwise neutral parties to their point of view. Stress levels increase while productivity decreases. At such junctures, mediation may be required (Fraser, 2001; Saravia, 1999). A neutral third party is invited to facilitate the process. The mediator begins by developing a rapport with the parties in conflict. Once the conflict is defined, alternative solutions are generated with each possible solution considered until an agreement can be reached (Fraser, 2001; Liberman, Rotarius, & Kendall, 1997; Marcus et al., 1995; Rotarius & Liberman, 2000).

To be successful, individuals cannot blame one another. They must carefully listen to understand all issues in the disagreement. The bottom line is that everyone agrees to accept and implement the decision.

## SUMMARY

This chapter described the importance of communication and its relevance to health care. It is imperative to develop a rapport with a client in order to provide quality care. We reviewed the components of communication, which include being present in the moment, using and interpreting verbal and nonverbal communication, and the importance of active listening and understanding what the client is "truly" saying.

The use of appropriate and inappropriate humor in communication was described. Used effectively, humor can decrease tension and assist health care professionals in developing relationships with clients.

Barriers to effective communication, such as role uncertainty, sensory overload, physical appearance, voice and words, language comprehension, and perceptions, were discussed.

It was noted that serious disagreements, disputes, and/or conflicts do not usually develop suddenly. A lack of trust or sense that people are being treated unfairly over a period of time often contributes to conflicts in health care settings. Respecting differences is critical to developing rapport, trust, and respect. Listening to others and encouraging innovative decision making and goal setting promotes harmony, minimizes conflicts, and fosters effective communication (Davidhizar, 1994; Shendell-Falik, 1997; Strutton & Knouse, 1997).

As health care professionals, we try to understand the clients' viewpoints and promote their participation in developing goals and solving problems. We can also use these same strategies to resolve conflicts with colleagues and others. Rather than confronting or accusing someone, we can ask him or her to work with us to help solve our mutual problem. Asking open-ended questions that encourage people to reveal their true concerns helps us focus on the important issues and allows us to resolve conflict in its early stages (Rakley, 1999).

This chapter also defined and presented an overview of conflict. Sources of conflict were identified, and elements of conflict resolution were explored. The advantages and disadvantages of common approaches to managing conflict were discussed. Methods of alternative conflict resolution were introduced. As the need for continued interdependence and teamwork increases in health care, effective conflict management is needed to provide optimal client care.

## REFLECTIVE QUESTIONS

1. a. What are some of the factors that determine how our actions are interpreted?
   b. How will you know if your words or actions have had the desired effect?
   c. What can you do if you think a client received the wrong message?
2. a. When you are listening, what do you do to demonstrate that you are listening?
   b. How will you know if a client has heard what you intended to say?
   c. If you are not sure that your message has been correctly understood, what can you do to verify this?
3. a. Clients are not always able to express what they are thinking or feeling and cannot always ask the questions that are bothering them. What feelings may clients feel uncomfortable expressing?
   b. How would you facilitate discussion?
4. a. What are some factors that might interfere with your ability to listen effectively to clients and members of the health care team?
   b. What can you do to improve your effectiveness?
5. a. Describe a situation in which conflict was handled well. What elements contributed to the beneficial outcome?
   b. Describe a situation in which conflict was poorly handled. What elements contributed to the unsuccessful outcome?

## CASE STUDY

Jennifer Pennington, a 36-year-old mother of two, returned to school to become an occupational therapist after raising her children. Having completed her didactic course work, she is now on her final clinical education assignment. She is a "take charge" person who has always prided herself on being in control. Her clinical supervisor, Jim Waterman, is a quiet-spoken man of 28, who has been practicing in this clinical environment for five years and has instructed six students prior to Jennifer.

Although Jim is very knowledgeable and has excellent clinical skills, Jennifer is having problems interacting with him. She perceives that he does not include her in completing evaluations and developing treatment plans as much as she thinks he should. In addition, she feels that he never explains his rationale for using certain tests. She observes treatments but does not always understand procedures and goals. When she tries to talk with Jim, he averts his eyes and changes the subject.

As this is her final clinical experience, she believes she should be more actively involved in assessing clients' needs and developing care plans. She has done extremely well on earlier clinical assignments and achieved high levels of independence. Believing that she would learn a great deal at this clinic, she is quite frustrated but does not know how to address the problem.

1. What verbal and nonverbal communication strategies are contributing to the conflict between Jennifer and Jim?

2. a. If Jim uses avoidance as a strategy to manage conflict, and Jennifer uses a competitive strategy, what type of scenario might occur?

   b. What might be the outcome of this confrontation?

3. Describe different scenarios and outcomes if Jennifer and Jim use other strategies to manage conflict.

4. During the midterm conference, Jennifer and Jim disagree as to how well she is performing. She believes that she is competent and close to meeting the passing criteria. He believes that she has a long way to go and expresses uncertainty about her ability to successfully complete the clinical requirements within the allotted timeframe.

   a. What interventions should be taken at this time?

   b. What additional problems do you foresee with this scenario?

   c. What steps could have been taken earlier in the clinical experience to avoid this situation?

   d. Who might be able to serve as a mediator in this situation? What would be that person's role?

# REFERENCES

Adler, R. B., & Rodman, G. (1994). *Understanding human communication* (5th ed.). Orlando, FL: Holt, Rinehart and Winston.

Alper, S., Tjosvold, D., & Law, K. S. (1998). Interdependence and controversy in group decision-making: Antecedents to effective self-managing teams. *Organizational Behavior and Human Decision Process, 74*(1), 33–52.

Alpers, A., & Lo, B. (1999). Avoiding family feuds: Responding to surrogate demands for life-sustaining interventions. *Journal of Law, Medicine and Ethics, 27*(1), 74–88.

Ang, M. (2002). Advanced communication skills: Conflict management and persuasion. *Academic Medicine, 77*(11), 1166.

Attewell, A. (1998). Florence Nightingale's relevance to nurses. *Journal of Holistic Nursing, 16*(2), 281–291.

Barringer, B., & Glod, C. A. (1998). Therapeutic relationship and effective communication. In C. A. Glod (Ed.), *Contemporary psychiatric-mental health nursing: The brain–behavior connection* (pp. 47–61). Philadelphia: F. A. Davis.

Beckman, H. B., & Frankel, R. M. (1984). The effect of physician behavior on the collection of data. *Annals of Internal Medicine, 101*(5), 692–696.

Black, D. W. (1984). Laughter. *Journal of the American Medical Association, 252*(21), 2295–3014.

Conine, T. A. (1976). Listening in the helping relationship. *Physical Therapy, 56*(2), 159–162.

Coombs, M. (2003). Power and conflict in intensive care clinical decision-making. *Intensive Critical Care Nursing, 19*(3), 125–135.

Cousins, N. (1979). *Anatomy of an Illness as perceived by the patient.* New York: Norton.

Davidhizar, R. E. (1994). Using facilitation as a managerial technique. *Journal of Nursing Management, 2*, 193–196.

Davidhizar, R., Giger, J. N., & Poole, V. (1997). When change is a must. *Health Care Supervisor, 16*(2), 21–25.

Davis, C. M. (1998). *Patient practitioner interaction: An experiential manual for developing the art of health care* (3rd ed.). Thorofare, NJ: Slack.

Davis, H., & Fallowfield, L. (1991). *Counselling and communication in health care.* West Sussex, UK: Wiley.

Dove, M. A. (1998). Conflict: Process and resolution. *Nursing Management, 29*(4), 430–432.

Eason, F. R., & Brown, S. T. (1999). Conflict management: Assessing educational needs. *Journal for Nurses in Staff Development, 15*(3), 92–96.

Estabrooks, C. A., & Morse, J. M. (1992). Toward a theory of touch: The touching process and acquiring a touching style. *Journal of Advanced Nursing, 17,* 448–456.

Fraser, J. J. (2001). Technical report: Alternative dispute resolution in medical malpractice. *Pediatrics, 107*(3), 602–612.

French, P. (1994). *Social skills for nursing practice* (2nd ed.). London: Chapman & Hall.

Greenwald, A. G., & Banaji, M. R. (1995). Implicit social cognition: Attitudes, self-esteem and stereotypes. *Psychological Review, 102*(1), 4–27.

Hall, E. T. (1966). *The hidden dimension.* New York: Doubleday.

Harvey, L. C. (1998). *Humor for healing: A therapeutic approach.* San Antonio, TX: Therapy Skill Builders.

Hassed, C. (2001). How humour keeps you well. *Australian Family Physician, 1,* 25–28.

Hayes, J., & Cox, C. (1999). The experience of therapeutic touch from a nursing perspective. *British Journal of Nursing, 8*(18), 1249–1254.

Henkin, A. B., Dee, J. R., & Beatus, J. (2000). Social communication skills of physical therapist students: An initial characterization. *Journal of Physical Therapy Education, 14*(2), 32–38.

Henrikson, M. (1998). Managing through conflict. Harnessing the energy and power of change. *Association of Women's Health, Obstetric and Neonatal Nurses (AWHONN) Lifelines, 2*(4), 53–54.

Herdtner, S. (2000). Using therapeutic touch in nursing practice. *Orthopaedic Nursing, 19*(5), 77–82.

Houts, P. S., Bachrach, R., & Witmer, J. T. (1998). Using pictographs to enhance recall of spoken medical instructions. *Patient Education Counseling, 35,* 83–88.

Jadad, A. R., & Delamothe, T. (2004). What next for electronic communication and health care? *BMJ, 328,* 1143–1144. [Online]. Available: http://www.bmj.bmjjournals.com/cgi/content/full/328/7449/1143. Date accessed: 6/6/05.

Jensen, G., Gwyer, J., Shepard, K., & Hack, L. (2000). Expert practice in physical therapy. *Physical Therapy, 80*(1), 28–52.

Kabat-Zinn, J. (1994). *Wherever you go, there you are.* New York: Hyperion.

Krieger, D. (1979). *The therapeutic touch: How to use your hands to help or to heal.* New York: Prentice-Hall.

Kummervold, P. E., Trondsen, M., Andreassen, H., Gammon, D., & Hjortdahl, P. (2004). Patient-physician interaction over the Internet. *Tidsskr Nor Laegeforen, 124*(20), 2633–2636.

Leiber, D. B. (1986). Laughter and humor in critical care. *Dimensions of Critical Care Nursing, 5*(3), 163–165.

Liberman, A., Rotarius, T. M., & Kendall, L. (1997). Alternative dispute resolution: A conflict management tool in health care. *Health Care Supervisor, 16*(2), 9–20.

Lipcamon, J. D., & Mainwaring, B. A. (2004). Conflict resolution in healthcare management. *Radiology Management, 26*(3), 48–51.

Marcus, L. J., Dorn, B. C., Kritek, P. B., Miller, V. G., & Wyatt, J. B. (1995). *Renegotiating health care: Resolving conflict to build collaboration.* San Francisco: Jossey-Bass.

Martin, S. T. (1999). Language shapes thought. *PT—Magazine of Physical Therapy, 7*(6), 44–45.

McCann, K., & McKenna, H. P. (1993). An examination of touch between nurses and elderly patients in a continuing care setting in Northern Ireland. *Journal of Advanced Nursing, 18,* 838–846.

McCray, A. T. (2004). Promoting health literacy. *Journal of the Medical Information Association,* [Epub ahead of print].

Mentgen, J. L. (2001). Healing touch. *Holistic Nursing Care, 36*(1), 143–157.

Miller, B. J. (1998). The art of managing conflict. *Journal of Christian Nursing, 15*(1), 14–17.

Milstead, J. A. (1996). Basic tools for the orthopaedic staff nurse. Part II: Conflict management and negotiation. *Orthopaedic Nursing, 15*(2), 39–45.

Moody, R. A., Jr. (1978). *Laugh after laugh: The healing power of humor.* Jacksonville, FL: Headwaters Press.

Moore, C. (1996). *The mediation process* (2nd ed.). San Francisco: Jossey-Bass.

Nelson, H. W., & Cox, D. M. (2003). The causes and consequences of conflict and violence in nursing homes: Working toward a collaborative work culture. *Health Care Management, 22*(4), 349–360.

Nibler, R., & Harris, K. L. (2003). The effects of culture and cohesiveness on intragroup conflict and effectiveness. *Journal of Social Psychology, 143*(5), 613–631.

Northouse, L. L., & Northouse, P. G. (1998). *Health communications: Strategies for health professionals.* (3rd ed.). Stamford, CT: Appleton & Lange.

O'Day, B. L., Killeen, M., & Iezzoni, L. I. (2004). Improving health care experiences of persons who are blind or have low vision: Suggestions from focus groups. *American Journal of Medical Quality, 19*(5), 193–200.

Payton, O. D., & Nelson, C. E. (1995). Involving patients in decision-making. *PT–Magazine of Physical Therapy, 3*(12), 74–76.

Pettrey, L. (2003). Who let the dogs out? Managing conflict with courage and skill. *Critical Care Nurse, Feb* (Suppl.), 21–24.

Pillemer, K., Hegeman, C. R., Albright, B., & Henderson, C. (1998). Building bridges between families and nursing home staff: The partners in caregiving program. *The Gerontologist, 38*(4), 499–503.

Pore, S. (1995, April). I can't understand what my patient is saying. *Advance/Rehabilitation,* 49–50.

Purtilo, R., & Haddad, A. (1996). *Health professional and patient interaction.* Philadelphia: W.B. Saunders.

Rakley, S. M. (1999). When I stopped yelling, everybody started listening. *Medical Economics, 76*(19), 131, 134, 137–138.

Robinson, V. (1983). Humor and health. In P. E. McGhee & J. H. Goldstein (Eds.), *Handbook of humor research* (Vol. 2, pp. 109–124). New York: Springer-Verlag.

Robinson, V. (1991). *Humor and the health professions* (2nd ed.). Thorofare, NJ: Slack.

Rotarius, T., & Liberman, A. (2000). Health care alliances and alternative dispute resolution: Managing trust and conflict. *Health Care Manager, 18*(3), 25–31.

Routasalo, P. (1999). Physical touch in nursing studies: A literature review. *Journal of Advanced Nursing, 30*(4), 843–850.

Saravia, A. (1999). Overview of alternative dispute resolution in healthcare disputes. *Journal of Health and Law, 32*(1), 139–153.

Schmitt, N. (1990). Patients' perception of laughter in a rehabilitation hospital. *Rehabilitation Nursing, 15*(3), 143–146.

Schneider, J., Kaplan, S. H., Greenfield, S., Li, W., & Wilson, I. B. (2004). Better physician-patient relationships are associated with higher reported adherence to antiretroviral therapy in patients with HIV infection. *Journal of General Internal Medicine, 19*(11), 1096–1103.

Seroka, A. M. (1994). Values clarification and ethical decision making. *Seminars for Nurse Managers, 2*(1), 8–15.

Shendell-Falik, N. (1997). Tips, tools, and techniques: The art of negotiation. *Nursing Case Management, 2*(3), 107–108.

Siegel, B. (1986). *Love, medicine, & miracles*. New York: Harper & Row.

Spickerman, S., & Brown, S. T. (1991). Student conflict management: Before and after instruction. *Nurse Educator, 16*(6), 6, 11.

Strutton, D., & Knouse, S. B. (1997). Resolving conflict through managing relationships in health care institutions. *Health Care Supervisor, 16*(1), 15–28.

Studdert, D. M., Mello, M. M., Burns, J. P., Puopolo, A. L., Galper, B. Z., Truog, R. D., & Brennan, T. A. (2003). Conflict in the care of patients with prolonged stay in the ICU: Types, sources, and predictors. *Intensive Care Medicine, 29*(9), 1489–1497.

Sutcliffe, K. M., Lewton, E., & Rosenthal, M. M. (2004). Communication failures: An insidious contributor to medical mishaps. *Academic Medicine, 79*(2), 186–194.

Swain, J. (1997). Interpersonal communication. In S. French (Ed.), *Physiotherapy: A psychosocial approach* (2nd ed., pp. 252–253). Oxford: Butterworth-Heinemann.

Thomas, K., & Kilmann, R. (1974). *Thomas Kilmann Conflict Mode Instrument*. Tuxedo, NY: Xicom.

Trill, M. D., & Holland, J. (1993). Cross-cultural differences in the care of patients with cancer: A review. *General Hospital Psychiatry, 15,* 21–30.

Umbreit, A. W. (2000). Healing touch: Applications in the acute care setting. *American Association of Critical Care Nursing Clinical Issues, 11*(1), 105–119.

Umiker, W. (1997). Collaborative conflict resolution. *Health Care Supervisor, 15*(3), 70–75.

Vanderhoff, M. (2005). Patient education and health literacy. *PT–Magazine of Physical Therapy, 13*(9), 42–46.

Wall, J. A., & Callister, R. R. (1995). Conflict and its management. *Journal of Management, 21*(3), 515–558.

Williams, K., Kemper, S., & Hummert, M. L. (2004). Enhancing communication with older adults: Overcoming elderspeak. *Journal of Gerontological Nursing, 30*(10), 17–25.

Woltersdorf, M. (1998). Body language. *PT–Magazine of Physical Therapy, 6*(9), 112.

Wyatt, D. (1999). Negotiation strategies for men and women. *Nursing Management, 30*(1), 22–26.

Xu, Y., & Davidhizar, R. (2004). Conflict management styles of Asian and Asian American nurses: Implications for the nurse manager. *Health Care Management, 23*(1), 46–53.

Zweibel, E. B., & Goldstein, R. (2001). Conflict resolution at the University of Ottawa Faculty of Medicine: The pelican and the sign of the triangle. *Academic Medicine, 76*(4), 337–344.

# 3

# *Cultural Aspects of Therapeutic Care*

Working in an inner-city clinic is challenging in more ways than I expected. I knew that many of the clients would be poor and have social difficulties, but I never realized how many different ethnic groups and cultures I would see. I used to think that all Asians or Latinos were the same and shared common values, beliefs, and traditions. Since starting my clinical rotation here, it is obvious that many different races and cultures are represented within each ethnic group. I learned that although people from China, Cambodia, or Vietnam may all be classified as Asian, they are different from one another and very different from me. My roommate says that I should treat everybody "the same," but I know that if I do, I'll offend people. If that happens, they won't trust me to care for them. I'm really confused about what to say and do.

*—From the journal of Susan Hancock, social work student*

The United States has been largely settled and developed by people who have emigrated from another country. The first wave of settlers consisted of white Europeans, who came seeking religious or political freedom and economic opportunities. The culture and traditions they brought developed into what is currently the majority, or "American," culture. Immigrants continue to come to America for many of the same reasons as the early settlers, but it is likely that some are also escaping the impact of war, oppression, persecution, or other forms of violence. Recent immigrants are more likely to be from Asia, Africa, or South and Central America than from Western Europe (Spector, 1996).

These newer immigrants are often either called "people of color" because they are not white or "minorities" because they are not from the majority culture. This terminology is quickly becoming outdated, as minority populations continue to swell. It is predicted that minority populations and new immigrants will become the majority of the population between the years 2030 and 2050 (Sue & Sue, 1999). Traditional wisdom holds that the United States is a "melting pot" for immigrants who will all assimilate, blending into a homogeneous "stew," with all individuals sharing the same culture and lifestyle. The United States, however, is more like a tossed salad, where each "ingredient" retains unique characteristics and maintains a highly visible identity (Brice & Campbell, 1999).

In this chapter, we define culture and describe the many factors that contribute to an individual's cultural identity. The culture of medicine is also explained. Implications of cross-cultural conflict between health care providers and clients of minority populations is discussed. Strategies for overcoming barriers and developing more culturally sensitive practice is also provided.

# Race, Ethnicity, and Culture

The concepts of race, ethnicity, and culture are often confusing and defy simplistic definitions. Although race and ethnicity make a significant contribution to culture, they are not the only determinants. Traditionally, race has been perceived to be determined by genetically inherited traits that are identifiable by physical characteristics, such as skin color, facial features, and hair color and texture. Census surveys, college registration forms, and medical history questionnaires typically ask people to identify themselves as being members of a very short list of possible races. It is customary for people to be identified as the race they most resemble (i.e., anyone with a dark skin tone is called black). How does a person self-identify if he or she is racially or ethnically mixed? How can we classify someone with a Jewish father, American paternal grandparents, a mother who is Muslim, with a Greek maternal grandmother and Egyptian maternal grandfather? Prominent golfer Tiger Woods is an example of an individual who is racially mixed, whose race defies clear categories. It would appear that ethnicity, or ethnic grouping, may be a more valuable concept than race in understanding people.

Unfortunately, ethnicity is also a vague, complex, and ambiguous designation. Some characteristics that may be considered when describing ethnicity include geographic origin or residence; migration history; race; language or dialect; religion or spiritual beliefs; shared traditions, values, or symbols; occupation; sexual orientation; socioeconomic status; and politics (Loveland, 1999; Spector, 1996; Sue & Sue, 1999). Consider how an elderly woman who practices Buddhism and came to the United States on a crowded, leaky boat from Vietnam is culturally different from a college student who is Japanese, Christian, and came to the United States with her father's economic support. While both may be considered Asian, they are culturally different.

Culture can be defined as "the sum of beliefs, practices, habits, likes, dislikes, norms, customs, rituals that we learned from our families" (Spector, 1996, p. 68). A critical distinction between the concept of culture and race or ethnicity is that it is learned, not inherited. The learning occurs during the socialization process, beginning while children are very young. Culture consists of a largely unconscious framework that is used for organizing our daily behavior (Krefting, 1991). It determines *how* we interact with the world, and what physical, social, or cognitive behaviors are acceptable (Banja, 1996).

The concept of culture can be subdivided into two types, the material and nonmaterial cultures (Loveland, 1999). Material culture consists of items that can be seen, heard, or touched. When we go to a natural history museum, attend a Native American crafts show, or listen to an Italian opera, we are examining the material artifacts of a culture. Our food preferences, architecture, and holiday displays or decorations are also examples of material culture. It is easier to identify a person from a "foreign" culture if he or she comes to the clinic wearing a sari or turban. Nonmaterial culture, which includes religious beliefs, morals, ethics, and views about roles of family members, is not so easily observed. Ideas may be so deeply embedded that an individual is almost unaware that they exist and just assumes that this is how "everyone" thinks. Nonmaterial culture may be extremely difficult to change (Loveland, 1999).

Culture serves to organize three essential social functions. First, it defines the parameters of social relationships, such as gender and family roles, vocational and community relationships, and relationships with professionals. Second, culture provides individuals with paradigms that explain how the universe is ordered, including spiritual beliefs and explanations for natural phenomena, such as health and illness. A final function is to provide a guide to differentiate one social group from another. People who look different from one another or who have no shared genetic background could share the same culture, while two individuals who share the same race could have different cultural identities. Consider a middle-aged black physician who lives in the suburbs and teaches at a prestigious medical school. His culture is much more likely to be similar to that of white professionals, living in similar circumstances, than it is to be like the culture of a black adolescent, living in poverty and attending an urban high school.

# Subcultures

According to the revised standards of October 1997, the Office of Management and Budget (OMB) of the United States identified five racial categories and two categories for ethnicity. The racial categories are now American Indian or Alaskan Native, Asian, Black or African American, Native Hawaiian or Other Pacific Islander, and White. Two minimum categories are recognized to describe ethnicity—Latino or Hispanic and Not Latino or Hispanic. Of interest, people of Latino or Hispanic heritage may be of any race (U.S. Census Bureau, 2000).

These groups refer to cultural practices, racial and ethnic features, and historical and geographic origins. Americans with dark skin and origins in Africa are called African American or black. For this cultural group, geographic origins in Africa and the experience of slavery serve as unifying themes. This culture also may include people from the Caribbean islands, although some people from these regions might consider themselves Latino or Caribbean. Native American cultures encompass a vast number of different tribes of people indigenous to North America. White, Caucasian, or European individuals typically come from a European heritage and make up what is described as the mainstream or majority culture in America. Asian culture describes people who may come from China, Japan, Korea, Vietnam, or Eastern Asian countries, such as India, Pakistan, and Iran. Finally, individuals who are Latino or Hispanic share a common cultural origin (Spain) and language (Spanish) but more recently have likely emigrated from South America, Central America, or the Caribbean islands (Arredondo et al., 1996).

There is debate and controversy over the naming or labeling of cultural groups. Issues of politics, stigma, and discrimination over the choice of these group names are significant in defining a culture. In addition, over time, group preferences change, and what was once considered an appropriate label may become unacceptable. We have chosen to use the terminology identified above because it is most consistently used in the current literature. The reader should understand that this does not imply universal acceptance of these terms.

Placing all Americans into only five cultural groups seems contrary to a multifactorial approach to defining culture. Using only these broad categories to define cultures can lead to simplistic thinking about culture and stereotyping. Each large cultural group listed above contains many subgroups or subcultures. For example, in the United States there are more than twenty Latino or Hispanic subgroups and at least eighteen Asian subgroups (Leavitt, 1999). In addition to identifying a person as a member of one of the five major ethnic groups, other traits are used to understand the culture of an individual (Erlen, 1998).

"Subcultures are smaller units within a culture that share many of the cultural traits of the majority of people in the larger culture but are in some way(s) distinct from them" (Loveland, 1999, p. 18). Subcultures have their own sets of customs and beliefs that may differ from those of the larger culture. Individuals from a subculture may be unable to understand or relate to someone from a different subculture, even though both come from the same country (Erlen, 1998). For example, India is a country with a rigidly stratified caste system. Someone from the Brahmin caste would have virtually nothing in common with an individual who is considered an Untouchable. Unfortunately, some subcultures are viewed by mainstream culture as being odd, holding deviant beliefs, or engaging in unacceptable practices (Leininger, 1995).

Arredondo and colleagues (1996) have proposed a model for describing the dimensions of personal identity within a culture. The largest, most prominent dimension is termed the *A Dimension,* which describes characteristics that are largely predetermined and difficult or impossible to change. A Dimension characteristics include age, ethnicity, gender, primary language, physical disability, race, and class. The *B Dimension* includes traits that are much more likely to be under the individual's control, including education, geographic location, income, religion, work experience, and hobbies or recreational interests. The *C Dimension* encompasses historical, political, and economic contexts that frame an individual's life experiences and opportunities. While the Arredondo model was designed to help professionals conceptualize the values and beliefs that are relevant to individual clients, these factors are also important for defining or describing various subcultures. In all interactions with clients and families, we must remember to identify the values and beliefs of the individual and not make assumptions based on stereotypes.

## Acculturation, Assimilation, and Biculturalism

Another factor that affects an individual's cultural beliefs is the process of acculturation. Following immigration to a new country, a person must slowly adapt to the culture and lifestyle of the new home. "Acculturation is the process through which people in subcultures adopt traits of the larger, or normative, culture" (Loveland, 1999, p. 19). When people fully embrace the cultural traits of the new residence, they achieve assimilation. In the United States, it is generally assumed that it takes three generations to fully assimilate or accept the majority culture (Spector, 1996). Cultural practices and beliefs are strongly affected by the level of acculturation. For example, some patients may believe that an illness is a punishment for past behaviors or that there is an imbalance between the body and the spirit. As people acculturate, they slowly relinquish the "old ways" and begin to speak and behave in ways that are common for the majority culture.

The rate of acculturation is variable and affected by many factors. Perhaps the most significant factor is age, with younger individuals acculturating more quickly than older people. Some older people who immigrate never fully accept the culture of their new home and continue to speak their native language, practice traditional rituals, and socialize with others from their native culture. Other factors that affect the rate of acculturation include length of time in the new culture, place of residence (living with people from the native culture or the majority culture), language spoken at home, and amount of contact with the country of origin (Krefting, 1991). Assimilation is most likely to be complete when individuals are not physically different from the majority culture, when there is little contact with the native culture, and when there is little educational or physical segregation (Loveland, 1999). This would explain the lack of assimilation of the Hmong peoples from Southeast Asia, people from Puerto Rico, and Native Americans, who look physically different from the majority culture, tend to live in ethnically homogeneous settings, and maintain strong bonds with others from their culture of origin.

To determine the degree of acculturation, you can ask clients about the language spoken at home, the language of their media preference, their family roles, worldview, and frequency and type of social interactions with people from other cultural groups (Leavitt, 2001). Individuals may maintain strong connections to both the original culture and the majority culture. For example, they may dress, speak, and behave like others from the majority culture while at school or work. However, at home, they may speak their native language, eat traditional foods, and practice familiar rituals. These individuals are called bicultural (Krefting, 1991). Consider Mai Ling who was born in China and came to the United States to attend college. She is now a college professor and fits in easily with her U.S. peers at the university. However, she continues to feel that her cultural orientation is primarily Chinese. After many years away from China, she returned home for a visit. One day, her distraught mother confronted her and stated, "You are no longer Chinese! You do not behave the way a proper Chinese daughter is expected to act!" Mai Ling realized that culturally, she was neither fully American nor Chinese but had become bicultural, with strong values and beliefs from both cultures.

# Worldview

Values, beliefs, and assumptions about human behavior can be summarized under the concept of *worldview* (Sue & Sue, 1999). This concept refers to the values people use to form a cohesive picture of the world around them. It provides a model of acceptable beliefs and social behaviors (Leininger, 1995). People from cultures with different worldviews may find each other's behavior bewildering or even offensive. Before beginning to advise a client about how to maintain health or treat an illness, it is important to assess his or her worldview and adjust your recommendations accordingly. Time orientation, activity orientation and levels of environmental control, use of space, and social organizations, relationships, and communication between people are some important dimensions that can be included in worldview. See Table 3–1 for a summary of cross-cultural differences.

**TABLE 3–1** Cross-Cultural Differences in World View

*Majority or White European Cultures*

| Time | Social Organization | Communication | Health Beliefs |
| --- | --- | --- | --- |
| Future | Individualistic<br>Autonomous<br>Mastery<br>Nuclear family<br>Long-range goals | Speak loud and fast<br>Prolonged eye contact<br>  when listening<br>Quick responses<br>Objective, task-oriented<br>Standard English | Standard western<br>  medical model<br>Reliance on drugs,<br>  procedures, prevention |

*Black Cultures*

| Time | Social Organization | Communication | Health Beliefs |
| --- | --- | --- | --- |
| Present | Collectivist<br>Extended family<br>  and kinships<br>Immediate short-<br>  range goals<br>Strong religious values | Significant affect<br>Highly emotional<br>Prolonged eye contact<br>  when speaking<br>Interruptions<br>Nonverbal is important<br>Quick responses<br>Nonstandard English | Many traditional beliefs/<br>  practices<br>Spiritual or charismatic<br>  healings |

*Asian Cultures*

| Time | Social Organization | Communication | Health Beliefs |
| --- | --- | --- | --- |
| Past/present | Collectivist<br>Honors elders, traditions,<br>  and harmony<br>Avoids conflict<br>Loyalty<br>Hierarchical<br>Extended family networks | Speak softly<br>Avoid eye contact<br>Indirect, low key Asian<br>  language or non-<br>  standard English<br>Emotional restraint<br>Silence | Traditional folk beliefs<br>Herbalism<br>Balance of forces and<br>  energy |

*Latino/Hispanic Cultures*

| Time | Social Organization | Communication | Health Beliefs |
| --- | --- | --- | --- |
| Past/present | Group-centered<br>Collectivist<br>Values harmony<br>Respect for all<br>Extended family<br>Fatalismo<br>Strong church affiliations | Spanish-speaking<br>Speak softly<br>Avoid eye contact<br>Indirect, low key | Traditional folk beliefs<br>Health is a gift from God<br>Balance of natural forces |

*Native American Cultures*

| Time | Social Organization | Communication | Health Beliefs |
| --- | --- | --- | --- |
| Present | Collectivist harmony<br>  with nature and others<br>Noncompetitive respect<br>  for tradition<br>Strong commitment to<br>  extended family/tribe | Speak softly, slowly<br>Avoid eye contact<br>Indirect, low key<br>Tribal dialects<br>Delayed responses | Traditional folk beliefs<br>Illness caused by<br>  disharmony of physical<br>  and spiritual forces |

## Time Orientation

People from various cultures may have vastly different orientations to time. Some are present-oriented, while others focus primarily on the past or future. In the United States, people from the white majority culture are strongly focused on the future (Sue & Sue, 1999). They value precise "clock time," and being on time for appointments is highly valued (Leininger, 1995). This future orientation also affects our expectations for health care behavior. We expect our clients and colleagues to plan ahead, make and keep appointments, and take steps to maintain health or prevent future problems (Spector, 1996). Cultures with a focus on the future also tend to delay present pleasure to work for future gratification (Brice & Campbell, 1999; Davidhizar, Dowd, & Newman-Giger, 1997; Sue & Sue, 1999).

Other cultures do not necessarily share this future orientation. People who are part of some black or Native American cultures, for example, tend to be present-oriented (Sue & Sue, 1999). Because they may perceive time as "circular" or "flowing," dividing time into artificial segments becomes meaningless. Making and keeping schedules may also be construed as meaningless or disruptive. In addition, people who are present-oriented may value youth and beauty and choose to live in the moment, rather than planning for the future (Brice & Campbell, 1999; Davidhizar, Dowd, & Newman-Giger, 1997; Sue & Sue, 1999).

In contrast, people of cultures that are past-focused tend to value elders and honor traditions. Changes in traditional practices, beliefs, and behaviors are strongly discouraged. In Asian cultures, for example, people often have a past-orientation and rely on traditional healing practices, such as herbal treatments, acupuncture, and the use of traditional healers (Spector, 1996).

## Activity Orientation/Environmental Control

The culture influences the level of control people believe they have over their environment and how much they can affect their destiny. The majority culture in the United States is extremely action-oriented, with an emphasis on environmental control. Individuals are expected to master nature, overcome all obstacles, and control their own future. The Protestant work ethic dictates an achievement-oriented outlook, based on a belief that all problems have solutions (Parry, 1984; Sue & Sue, 1999). This may help explain why Americans tend to view themselves as a "can-do" society, where people who face challenges or adversity are expected to "pull themselves up by their bootstraps." Every problem is perceived as being solvable, if you work hard or long enough.

People from other cultures, particularly Asian, Latino, and Native American, sometimes reflect a feeling of powerlessness over nature (Parry, 1984; Sue & Sue, 1999). Harmony with the universe, rather than mastery or control of it, is valued. Behaviors that white Americans view as passivity, noncompetitiveness, or stoicism may actually be serenity or inner peace with one's place in the universe. For example, people in the Latino culture may believe that one's status in life is predetermined and that one cannot be held accountable for it because this is the state into which a person is born.

Incompatibility of beliefs between health care providers and clients can lead to significant conflict if they hold opposing ideas about the optimal level of activism and environmental control (Gannotti, Handwerker, Groce, & Cruz, 2001). Consider Emilio, a young child with cerebral palsy, living in a traditional Puerto Rican family. The medical staff believes that it is important for the family to perform daily exercises with Emilio, practice new skills, and encourage him to work hard to maximize function. They are frustrated by the family's apparent lack of motivation and follow-through with their recommendations. The family decided to discontinue medical care because they felt uncomfortable with the health care providers' emphasis on their taking control of the situation.

## Use of Space

Cultural space refers to the ways different cultures use the body and regard visual, territorial, and interpersonal distance to others (Leininger, 1995). Health care professionals must often cross clients' physical boundaries in order to examine or treat clients. We may innocently assume that everyone maintains the same boundaries that "we" do or that all clients will accept the suspension of boundaries in order to receive care. This is not so. For example, a young female health care provider was assigned to treat a gentleman who practiced Islam. When she extended her hand to greet him, he politely declined, and told her, "If I shake your hand, I will be obliged to marry you." The therapist asked him if he would prefer a male therapist to treat him, and he gratefully accepted the offer.

Territorial space describes the larger area that is occupied or defended by a group or about which that group holds strong emotional ties (Leininger, 1995; Spector, 1996). Personal space refers to the space immediately surrounding the body. What is comfortable for one may be unacceptable for another. Violating personal space preferences can lead to stress, anger, and conflict. In the majority American culture, the intimate zone extends to about 18 inches from the body and allows individuals to have very close personal contact. Only close personal associates are allowed to enter this space. Entering without permission may be viewed as an act of aggression (Leininger, 1995; Spector, 1996; Sue & Sue, 1999).

## Social Organization and Relationships

The majority culture in the United States is individualistic and values autonomy. Each person has the primary responsibility for his or her actions and is viewed as a social unit. Independence and personal autonomy are both highly valued and rewarded (Sue & Sue, 1999). We expect our young people to sleep in their own beds, live apart from parents and other family members as adults, and be financially independent. The family is considered to be the nuclear unit, with little consideration for collateral relationships and the connections to ancestors (Sue & Sue, 1999). Direct communication is valued, and communication with strangers is easily established (Brice & Campbell, 1999).

For people living in many minority cultures, the situation is often the opposite. The family is the psychosocial unit, with dependence and connectedness to the group strongly valued (Brice & Campbell, 1999). These cultures have a collective or group orientation. People do not make decisions based on what is good for the individual, but rather by what is best for the family or the social group. In collectivist cultures, the family unit may be much broader than the nuclear family and include aunts, uncles, cousins, or tribal elders. For example, in the Confucian value system practiced by many Asians, loyalty and harmony with the family lead to harmony with the environment and within the self (Sue & Morishima, 1982). Children are expected to be well-behaved and achieve in school because it will bring honor to the family. "Saving face," protecting one's honor, and "giving face," or showing respect for others, are also highly valued behaviors. Being disrespectful is not tolerated (Brice & Campbell, 1999).

While the majority U.S. culture values solving problems directly, collective cultures take a different approach. Problems are solved indirectly by suggestion or guidance. Confrontation is not only avoided but is considered unacceptable. Parents will discipline children using indirect guidance rather than punishment (Sue & Sue, 1999).

## Communication

Communication forms the basis for human interaction. In Chapter 2, we discussed the significance of different types of communication and factors that have an impact on its effectiveness. Communication is typically based on a formal language structure and also includes nonverbal communication, paralanguage (tone of voice, inflection, speed), and other factors. There is a strong reciprocal relationship between culture and communication, with each exerting a powerful influence on the other. The language we use is influenced by our culture, and the words that are available in our language help to shape perceptions of reality and convey our ideas (Brice & Campbell, 1999). The language that we acquired as children influences our worldview and our beliefs (Brice & Campbell, 1999). As our culture develops, words and phrases are developed or "coined" to describe new phenomena. Consider the rapid growth in the use of computers, which has spawned a new language of computer-related words and acronyms.

In the health care setting, communication is the means by which health care practitioners and clients develop a relationship. When communication is impaired due to language or cultural barriers, client care can suffer (Duffy & Alexander, 1999). Unfortunately, many health care providers in the United States speak only English, while clients from other cultures may have limited English skills. Differences in the structure and formation of language can make it difficult or impossible for languages to achieve direct translation of ideas or social reality. Clients who are bilingual may have difficulty with complex medical terms or be unable to describe their symptoms accurately. In the United States, where everyone "shares" the English language, it is assumed that we all understand each other, but research indicates that this is not so (Favazza & Oman, 1978).

Mr. Chang, who is Chinese, is my newest client, and I just can't seem to figure out how to communicate with him. He has chronic obstructive pulmonary disease and is coming to our center for rehabilitation. His family seems very supportive, and his wife and daughter often come to his appointments with him. They seem very interested in his health, sitting quietly in the room while he goes through his program. However, I don't have a clue whether anyone understands a word I'm saying! They always seem to listen attentively, nod, and smile.

When I ask if they have understood, they politely say "yes" and never ask any questions. Mr. Chang doesn't seem to be improving, and I suspect that he is not following his exercise program at home. However, when I ask if there are any problems or if they would like me to make some changes, they state that everything is fine. I wish I could figure out what to do differently.

*—From the journal of Sean Murphy, exercise physiology student*

In the above journal entry, there are many possible explanations for the client's and family's behavior. They may not be sufficiently proficient in English to understand what is being explained. As mentioned earlier, in Chinese culture, protecting one's honor is highly valued. The client and his family may have been too embarrassed to admit their lack of comprehension. Respecting others, especially those in positions of authority, is also important. Asking questions is considered a sign of disrespect. In Asian cultures, health care providers are considered to hold positions of high esteem and authority. They may have been respecting the honor of the health care professional by not wanting to embarrass him for not explaining well. The student could have provided pictures, diagrams, or instructions in the client's native language. Asking the client to demonstrate the exercises would be another way to assess understanding. Chinese families traditionally maintain a high level of involvement in health care situations, and the student may have been able to find a way to tactfully engage them in supporting Mr. Chang's treatment.

Language and communication differences present significant barriers to providing effective health care to clients and families from minority cultures (Choi & Wynne, 2000; Flores, Abreu, Olivar, & Kastner, 1998). In a study of Latino parents, 26 percent stated that language problems were the greatest barrier to obtaining health care for their children. Many families indicated the wrong diagnosis was made or incorrect treatment was received because the health care provider and the client did not understand each other.

While language is a significant component of communication, it is not the only factor. Style and content of interactions are also significant. An important concept used to describe the culturally mediated style of communication is the designation of a culture as high or low context. Context refers to the amount of environmental or social cues that are available to help frame the exchange of information. "Low-context communication relies little on the surrounding context for interpretation" (Brice & Campbell, 1999, p. 86). It tends to be explicit and highly descriptive. Low-context communication also assumes that words must be used to explain everything because little is implicitly understood. This communication is most commonly seen in individualistic cultures that prefer a very direct style of communication.

In contrast, high-context communication is highly dependent on nonverbal interactions, strong group identification, and understanding of the interaction. It relies on shared group experiences, history, and customs, rather than verbal communication, to express ideas (Lynch, 1992). Nonverbal cues and messages are used extensively to convey meaning. This type of interaction is most often seen in collectivist cultures (Sue & Sue, 1999); for example, black cultures tend to be high-context. Members of these cultural groups often use body movements, facial expressions, and culturally relevant phrases to express ideas using few words. Asian cultures also tend to be high-context. Communication is very indirect, with individuals rarely stating exactly what they mean or what they want. Instead, meaning is conveyed from the context of the situation.

Low-context language tends to be logical and linear, while high-context communications are indirect and less explicit. It is easy to see how cultural misinterpretations can occur. Members of low-context cultures may view individuals who use high-context forms of expression as being less intelligent or less educated because they use fewer words. Individuals who prefer high-context communication can be offended by overly direct statements made by those who use a low-context communication style. They prefer suggestion and guidance rather than forceful declarations.

## Poverty as a Cultural Issue

I had heard that there are disparities in the way health care is delivered to people who are poor or in a minority subculture as compared to those who are middle-class or from the mainstream culture. I always found this difficult to believe because I know that health care providers are caring and ethical professionals.

Today, I noticed something that left me sad and confused. My clinical instructor and I have been treating several patients who have had total joint replacements. Two of the patients, who are about the same age, had the same surgery for the same diagnosis. While reviewing our billing logs, it struck me that although their plans of care are the same, the patient who has private health insurance is receiving longer treatments than the other who is receiving free care.

*—Melissa Ferris, physical therapist student*

Poverty and minority status play a significant role in determining who will get sick and how they will respond when they become ill (Freeman, 2004). These two conditions often coexist because people of color are more likely to live below the poverty line than people who are white. According to 2003 data, the rate of poverty was 11 percent for Americans who are white, 33 percent for those who are black, 30 percent for those who are Latinos, and 20 percent for people in other categories (Kaiser Family Foundation, 2005). Poverty and the effects of living in poor areas compound the cultural differences between those who are from the mainstream culture and people of color.

Poor inner city neighborhoods have higher levels of crime, drug use, and single-parent households. The combined effects of poverty and race can marginalize residents and create barriers to assimilation and movement into mainstream culture and better-paying jobs. For example, youth living in areas where poverty rates are high lack role models and mentors who can assist them in moving into well-paid jobs and stable employment (Williams, 1999). Job applicants who are from minority subcultures or live in impoverished areas may be unable to acquire jobs due to discrimination and racism (Bauder, 2002). In addition, psychosocial stressors, such as family dysfunction and reduced social support, more frequently create barriers to upward mobility for people with low incomes (Fiscella, 1999). Lack of education and poor job skills present barriers for mothers who are attempting to move away from public assistance (Fiscella, 1999). Education and social infrastructures, such as affordable day care, job training, and access to jobs with insurance, are usually unavailable to women attempting to transition from public assistance to stable employment (Anderson, Halter, & Gryzlak, 2004).

Unfortunately, poverty is also a significant factor for poor health. Although we believe that we deliver health care services equitably to all individuals, regardless of income level, race, or ethnicity, the reality is that this is not always true (Institute of Medicine, 2001). A substantial body of research demonstrates that there are significant disparities in health outcomes between people who are middle-class or affluent and people who are poor. Death from cancer, heart disease, diabetes, and many other disorders occurs disproportionately in those who are poor and who are from racial or ethnic minority groups (Benson, 2000; Freeman, 2004; Institute of Medicine, 2001). In 2003, the death rate per 100,000 people was

833 for Americans who are white versus 1099 for Americans who are black. Further, people of racial and ethnic minority groups have higher rates of illness and death than for those who are white, even when socioeconomic status, insurance, and co-morbidities are factored in (Institute of Medicine, 2001). Racism and discrimination are also considered powerful deterrents to equitable care for all (Institute of Medicine, 2001).

There are many variables that contribute to the diminished health status of people who are poor, such as institutional barriers that limit access to care. People with low income may not have health insurance and may not be able to afford the premiums even if it were available. Many people do not seek health care if they know they cannot afford it (Freeman, 2004). Service delivery models do not always employ health professionals who are multilingual or who provide culturally sensitive care (Institute of Medicine, 2001).

A study of barriers to health care for children from families of Latino origin provides evidence of additional factors that limit access to quality medical care (Flores et al., 1998). In this study, most families were not fluent English speakers. Spanish was the primary language spoken at home in 86 percent of the families. Median family income was $11,000. Only 57 percent of the children had health coverage. The most significant barrier to health care was the lack of a common language, followed by long waits at the doctor's office and no insurance and/or difficulty paying for care. Transportation was listed as the most significant reason why they did not bring a sick child for medical care. What is particularly troubling about this study is that 11 percent of the families stated that language and cultural barriers kept them from bringing the sick child for care.

Health disparities for people who are poor and/or who are among ethnic minority groups are not only due to institutional barriers. Poor neighborhoods are more likely to have substandard housing, resulting in increased contagion from infectious diseases and incidence of asthma. Noise and crowding generate physiological stress that are predisposing factors for cardiac disease and hypertension (Ulrich, 2002). Air and water quality are more apt to be poor and cause a plethora of illnesses, including cancer.

It is important for health providers to understand that poverty is a powerful predictor of health behaviors and adherence to health regimens. Smoking, alcohol and substance abuse, unhealthy diets, and lack of exercise are risk factors for ill health that occur at higher rates among people who are poor and poorly educated (Fiscella, 1999). It is more challenging for people to engage in health-promoting behaviors, such as eating healthy diets, when fresh fruits and vegetables may not be affordable or available. Struggling with the day-to-day stresses imposed by poor living conditions can make investment in future good health seem overwhelming. In addition, people who are poor have higher rates of mental illness, including depression, which leads to a rate of nonadherence to health care regimens that is three times higher than in clients who are not depressed (DiMatteo, Lepper, & Groghan, 2000).

Elimination of health disparities has been identified as a major target for health professionals. "Healthy People 2010" is a public health initiative, sponsored by the U.S. Department of Health and Human Services, to meet this challenge because the health of the community is dependent on the health of each individual (U.S. Department of Health and Human Services, 2005). As health providers, it is important to consider the variables that affect the outcome of all clients, regardless of financial status or racial or ethnic background. Understanding the factors that cause burdens of disproportionate illness on underserved populations is an important first step to providing comprehensive and ethical care.

# Explanatory Models of Health and Illness

While culture strongly influences the health beliefs and practices of the client, there are multiple variations within each culture. Clients integrate cultural, personal, family, and "popular" beliefs, personal experiences, and biomedical information to explain health and illness. "Personal experiences, family attitudes, and group beliefs interact to provide an underlying structure for decision-making during illness" (Pachter, 1994, p. 690). Kleinman (1978) has termed this system of personal beliefs the client's "explanatory model of illness." This model is used to describe a specific illness, rather than providing a belief system for general health and sickness. It is grounded in strong emotions and may be difficult for the client to identify or describe.

Explanatory models provide a mechanism for the client to conceptualize the cause, time of onset, course of symptoms, the pathophysiology or mechanism of the illness, and expected treatment. It also prescribes the accepted roles and behaviors of the client and health care provider (Kleinman, 1988; Pachter, 1994; Reifsnider, Allen, & Percy, 2000). The health care practitioner and the client both have explanatory models of illness, and it's important to assess how the client explains his or her illness so that meaningful communication can be established. When the health care provider understands the client's explanatory model, he or she can negotiate with the client to find ways to provide effective care that is mutually acceptable (Kleinman, 1988).

# Health Beliefs and Practices

Cultures profoundly influence health and the response to illness (Kleinman, 1978). They determine how people define health and illness, explain the causes of illness, describe how to maintain health, and outline how to restore health when illness occurs (Groce, 1999; Spector, 1996; Vanderhoff, 2005). The ways people behave when they are ill are culturally determined and are governed by cultural norms (Banja, 1996). Clients who appear in the medical setting complaining of "high blood," "nerves," "wind," "evil eye," or "soul loss" may strike the provider as ignorant or poorly educated individuals who need to be taught about the facts and true nature of their health problems. Instead, these complaints alert the provider that the individual may have recently immigrated or be someone who maintains traditional health care practices or beliefs. Health care providers need to be sensitive to their clients' cultural beliefs and practices (Kleinman, 1988).

To illustrate some salient health beliefs and practices, we will discuss those held by the four largest minority cultures in the United States: Native American, Asian, Latino/Hispanic, and black. While each of these cultures is unique, and each subculture within the larger culture even more individualistic, there are several important beliefs that tend to be consistent. They must be recognized and understood because, in many cases, these beliefs are strikingly different from those held by practitioners of Western medicine. These beliefs include:

- Health is believed to result from a harmony of mind, body, and spirit.
- Disharmony will result in illness.

- Healing practices are based on restoring balance or harmony.
- The role of the health care provider is to restore this balance.
- The personality or social style of the health care professional is extremely important.

## Native American Cultures

Native American cultures are closely tied to a belief in spiritual forces and the traditions of the ancestors. Rehabilitation and healing are bound by sacred religious narratives and rituals. Because a person has three dimensions—mind, body, and spirit—all must be treated in order for healing to occur. The spirit is considered to be the most important element in Native American cultures, and spiritual distress is manifested by physical symptoms. The mind links the body and spirit, and wellness is achieved when all three are in harmony (Pichette, Garrett, Kosciulek, & Rosenthal, 1999).

Native Americans do not traditionally speak about illness, disability, or death because it is believed that this may cause the spirit to manifest the problem in the body. This belief has significant implications for Western health care practitioners who are trained to educate clients by explaining diseases and treatments in great depth. Health care interactions are further complicated by the fact that people of these cultures typically speak little, avoid smiling, and believe that making eye contact is a sign of disrespect. These factors may lead the health care provider to believe that the client is disinterested or noncompliant (Pichette et al., 1999; Sue & Sue, 1999).

## Asian Cultures

People from traditional Asian cultures believe that health results from a harmony between the body and the spirit. They view the universe as an indivisible whole, with each person interconnected to all others in a state of harmonious balance. It is believed that a disruption of this state of balance leads to illness. There must be a balance between the forces of yin and yang that are found within each person. Yin signifies forces that are static, internal, downward, dull, or low activity. In contrast, dynamic, external, upward, and brilliant forces manifest yang. Imbalance or predominance of either force, yin or yang, causes specific, identifiable diseases, which are treated by restoring balance (Spector, 1996).

As discussed earlier, Asian cultures value authority figures and expect the medical practitioner to provide the "best" treatment, rather than discussing options and offering choices. Asian people tend to be reserved, and it is unusual to openly discuss feelings or display emotions. Unfortunately, this may lead to the mistaken notion that they have a high tolerance for pain, when in fact, they may be too embarrassed to admit having pain or too polite to ask for pain medication when it is not offered. In addition, Chinese clients often prefer to use traditional healing techniques, such as acupuncture or herbs, instead of, or in addition to, Western health interventions (Tang & Cheng, 2001).

## Latino/Hispanic Cultures

People from traditional Latino cultures tend to have strong religious beliefs (Nava, 2000). Good health is regarded as good luck or a gift from God. Poor health is the result of fate and is not under the active control of the client or family. Disease or disability may also be perceived as punishment for sins or transgressions or as a result of negative spiritual forces, such as the "evil eye." Similar to the other cultures discussed, people from Latino cultures do not separate the natural and spiritual worlds, and therefore, body and soul are not separate entities (Salimbene, 2000). For example, *susto* (soul loss) is an illness that can develop after a serious fright or trauma and occurs when the soul leaves the body and wanders freely. The symptoms of this disorder are similar to depression or anxiety and include disruptions in sleep patterns, as well as loss of energy, interest, and weight (Spector, 1996).

The personality and social skills of the health care provider are extremely important to the Latino client. An essential element in providing care is *respeto* (respect). All people, regardless of age, education, or social class, expect to be treated equally with regard to dignity, formality, and respect. A warm, caring personality is also anticipated, *personalismo*, with the health professional shaking hands, making eye contact, warmly greeting the client, and showing a genuine interest in the individual. Finally, the family tends to be involved in the client's care and expects to be included in decision making. It may be alarming for health professionals to see so many family members participate in medical appointments or visit during recovery, providing noisy and enthusiastic support for the clients (Leavitt, 2001; Nava, 2000; Salimbene, 2000).

## Black Cultures

Traditional beliefs about health care in black cultures do not separate mind, body, and spirit. Health results when these forces are in harmony. Clients of these cultures may believe that one can positively influence the future by the appropriate use of behavior and knowledge. This belief in the power to effect a positive change may lead to a person refusing to accept a diagnosis of a terminal illness or incurable disease. In the face of a negative health care assessment or prognosis, the client and family may seek alternate health care, believing that all problems have a solution. Sometimes it is held that misbehavior by an adult may be punished by God, causing illness in the adult or his or her child. The only way to release or heal these illnesses is through prayer or repentance (Salimbene, 2000; Spector, 1996).

The first black people who were brought to America were sold as slaves. Families were disrupted, native cultures destroyed, and human rights ignored. Although more than a century has passed since the U.S. Civil War and the emancipation of the slaves, the experiences of slavery and the discrimination that followed continues to exert powerful influences on the black community. This may cause distrust of individuals from other cultures and the expectation of discrimination. These influences must be acknowledged and appreciated by health care professionals (Spector, 1996). This historical perspective, combined with the cultural beliefs that all problems are solvable, can lead to distrust of white health care providers.

# The Culture of Medicine

In the Western medical system, health care providers are trained in a biomedical approach to health. Sickness is viewed as a biological process gone awry, with scientific explanations for the various disorders and their treatments. As children, we are socialized by our families to acquire the norms, beliefs, values, rituals, language, and practices that are consistent with our culture of origin. During the educational process to become health care providers, we are acculturated to acquire the beliefs and attributes of the Western health care system. We set aside the health-related beliefs of our native culture and families as we learn to identify ourselves as health care providers and acquire the culture of medicine (Spector, 1996).

In the context of the work setting, health care providers constitute a cultural group. We have many common beliefs and practices, including:

- A core of knowledge and beliefs that defines health, describes disease, identifies causes of illness, and prescribes acceptable treatment methods.
- A common language (medical terminology and jargon) that is not understood by outsiders.
- Rituals, such as hand-washing, sterile procedure, bed-making, and performing the physical exam.
- A formalized style of interaction that is governed by rules of communication and professional behavior.
- Values and norms, such as promptness, cleanliness, compliance, orderliness, and a hierarchy of responsibility (Pachter, 1994; Spector, 1996).

Every encounter between health care providers and clients has four potential cross-cultural components: (1) the native culture of the health care provider, (2) the native culture of the client, (3) the culture of the majority health care system, and (4) the medical culture of the client. Health care providers must be continuously aware of the potential for conflicts between one or more of these cultural intersections. The complexity and sensitivity of our interactions with clients present opportunities for misunderstanding and miscommunication. We must develop effective communication (see Chapter 2) to be able to bridge these differences (Simpson, Mohr, & Redman, 2000).

# Barriers to Effective Cross-Cultural Health Care

In this chapter, we identified several barriers to effective interactions with clients in the health care setting. Language and communication differences are among the most significant barriers. Unfortunately, many clients expand the health professionals' inability to understand the clients' language to a general inability to understand the clients' needs or their illnesses. The client may feel that the medical provider "does not understand me." The use of silence or high-context communication style by clients may frustrate Western health care providers' attempts to gather information about symptoms or problems. Silence may also be interpreted as hostility (Sung, 1999). When the client and practitioner do not speak the same language, literally or figuratively, it is difficult to establish trust and share critical information. It is more challenging to develop empathy for someone whom you do not know.

Ethnocentrism also creates a barrier to establishing a relationship with clients and presents significant implications for effective practice. This belief that your worldview and cultural practices are "correct" makes others inferior and less worthy of respect (Sue & Sue, 1999). "It is exceptionally difficult to describe or comprehend the extent to which ethnocentrism and racism have been woven into the fabric of our health care system" (Tripp-Reimer, Choi, Kelley, & Enslein, 2001, p.14).

Health care providers in the United States have been socialized that Western medicine, as taught and practiced in medical schools and hospitals, provides the answers to meet everyone's health care needs (Spector, 1996). This belief, however, is not shared by all clients. It also poses significant barriers to providing appropriate health care to people from different cultures who may have conflicting beliefs. Clients intuitively believe that when the health care provider rejects their view of health and illness, they are also rejecting all of the clients' cultural beliefs. They need to feel valued and respected by health professionals in order to develop a relationship (Sung, 1999). Therefore, health care providers need to learn how to assess the cultural beliefs and practices of clients so that services can be delivered in a manner that is both sensitive and respectful of cultural norms. This practice may be called culturally sensitive care or cross-cultural competency (Arredondo et al., 1996).

Most health providers are committed to providing high-quality care to all clients and treating them with dignity and respect. However, unless the provider has been trained in culturally sensitive care practices, he or she may feel bias or disrespect for certain cultures' health beliefs or practices. Lack of understanding of a culture can lead to fear or hostility toward that group. The client may be aware of the provider's feelings of hostility, disdain, or contempt, regardless of how well the practitioner attempts to appear nonjudgmental. Effective clinical encounters are based on trust, and when this trust does not exist, the likelihood of an effective relationship is affected (Thomas, 1999).

The client's and family's ethnocentrism may also create barriers to effective health care delivery (Banja, 1996). People from Asian, Latino/Hispanic, black, and Native American cultures may have health care beliefs that differ from those held by most Western medical practitioners. This may lead to refusal to seek health care or to client nonadherence with the recommended treatment (Canlas, 1999; Stell, 1999; Sung, 1999). Although health practitioners may believe that poor adherence is solely the clients' problem, failure to present the medical problem and its treatment in a manner that is congruent with the clients' beliefs is also the providers' problem (Tripp-Reimer et al., 2001).

# Creating Solutions to Cross-Cultural Health Care

Solutions to improving effective cross-cultural health care are both simple and complex. The key to eliminating fear and distrust of people of other cultures is to develop knowledge about, and respect for, their traditions (Canlas, 1999). In addition, this includes using many frames of reference when interacting with others and understanding that there is no one "right" way to provide health care. This ability to embrace and effectively use multiple cultural paradigms has been termed "cultural competence" (Nuñez, 2000).

Arredondo and colleagues (1996) have identified three core sets of skills that must be developed to deliver culturally competent care. They are self-awareness, knowledge about clients' cultures, and skill in delivering care. The first step in becoming culturally competent is developing an awareness of our own cultural identity and beliefs so that we can identify stereotypes or prejudices. As we discussed in Chapter 1, the ability to recognize how our background and experiences shape our attitudes, beliefs, and biases about others is an essential step in the process of eliminating any that may interfere with client care.

Once we have become aware of our own cultural values and how they affect our behavior with clients, the next step in developing culturally competent care is to be knowledgeable about other cultural traditions and beliefs. Although it is impossible for health care providers to be knowledgeable about all minority cultures, they can acquire specific information about the groups of people they most frequently treat. This information may be obtained from consulting colleagues, reading professional literature, participating in cultural events, and asking the clients directly.

The third core set of skills that must be developed to deliver culturally competent care is demonstrating receptive and respectful behaviors during professional interactions. This includes respect for spiritual beliefs, psychosocial functioning, expressions of distress, and beliefs about health, illness, and healing. Nuñez (2000) prefers the term "cross-cultural efficacy" to cross-cultural competence because it implies that the health care provider is not only knowledgeable but also effective in providing sensitive care. This health professional would have an "ethnorelative," rather than ethnocentric, point of view, and understand that there can be many valid interpretations of behavior. A culturally competent health care provider perceives that all cultural beliefs and practices have equal value or worth. In addition, he or she is vigilant about seeking the clients' perspective and providing care that is respectful of their beliefs and meets their medical needs.

## Culturally Competent Practices

Culturally competent health care providers recognize that they must alter their natural communication style to be acceptable to clients from minority cultures. We need to determine how to demonstrate respect in our interactions, which may include learning to use an indirect rather than a direct style. We can also learn to use conversational styles that are comfortable to the clients, such as extended greetings, expressing concern about the family, altering the speed or pacing of the conversation, and valuing silence (Tripp-Reimer et al., 2001).

For clients who do not speak English, we need to either become proficient in their native language or utilize a trained interpreter. If possible, it is desirable to have interpreters who are bicultural as well as bilingual (Fadiman, 1997). Due to the expense and difficulty in obtaining interpreters, bilingual family members and staff may be used, but this may present difficulties. A client may not feel at ease revealing personal information to a younger family member or a spouse who is acting as the interpreter. The client may also not want the family member-interpreter to know the seriousness of the problem. Conversely, the family member-interpreter may choose to withhold vital information from the health care provider or to "protect" the client by not revealing the truth about the medical condition. There are issues of confidentiality, norms about appropriate topics of conversation between generations, and a possible reversal of family roles when the child or spouse is asked to become the family spokesperson. In addition, the bilingual family member may have difficulty understanding or interpreting complex medical information (Tripp-Reimer et al., 2001). Multilingual client literature, videotapes, signs, and directions can be beneficial (Duffy & Alexander, 1999).

It is unwise to assume that all people from a particular neighborhood, ethnic group, or culture have the same values or feel comfortable with the same health care practices. Therefore, it is important to carefully assess the cultural beliefs and behaviors of each client and family. In Chapter 15, we included questions to determine how clients perceive their illness and to help develop a plan of care. Similar questions can be used to determine the client's explanatory model of illness. Kleinman (1978, p. 106) proposes that we ask:

- What do you call your problem? What name does it have?
- What do you think has caused your problem?
- Why do you think it started when it did?
- What does your sickness do to you? How does it work?
- How severe is it? Will it have a long or a short course?
- What do you fear most about your illness?
- What are the chief problems your sickness has caused for you?
- What kind of treatment do you think you should receive? What are the most important results you hope to receive from the treatment?

We need to go beyond these questions, though, to understand how the client and family would like us to interact and what practices are comfortable. For example, we can ask, "Who makes the health care decisions in the family? Who would they like us to address? How much information should the client be given?" (Simpson et al., 2000). It may not feel "right" to us to ask the family's permission to give information to the client, but it may be right for them. It is important to attentively listen to the messages family members are giving. Carefully assess the client and family understanding of the illness and the plan of care you are recommending. Ask them to explain it to you in their own words or demonstrate the technique (Wilson & Robledo, 1999).

It may also be useful to ask the client and family about the health care practices they use at home. You may mention that you have met other clients who call their condition_____ and treat it by using_____. You can follow by asking if this is what they call the illness or if this is a treatment they would use. The effect of a traditional measure can be a powerful adjunct to care. If folk remedies are benign, they can be included in the client's treatment plan, but the health care provider first needs to be knowledgeable about potential outcomes. If possible contraindications for the folk remedy are explained, clients will often accept the care provider's recommendations if they are made respectfully and the negotiation is handled sensitively. It may also be appropriate to incorporate or accept folk healers into the overall plan of care. The health care provider can support the client's practices, while educating them about the benefits of adding Western medical interventions (DiCaprio, Garwick, Kohman, & Blum, 1999; Pachter, 1994; Wilson & Robledo, 1999).

When conflict arises about the most effective form of treatment, the health care provider must determine what components of the intervention are absolutely essential and be prepared to compromise everything else. For example, taking antibiotics to treat an infection may save the client's life, but the wisdom of drinking large volumes of water and resting may be of lesser importance. Encouraging the client to engage in practices they traditionally use, such as massage, acupuncture, or herbal treatments, in addition to Western medical treatments, demonstrates respect for the client's beliefs and facilitates collaboration. At times, hope can be nurtured and supported by incorporating traditional practices into Western care (Brice & Campbell, 1999, Fadiman, 1997). This strategy may take more time than seems available, but an inability to listen and compromise sends the message that information is not important and diminishes the provider's credibility. In reality, this becomes time well-spent when client adherence and satisfaction improves.

## SUMMARY

In this chapter, we summarized important concepts in providing sensitive, effective care to clients from other cultures. The concept of worldview and characteristic beliefs or behaviors were described. Examples were provided to facilitate understanding of how people from various cultures can respond differently to similar events. We also presented information about the culture of medicine and the values and beliefs that we accept as we acculturate as health care professionals.

Barriers to providing effective health care to people from minority cultures were presented. Many of these barriers arise from ethnocentrism and our lack of awareness of our own cultural beliefs and biases. Strategies were offered to help readers begin to develop cultural competence. The key concept is our responsibility to be open to and respectful of all cultural practices during interactions with clients.

## REFLECTIVE QUESTIONS

1. Describe the derivation of your name.
2. What are the beliefs, attitudes, and practices that you acquired from your family's cultural heritage regarding:
   a. religious or spiritual beliefs
   b. holiday traditions
   c. time orientation
   d. activity orientation/environmental control
   e. use of space
   f. social organization and relationships
3. Think about your cultural communication style.
   a. Is it high-context or low-context? Give examples.
   b. Is it direct or indirect? Give examples.
4. a. Describe the roles of your family members.
   b. Imagine working with a family whose roles are different from your own. What might feel comfortable or uncomfortable to you?
5. Consider working with clients from a culture different from your own. What specific actions can you take to increase your knowledge of this culture and improve your effectiveness working with people of this culture?

## CASE STUDY

Mark Sciano is a therapist who works in an urban home care setting, treating many clients who are recent immigrants to the United States, including Mrs. Giovanni from Guatemala. She is living with her son, daughter-in-law, and grandchildren, who treat her with great respect and patience, even though her stroke has made her care more challenging.

On occasion, the family is not ready for Mark when he arrives or no one answers the doorbell or telephone, and he is unsure if they are home. When they do connect, Mark wants to get to work right away because of his busy schedule, but the family always offers him coffee and food and talks with him, in limited English, about most things that have nothing to do with Mrs. Giovanni. They ask what Mark considers to be personal questions and talk about so many things, except for matters of why he is there.

After initially assessing Mrs. Giovanni, Mark had developed a plan of care, and he is surprised that although the family shows her love and tenderness, no one seems particularly interested or adherent in his program, including his client.

1. Given that the Giovanni family has recently immigrated and speaks limited English to Mark's limited Spanish, how can he best communicate and develop an effective collaborative relationship and plan of care?
2. Consider some general guidelines about cultural norms of people from Latino cultures.
   a. What are the differences between the Giovanni family and Mark?
   b. What barriers may these differences create?
3. What value do you think the Giovanni family might place on medical intervention to improve the health or independence of Mrs. Giovanni?
4. How might Mark modify his intervention, attitude, and behavior to create a more positive collaboration with Mrs. Giovanni and her family?

# REFERENCES

Anderson, S. G., Halter, A. P., & Gryzlak, B. M. (2004). Difficulties after leaving TANF: Inner-city women talk about reasons for returning to welfare. *Social Work, 49*(2), 185–194.

Arredondo, P., Toporek, R., Brown, S. P., Jones, J., Locke, D. C., Sanchez, J., & Stadler, H. (1996). Operationalization of the multicultural counseling competencies. *Journal of Multicultural Counseling and Development, 24*, 42–78.

Banja, J. D. (1996). Ethics, values, and world culture: The impact on rehabilitation. *Disability and Rehabilitation, 113*(6), 2279–2284.

Bauder, H. (2002). Neighborhood effects and cultural exclusion. *Urban Studies, 39*(1), 85–93.

Benson, D. S. (2000). Providing health care to human beings trapped in the poverty culture. *Physician Executive, 26*(2), 28–33.

Brice, A., & Campbell, L. (1999). Cross-cultural communication. In R. L. Leavitt (Ed.), *Cross-cultural rehabilitation* (pp. 83–94). London: W. B. Saunders.

Canlas, L. G. (1999). Issues of health care mistrust in east Harlem. *Mount Sinai Journal of Medicine, 66*(49), 257–258.

Choi, K. H., & Wynne, M. E. (2000). Providing services to Asian Americans with developmental disabilities and their families: Mainstream service providers' perspective. *Community Mental Health Journal, 36*(6), 589–595.

Davidhizar, R., Dowd, S. B., & Newman-Giger, J. (1997). Model for cultural diversity in the radiology department. *Radiologic Technology, 68*(3), 233–239.

DiCaprio, J. J., Garwick, A. W., Kohman, C., & Blum, R. W. (1999). Culture and the care of children with chronic conditions. *Archives of Pediatrics and Adolescent Medicine, 153*(10), 1030–1037.

DiMatteo, M. R., Lepper, H. S., & Groghan, T. W. (2000). Depression is a risk factor for noncompliance with medical treatment: Meta-analysis of the effects of anxiety and depression on patient adherence. *Archives of Internal Medicine, 160*(14), 2101–2107.

Duffy, M. M., & Alexander, A. (1999). Overcoming language barriers for non-English speaking patients. *Annals of the National Nursing Association, 26*(5), 507–513.

Erlen, J. A. (1998). Culture, ethics and respect: The bottom line is understanding. *Orthopedic Nursing, 17*(6), 79–83.

Fadiman, A. (1997). *The spirit catches you and you fall down.* New York: Farrar, Straus, and Giroux.

Favazza, A. R., & Oman, M. (1978). Overview: Foundations of cultural psychiatry. *American Journal of Psychiatry, 153*(3), 293–301.

Fiscella, K. (1999). Is lower income associated with greater biopsychosocial morbidity? Implications for physicians working with underserved patients. *Journal of Family Practice, 48*(5), 372–377.

Flores, G., Abreu, M., Olivar, M. A., & Kastner, B. (1998). Access barriers to health care for Latino children. *Archives of Pediatrics and Adolescent Medicine, 152,* 1119–1125.

Freeman, H. P. (2004). Poverty, culture, and social injustice. *CA Cancer Journal Clinics, 54,* 72–77.

Gannotti, M. E., Handwerker, W. P., Groce, N. E., & Cruz, C. (2001). Sociocultural influences on disability status in Puerto Rican children. *Physical Therapy, 81*(9), 1512–1523.

Groce, N. E. (1999). Health beliefs and behavior towards individuals and people with disabilities. In R. L. Leavitt (Ed.), *Cross-cultural rehabilitation* (pp. 37–48). London: W. B. Saunders.

Institute of Medicine. (2001). *Unequal treatment: Confronting the racial and ethnic disparities in healthcare.* Washington, DC: National Academies Press.

Kaiser Family Foundation. (2005). *State health facts.* [Online]. Available: http://www.statehealth facts.org. Date accessed: 6/6/05.

Kleinman, A. (1978). *Patients and healers in the context of culture.* Berkeley: University of California Press.

Kleinman, A. (1988). *The illness narratives.* New York: Basic Books.

Krefting, L. (1991). The culture concept in the everyday practice of occupational and physical therapy. *Physical and Occupational Therapy in Pediatrics, 11*(4) 1–16.

Leavitt, R. L. (1999). Introduction. In R. L. Leavitt (Ed.), *Cross-cultural rehabilitation* (pp. 1–9). London: W. B. Saunders.

Leavitt, R. L. (2001). Special considerations when working with individuals of Hispanic origin. *GeriNotes, 7*(6), 20–23.

Leininger, M. (1995). *Transcultural nursing.* New York: McGraw-Hill.

Loveland, C. (1999). The concept of culture. In R. L. Leavitt (Ed.), *Cross-cultural rehabilitation* (pp. 15–26). London: W. B. Saunders.

Lynch, E. W. (1992). From culture shock to cultural learning. In E. W. Lynch & M. J. Hanson (Eds.), *Developing cross-cultural competence* (pp. 19–33). Baltimore: Paul Brookes.

Nava, Y. (2000). *It's all in the frijoles.* New York: Fireside Books.

Nuñez, A. E. (2000). Transforming cultural competence into cross-cultural efficacy in women's health education. *Academic Medicine, 75,* 1071–1080.

Pachter, L. P. (1994). Culture and clinical care: Folk illness beliefs and behaviors and their implications for healthcare delivery. *Journal of the American Medical Association, 271*(9), 690–694.

Parry, K. (1984). Concepts from medical anthropology for clinicians. *Physical Therapy, 64*(6), 929–932.

Pichette, E. F., Garrett, M. T., Kosciulek, J., & Rosenthal, D. A. (1999). Cultural identification of American Indians and its impact on rehabilitation services. *Journal of Rehabilitation, 65*(3), 3–8.

Reifsnider, E., Allen, J., & Percy, M. (2000). Low-income mothers' perceptions of health in their children with growth delay. *Journal of the Society of Pediatric Nursing, 5*(3), 122–129.

Salimbene, S. (2000). *What language does your patient hurt in?* Rockford, IL: EMC Paradigm.

Simpson, G., Mohr, R., & Redman, A. (2000). Cultural variations in the understanding of traumatic brain injury and brain injury rehabilitation. *Brain Injury, 14*(2), 125–140.

Spector, R. (1996). *Cultural diversity in health and illness.* Stamford, CT: Appleton & Lange.

Stell, L. K. (1999). Diagnosing death: What's trust got to do with it? *Mount Sinai Journal of Medicine, 66*(4), 229–235.

Sue, D., & Morishima, J. K. (1982). *The mental health of Asian Americans.* San Francisco: Jossey-Bass.

Sue, D., & Sue, D. W. (1999). *Counseling the culturally different.* New York: Wiley.

Sung, C. L. (1999). Asian patients' distrust of Western medical care. *Mount Sinai Journal of Medicine, 66*(4), 259–262.

Tang, S. H., & Cheng, S. Y. (2001). Chinese culture and health practices. *GeriNotes, 7*(6), 15–16.

Thomas, L. M. (1999). Trusting under pressure. *Mount Sinai Journal of Medicine, 66*(4), 223–228.

Tripp-Reimer, T., Choi, E., Kelley, L S., & Enslein, J. C. (2001). Cultural barriers to care: Inverting the problem. *Diabetes Spectrum, 14*(1), 13–26.

Ulrich, C. (2002). High stress and low income: The environment of poverty. *Human Ecology, 30* (4), 14–20.

U.S. Census Bureau, Population Division, Special Population Staff. (2000). *Racial and ethnic classifications used in Census 2000 and beyond.* [Online]. Available: http://www.census.gov/population/www/socdemo/race/racefactcb.html. Date accessed: 6/6/05.

U.S. Department of Health and Human Services. (2005). *Health People 2010.* [Online]. Available: http://www.healthypeople.gov. Date accessed: 6/6/05.

Vanderhoff M. (2005). Patient education and health literacy. *PT-Magazine of Physical Therapy, 13*(9), 42–46.

Williams, D. (1999). Race, socioeconomic status, and health: The added effects of racism and discrimination. *Annals of New York Academy of Science, 896,* 173–188.

Wilson, A. H., & Robledo, L. (1999). Listening to Hispanic mothers: Guidelines for teaching. *Journal of the Society of Pediatric Nurses, 4*(30), 125–127.

# 4

# *Understanding Family Needs, Roles, and Responsibilities*

Mrs. Casey paced back and forth in the waiting room. Her husband was seated in a wheelchair, breathing heavily and in apparent pain. I watched as she approached the clerk at the emergency room desk for the third time. She said, "We've been waiting over an hour. My husband's blood pressure is very high. I'm afraid he might be having a heart attack. When will somebody see him?" The clerk, obviously annoyed, responded, "We'll see him as soon as we can. Please be seated and stay out of the corridor." As her husband lowered his head and closed his eyes, Mrs. Casey looked even more distressed. She saw a nurse walking by and shouted, "Please help my husband! I'm afraid he's having a heart attack!" I could see the nurse wasn't happy about this and grudgingly decided to take the client into the examination room. When Mrs. Casey started to come with him, the nurse held up her hand, stopping her. She actually told his wife to sit down until she was called. His wife began to shake. She tried to explain that she had his nitroglycerin with her if he needed it. The nurse curtly told her that they had their own and repeated that she should sit down. Exasperated, Mrs. Casey found a seat in the waiting room, where she waited for the next two hours.

Observing this whole interaction made me feel very uncomfortable. I didn't know what to do. I knew the doctors and nurses were busy with other clients and had to establish priorities. It was just that Mrs. Casey reminded me of my grandmother. I understood her worry and concern. She was trying to help and protect her husband and was afraid of losing him. I wished there was something I could have done to comfort her.

*—From the journal of Rebecca Soren, social work student*

Family caregivers play a significant role in the health care system in emotional, practical, and economic terms. Illness or injury of one member affects the entire family system. This chapter discusses the resulting changes in members' roles and responsibilities, client and caregiver needs, and caregiver burden. Strategies to develop caregiver skills and minimize burnout are explored.

# Family Systems

The "nuclear family" of the 1950s has become mobile and varied. Children grow up and move away from old neighborhoods. Grandparents may not be nearby to assist in raising grandchildren. Blended families from remarriages and nontraditional family groupings have become more common.

In defining the family, Randall and Boonyawiroj (1999) discuss both the family of origin and the family of creation. The family of origin is the social group into which a person is born or adopted. In contrast, the family of creation is the social group that an individual develops outside the fold of the family of origin. Families of creation include friends, significant others, roommates, coworkers, and other individuals with whom one develops a relationship. These families of creation may be as important as those of origin in assuming caregiver responsibilities. When evaluating client problems, health providers need to assess family relationships and determine availability of caregivers.

The family system is comprised of a group of individuals who work together to process information and adapt to outside influences. Individuals relate to each other in predefined ways. Power and decision-making responsibilities are understood among all group members. Illness, injury, or disability of one family member affects the entire family and may cause increased stress among all members. This may necessitate reassigning roles and changing established communication patterns. In an attempt to maintain a sense of equilibrium, group members may resist change, which can further increase tension. Disagreements regarding individual autonomy and family responsibility may lead to conflict, which may negatively affect client care (Randall & Boonyawiroj, 1999).

Health care professionals need to view family members as partners in the health care delivery system. As such, they need to be educated about how they can best assist in the healing process. Early collaboration with family members can reduce conflict, increase adherence with treatment protocols, and improve continuity of care. The value of family caregiving cannot be underestimated. However, health care providers and family caregivers often have conflicting opinions about what is best for the client.

## Working Together, Working Apart

Busy health care professionals may view family members as being overly concerned and "in the way." Conversely, family members may view health care providers as being aloof and uncaring. Although health professionals and family members want what is best for the client, they may have different views, which can place them in adversarial roles. Professionals value medical and technical expertise and may fail to recognize that family members can also be experts about their loved one's problems. Family members may be the first to note changes in a client's condition, based on knowledge developed over years of caring. Yet they may be perceived as challenging a hospital's and doctor's authority, policies, and procedures, especially if they assert themselves and disrupt the routine of care.

Consider Mrs. Brown, who has been assisting her 95-year-old father with his activities of daily living for twenty years because he has had multiple cerebrovascular accidents. Whenever she accompanies him to visit a new care provider, she encounters the same scenario. Because he cannot hear, she offers to accompany him into the examination room and assist with communication. Over the years, many well-meaning health providers have informed her that they need to talk directly to her father and ask her to remain in the waiting room. Repeatedly frustrated, she no longer argues and waits until they discover that they are unable to communicate with him. When they later ask for her assistance, she enters the treatment room, and the examination is able to begin.

When a client is ill or dying, health care providers are often uncomfortable surrounded by the emotions that families express. They may prefer to distance themselves from emotional involvement and move on to treat others who can be helped. In today's society, some health providers fear litigation from family members and avoid communication at all costs (Levine & Zuckerman, 2000). However, health care professionals may need to rely on family members. For example, as the acuity level of hospitalized clients increases, nurses are required to spend most of their time attending to the needs of those who are critically ill. As clients are transferred from specialized units, such as intensive care or coronary care, family members become more important in providing comfort measures and monitoring the needs of their loved ones. Although hospitals frequently post limited visiting hours, staff members often encourage the family to come in early or stay late to assist clients with activities of daily living. Their help alleviates the staff of some of these responsibilities and allows them time to care for complicated, medically ill clients.

As the lengths of hospital stays decreased and managed care increased, clients began to be discharged home sicker than ever before. Health care professionals now depend on family members to carry out procedures at home that previously were performed only by licensed personnel (Biegel, Sales, & Schulz, 1991; Levine & Zuckerman, 2000; Nottingham, 1995; Phillips, 1995). Family members are expected to provide wound care, monitor respirators, administer medications, give injections, and complete chemotherapy infusions. These "home care providers" are often not well-educated for these tasks and may be terrified that their lack of expertise will adversely affect their loved one's health. The responsibilities also increase the burden of family members who may already be overextended with household chores, child care, and work. In addition, the worry and concern they may experience can further drain the family's emotional resources.

## Family Caregivers: Who Are They? Where Do They Come From?

Anyone can become a family caregiver. While some people are prepared to assume this responsibility and plan ahead, others assume this role quite unexpectedly. A sudden car accident, stroke, or diagnosis of peripheral vascular disease can lead to the need for someone to assume the caregiver role. When asked how they became a caregiver, people often respond, "I had to. There was no one else available." Caregiving has been described as a "career," often an unintended, unplanned, and unselected career. There are no wages, no raises, and the caregivers cannot resign, even if they prefer to do so (Pearlin & Aneshensel, 1994).

When the need arises, one family member usually assumes the role of primary caregiver (Phillips, 1995). Some spouses and children may be willing to shoulder this responsibility because of family solidarity, love, and lifelong commitment. Who gets to be the caregiver often follows a substitution principle. In the United States, most caregivers are women. Responsibilities first go to the wife, if one is available. If a wife is not present, the eldest daughter or wife of the eldest son is usually tapped to serve. Other female children or female children-in-law in their birth order follow. However, husbands or sons may also become primary or secondary caregivers. When sons do assume caregiving responsibility, they usually provide financial advice and management rather than assisting with activities of daily living.

Studies show that husbands and sons report less caregiver burden than wives or daughters. This may be because men tend to be less emotional about caregiving and use a problem-solving approach. They may see their new role as a continuation of their role as a provider and authority figure within the family. It is also likely that many sons are married and that their wives assume a share of the caregiver duties (Faison, Faria, & Frank, 1999; Hoffmann & Mitchell, 1998; Laditka & Laditka, 2000).

Adult children often become caregivers. Some may do this as a way of showing gratitude for all their parents have done. Conversely, others may want to "make up" for the way they treated their parents when they were growing up. However, caregiving does not just happen.

Family roles are implicitly or explicitly assigned, and children learn them beginning in childhood (Phillips, 1995). Parents often choose their primary caregiver early in life, long before the child needs to assume the role. They educate the child about the necessity of assuming caregiver responsibilities, often role-modeling this behavior with their own parents. When the need arises, the designated primary caregiver assumes major responsibilities for all care. He or she serves as the family spokesperson and enlists the aid of other family members as needed.

While one child may be groomed for the role of primary caregiver, others are given different paths. Parents teach some children that they are not responsible for providing care, inadvertently or purposely assigning them the role of "abdicator." In doing so, parents give these people permission to continue as if there is nothing wrong. This can result in conflict among other family members who would prefer this role. Because these other people want to be the primary care provider but were not selected for that role, they may become a "pretender." They may be critical of and often disagree with the primary caregiver's decision making (Phillips, 1995). When working with families, it is imperative that health care providers determine who the primary caregiver is, so they can communicate and work with that person to develop appropriate care plans. Sometimes, working with the "wrong" person may increase family conflict and negatively affect client outcomes.

## Economics of Family Caregiving

One of the trends in health care reform focus on cutting costs by decreasing lengths of hospital stays. This results in a shift of care from the hospital to the home setting. While it may appear that this system is more efficient and cost-effective, the effect on family caregivers and their employers needs to be considered. As a result of this shift in care, clients and family caregivers often suffer financially, physically, and emotionally (Pasacreta, Barg, Nuamah, & McCorkle, 2000).

While the true value of receiving care in the home rather than in an institution may be difficult to measure, some attempts to determine the economic value of family caregiving have been made. The following estimates characterize the financial impact of family care providers:

- 25 million U.S. family caregivers
- 24 billion hours of service
- $196 billion worth of unpaid labor

Compare this to the estimates of the costs of professional home health and nursing home care:

- Home health care: $32 billion
- Nursing home care: $83 billion
- Total: $115 billion (Arno, Levine, & Memmott, 1999).

The estimated value of informal caregiving is approximately 13 percent of the total national health care spending of $1.1 billion. This economic study should not detract from the "emotional, cultural, and societal values expressed through informal caregiving. It enhances their importance by providing a tangible measure of the vast, but vulnerable, base upon which our chronic care system rests" (Arno et al., 1999, p. 186).

Most of the nation's caregivers are adult daughters who continue to be employed in the workplace (Marosy, 1997). As a result of their caregiving responsibilities, these women experience added stress and pressure, which often results in decreased productivity at work, absenteeism, workday interruptions, elder care crisis, and burnout. As employees they tend to use health care plans more frequently than other workers, resulting in additional costs to employers for mental and physical health problems related to anxiety and depression. Coberly and Hunt (1995) estimate that employees who are caregivers for elderly relatives cost employers an additional $3,100 per year.

The fastest growing age group in the United States is people over the age of 85. An estimated 13 million people will be older than 85 by the year 2037. Many of these individuals will be dependent upon others to assist them with their daily lives. With the increasing life expectancy and a declining birth rate in the United States, fewer family members will be available to care for elderly people at home (Bird et al., 1998). Employers need to start planning now to offer employees leaves of absences, flexible work schedules, job-sharing, and onsite family day care if they want to attract and retain future workers who have caregiving responsibilities (Marosy, 1997; Spillman & Pezzin, 2000).

As the population ages, the prevalence of illness increases. For example, it is estimated that nearly 50 percent of individuals over age 85 are diagnosed with Alzheimer's disease. More than 22 million people worldwide will be diagnosed by the year 2025. This disease currently costs the United States $100 billion per year. The cost to U.S. businesses exceeds $33 billion each year, $26 billion lost due to decreases in caregivers' productivity and $7 billion related to costs for health care benefits. Seven out of ten clients with Alzheimer's disease are cared for at home. Since Medicare and most private insurance companies do not cover the long-term care needed by these clients, caregivers spend approximately $12,500 per year caring for family members (Alzheimer's Association, 2001).

# Caregiver Needs

A review of the literature indicates that caregivers of long-term clients seek information, education, trust, and understanding from their health care providers. They further need support systems, the ability to speak on behalf of their family members, and assistance navigating the health care system (Smith & Smith, 2000). Health care professionals need to recognize these issues and provide clients and family caregivers with mechanisms to obtain what is required to improve care.

## Information and Education

Family caregivers want and seek honest information about their loved ones' diagnoses and prognoses. They want to understand care plans and what the future holds. It is wise to individualize this information, based on client and family needs and questions (Harrington, Lackey, & Gates, 1996; Pasacreta et al., 2000). Many caregivers indicate that they were given information in the hospital but do not remember much because of the stress of the moment. It was left up to them to follow through and obtain additional information or to ask questions. Lack of knowledge results in a sense of fear and feelings of frustration (Smith & Smith, 2000; Zwygart-Stauffacher, Lindquist, & Savik, 2000).

Health care professionals may provide clients and family members with written information regarding diagnoses and treatment plans. Is this an effective educational tool? As discussed in Chapter 6, timing is important. Providing too much information to clients or family members when they are under stress will probably be ineffective. Another consideration is their literacy level. A national study by the Department of Education found that nearly half of the adults in the United States were poor readers. Surprisingly, some individuals who read poorly believe they read and comprehend information well (Kirsch, Jungeblut, Jenkins, & Kolstad, 1993). They will be unlikely to ask questions about information they do not understand.

According to Kirsch and colleagues (1993), "literacy includes: prose literacy, the ability to understand written news stories, poems, and editorials; document literacy, the ability to understand bus or train schedules, charts, maps, and graphs; and quantitative literacy, the ability to use numbers, balance a checkbook, and understand fractions" (p. 108). To understand most client education materials, an individual must be competent in all three dimensions of literacy. The percentage of individuals over the age of 65 with a fifth-grade education is more than double that of the general population (Hanson, 1995). This is important information for health care providers who work with clients whose caregivers are over 65.

In a study of clients in home settings, Wilson (2000) determined that 85 percent of written client educational materials were inappropriate. Presented in a full text format, they did not identify or emphasize "need-to-know" information first. Instructions were not summarized and were handwritten and difficult to read. When interviewing clients and caregivers, it is important that health care professionals assess their ability to read and understand written instructions. Materials should be in larger print, and writing should be at a fifth- or sixth-grade reading level to ensure consumer comprehension (Wilson, 2000).

Zwygart-Stauffacher and colleagues (2000) note that health providers, clients, and their caregivers may disagree about the type of knowledge needed. While health providers want to disseminate factual information, clients and family caregivers may want information on alternative therapies. A needs assessment survey for clients and family members can help determine what type of information is desired.

Family members also report that health professionals do not understand or address the families' fear of the future and the unknown. They stressed the need for continuity of care so they could develop a relationship with their health providers. Because clients and family members often think of questions once they are home, new methods of communication, such as email, telephone hot lines, listservs, and websites, can augment information disseminated in the acute care and rehabilitation settings (Zwygart-Stauffacher et al., 2000).

Educational workshops and peer support groups for family caregivers after the client has returned home are also effective. They provide additional information as problems arise and improve communication and cooperation among family members. In addition, they help caregivers develop confidence in their skills and abilities. Providing a day care center for clients to attend, concurrent with the workshop sessions for their caregivers, reduces stress and allows caregivers the opportunity to participate, without needing to find someone else to care for their family member (Ostwald, Hepburn, Caron, Burns, & Mantell, 1999).

## Trust

Family caregivers want to be able to trust their health providers. However, in today's busy health care environment, families are often afraid to leave their loved ones alone in the hospital. There are many publicized and observed errors of judgment and practice. In addition, overlooking basic elements of a nurturing environment and the failure of professionals to respond to clients' needs in a timely manner and elicit meaningful responses all can create distrust. This is especially true when clients have been diagnosed with neurological conditions that may leave them unable to protect themselves (Smith & Smith, 2000).

Consider Mr. O'Donnell, an 84-year-old man who has been caring for his wife of 57 years since she began showing symptoms of dementia during the past several months. Following abdominal surgery, she was transferred from the intensive care unit to the surgical floor. The nurse left her sitting in a chair and said she would return. Two hours later, when Mrs. O'Donnell told her husband that she was in severe pain, he contacted the nurse and asked her for medication. When the nurse asked the client how she felt, she responded, "Fine." The nurse indicated that, based on the client's response, no pain medication was needed. Mr. O'Donnell became agitated. "You don't understand. I know my wife. She needs medication! She just doesn't want to complain." The nurse was also becoming frustrated, knowing she had a busy schedule. She then asked the woman to rate her pain on a one-to-ten scale. When Mrs. O'Donnell replied, "Ten," the nurse agreed to the medication. After this incident, Mr. O'Donnell was very anxious about leaving his wife alone. He did not trust the nursing staff to provide the care he felt his wife needed.

How can we instill trust in clients and family caregivers in the current health care climate? Beneficial strategies are more fully explored in other discussions in this book, such as those addressing communication, rapport, and the client–provider relationship.

## Advocacy

Because Mr. O'Donnell believed he could not trust the hospital staff to adequately care for his wife, he became an advocate for her. Many caregivers need advice and guidance on how to advocate for their family members.

Elements of effective advocacy include a knowledge of federal, state, and local regulations regarding health care services, insurance, and special education delivery; assertive communication skills; negotiation; and conflict resolution. Because it is challenging to advocate for clients' welfare when dealing with bureaucracies, caregivers benefit from encouragement, as well as emotional and social support.

Some caregivers may need to become surrogate decision makers if, for example, the people in their care are under the age of 18, are frail, elderly, or diagnosed with dementia, or have physical, cognitive, and/or emotional deficits rendering them unable to make their own decisions. Caregivers' decisions may conflict with the goals and desires of other family members or even with those of the client. Clients with cognitive or emotional deficits may have unrealistic goals or behavior problems, which require caregiver involvement (Smith & Smith,

2000). If the client is over the age of 18, a legal process may be required to allow the family member to assume decision-making responsibilities.

Consider the case of Denis Rockwell and his 16-year-old son. Continually "acting out" in school, Jeff had been suspended several times before finally being expelled. He had been arrested for shoplifting on numerous occasions and attacked his mother, causing her to leave the family home. When Jeff began talking about suicide, Mr. Rockwell tried to discuss his concerns with school professionals and the family doctor. They considered Jeff a "problem child," who only needed more structure in his life. Mr. Rockwell, however, believed that something more serious was being overlooked. He continued to be an advocate and found a doctor who admitted the young man to a psychiatric hospital, against his son's wishes. While there, he was diagnosed with depression, placed on medication, and attended counseling sessions and peer support groups. When he returned home, his father needed to advocate with the school system to provide appropriate educational support so that Jeff could successfully complete high school. This would not have been possible had Mr. Rockwell not served as his spokesperson and advocated for him, obtaining the necessary medical interventions.

## Identification of Resources

Another need expressed by family caregivers is assistance in dealing with the health care system and obtaining necessary supportive resources (Findeis, Larson, Gallo, & Shekleton, 1994; Smith & Smith, 2000). Family members who wish to or must provide home care need professional advice and coordination. For example, the Visiting Nurses Association or other home care agency may provide medical care, including nursing and rehabilitation services. A home health aide can be enlisted to assist clients with activities of daily living. Programs like Meals on Wheels serve hot, nutritious, meals daily. A raised toilet seat, grab bars in the hallway, or other accommodations may be installed to assist the client in safely ambulating in the home. It is the role of the health care team to identify needs and collaborate with the client and family caregivers to help them navigate the health care system and acquire needed resources.

As time progresses, the needs of clients and family caregivers may vary. Health providers need to remain in contact with clients and family caregivers to assist them in identification of these changing needs. For example, if a client is no longer able to independently remain at home, family members may require counseling in how to adapt to this new situation. Perhaps it will be necessary for the client to move in with a family member and attend a day care center while the family member is at work. Depending on the client's and family's situation, a long-term care facility may be more appropriate. It is difficult for families to make these decisions. They rely on expert advice from health care professionals to assist them with these transitions (Findeis et al., 1994).

# Developing Caregiver Skills

In order to become licensed, health care professionals must complete lengthy educational programs and pass examinations; yet there are no such requirements for family caregivers. Imagine how family caregivers may feel when first put in the situation of caring for a loved one. Years ago, the role of family caregivers was similar to that of a nurse's aide. Today, they are expected to complete complicated, highly skilled tasks, but have limited training and sometimes few resources (Pasacreta et al., 2000; Phillips, 1995).

Alone with their "client" in the home setting, caregivers may not know what to do. They may wonder, "Is nausea and vomiting to be expected?" or "How soon should I expect my son to be able to dress independently?" The client may lack an appetite and not want to eat or drink. Respecting his or her wishes, a family caregiver may unknowingly allow the client to become dehydrated.

While some family caregivers may telephone health care professionals daily, asking questions and clarifying concerns, others are reluctant to call, afraid that they are being bothersome. How do we respond to these individuals? Do we lose patience with constant callers, or do we educate them to alleviate their concerns? Do we become angry at the person who failed to call, unwittingly putting a family member at risk? We need to understand the dynamics. Consider that 65 percent of caregivers taking part in one psychoeducational intervention program stated they had difficulty watching their family members become sicker and not knowing how to help. Seventy-four percent were concerned about how to handle future problems (Barg et al., 1998).

Developing caregiver skills requires education, time, patience, and practice. Caregiving demands that they:

- monitor clients
- observe subtle changes
- interpret verbal and nonverbal cues
- analyze the information and make decisions for action
- keep track of what to do and when to do it
- provide direct care, making necessary adjustments
- manage treatment schedules
- administer medications
- identify appropriate resources
- seek outside help as needed
- negotiate the health care system (Schumacher, Stewart, Archbold, Dodd, & Dibble, 2000)

Competent caregiving involves understanding health care plans. Most family caregivers want to provide excellent care. It is the role of health care professionals to determine what skills caregivers need and work with them to develop these skills so they can provide care efficiently and effectively (Schumacher et al., 2000).

# Roles and Responsibilities within the Family System

Within each family system, everyone has specific roles and responsibilities. Each member intuitively knows what is expected and reacts to other family members according to his or her defined role. However, when a member of the family becomes ill or has limitations, impairments, or disabilities, responsibilities and roles change. It is important to note the difference between these terms. Responsibilities are jobs that family members perform, such as cooking meals, paying bills, doing laundry, and going to school. Roles are more complex and difficult to define. Established over many years, they include who you are, how people see you, and what people expect of you. Roles include that of parent, money manager, head of the household, child, and caregiver (Mace & Rabins, 1991). While someone may be able to afford to hire people to fulfill household responsibilities, it is much more difficult to adjust to role changes within the family system.

## Caring for a Spouse or Partner

When a husband, wife, or partner becomes ill or disabled, their marital relationship is altered. Responsibilities change, and each may assume a new role. Sometimes individuals must give up their independence. For example, if an individual who becomes ill had been responsible for paying the bills and managing the household, the person who is well may feel overwhelmed when he or she must assume these activities. The partner who is ill or disabled may not realize his or her deficits and/or not want to relinquish responsibilities. He or she may feel that the partner is "taking over." It takes everyone in the family, including the person who is ill or disabled, time to adjust. As they grieve, they try to adjust to the new "self" and the changing roles and responsibilities within the family system.

Consider Mrs. Benedetto, a 35-year-old woman, who sustained a traumatic brain injury (TBI) in a motor vehicle accident. It is not surprising that her husband and two young children are devastated. In addition, he is angry with her for driving, contrary to his advice, to an aerobics class during a snowstorm. Her health status and inability to work add considerable financial strain on the family. Secondary to the TBI, she sometimes behaves inappropriately, causing great embarrassment. The children do not have their friends visit, and her husband is uncomfortable taking her out in public. They see their friends less often and are becoming socially isolated. Mr. Benedetto misses the companionship and intimacy of his partner. They are both depressed, and the marriage is breaking apart.

Individuals may experience "personality changes" as a result of a TBI. Family caregivers frequently find these changes extremely difficult, if not impossible, to accept. Separation and divorce are common (Webster, Daisley, & King, 1999). The noninjured spouse may experience grief, anger, and chronic sorrow, as described in Chapter 13. Although he or she has "lost" the partner once known, the spouse is still alive, and there is no sense of closure. Counseling has been shown to be effective in helping couples deal with anger management following TBI; however, it has not assisted in improving marital adjustments (Perlesz & O'Loughlan, 1998). These problems are not unique to TBI. They are universal responses to loss and change within the family system.

When treating families who are in transition and conflict, health care professionals must remain objective. They need to understand roles and responsibilities so they can maintain client confidentiality, support the client and family, and provide effective care for individuals undergoing family breakdown (Webster et al., 1999).

According to Banja (1992), health care providers need to integrate the psychosocial dimensions with the clinical phenomenon. "Patients and families who are in the midst of tragedy not only will want superior clinical skills, they will want the company of providers who have opened themselves up to the experience of tragedy and who are willing to share their humanity in the rehabilitation process. Misfortune can be overcome, but tragedy never can. It can only be accommodated" (p. 114). When clients and family members appear to be "difficult" or unmotivated, we must try to understand the changes they are experiencing and work with them to help them adjust to their new roles and responsibilities. Accommodation takes time.

Health care providers need to understand that caring for a spouse or partner who is terminally ill often requires round-the-clock coverage and can be intensely emotional. In addition to helping the spouse or partner with required physical and emotional assistance, the healthy individual is attempting to deal with his or her anticipated future loss of companionship and changing lifestyle. While symptoms of depression are common, some positive outcomes have also been shown to occur.

In a two-year longitudinal study of over 270 gay men caring for a partner who was terminally ill, Folkman (1997) identified four coping processes associated with positive psychological states. She defined these mechanisms as positive reappraisal; goal-directed, problem-focused coping; spiritual beliefs and practices; and the infusion of positive meanings into ordinary events.

Positive reappraisal refers to reframing an event to see it in a more positive light. In Folkman's study (1997), although they were often exhausted, partners stated that they felt proud that they could comfort their loved ones and help them cope. A second coping process, problem-focused coping, includes developing individual strategies, such as gathering information, planning ahead to foresee and manage problems, and making decisions about future courses of action. In addition, the men in the study reported that spiritual beliefs were extremely important in helping them cope with loss. Finally, they indicated that simple activities, like going to a movie or party or taking a trip, were extremely important. They distracted them from their everyday caregiving and made them feel mutually cared about and connected.

These positive coping mechanisms help people find meaning in life, clarify goals, and establish new priorities (Folkman, 1997). Health care professionals can assist clients and caregivers in developing similar coping strategies and aid in their process of rediscovering purpose and meaning in their lives.

## Caring for a Parent

In today's society, women often postpone childbearing to continue careers. As these women age and begin families, they may find themselves caring for older parents at the same time they are caring for their own young children. They are what has become known as the "sandwich generation" (Marosy, 1997; Spillman & Pezzin, 2000). Conflicting responsibilities may increase stress within the family. Husbands may resent time their wives spend away from home caring for parents. Women may feel guilty—either they are not spending enough time at home or not spending enough time with parents. Chronic sorrow may be experienced, as described in Chapter 13 (Lindgren, Connelly, & Gaspar, 1999). The same is true for sons as caregivers. These adult children may have difficulty taking over the roles and responsibilities their parents once performed. While they "grew up" depending on their parents, their parents may now be the dependent ones. Their own children may sense tension in the home, feel neglected, or "act out," seeking attention. As a result, caregivers may develop their own health care problems.

When a younger parent becomes ill or disabled, more responsibilities may be placed on children who still live at home. They may be expected to care for both their parent and younger siblings. This may also increase family tension. Adolescents may be angry and resentful of time taken away from their social life to help with family chores. They may also feel guilty because of this anger and sadness as they grieve the loss of the parent they once knew (Dunn, 1993).

When a younger parent experiences a chronic illness, it highly influences the lives of the children (Steele, Forehand, & Armistead, 1997). Family dynamics and relationships are adversely affected. Both parents frequently experience depression and conflict is not uncommon. As a result, children may internalize their own problems and develop maladaptive coping behaviors. These children may either keep their feelings to themselves or express anger toward others. Health care professionals can assist these families by encouraging discussion among members. Parents need to be open with children, providing them with accurate information about an illness or disability. Family counseling and support groups may be recommended. Parents also need to recognize that their depression and conflict affects their children. Therefore, they need to be encouraged to seek help to deal with their own feelings, for the benefit of the entire family.

## Caring for a Child

I was so excited this morning! It was my first day on the maternity ward. I love babies, and I was really looking forward to being a part of the birthing process. This would be a happy rotation, filled with expectant mothers and fathers looking forward to experiencing the birth of an infant. My days would fly by, and I'd be anxious to return to work the next day.

Boy, was I wrong! My very first client was in trouble. She had been in labor for a long time and was in severe pain. The doctor finally determined that she would have to perform a cesarean section. Although the baby was safely delivered, the umbilical cord was wrapped around his throat. Instead of handing the child to the mother to breastfeed, the doctors rushed the baby into the neonatal intensive care unit for further evaluation. Rather than experiencing tears of joy, the parents were sobbing uncontrollably, awaiting some word of their child's status. I quietly stood in the background, not knowing what to say or do.

*—From the journal of Michelle Crowley, nursing student*

Men and women enter parenthood with the expectation that they will love and raise healthy children who will grow up to be independent and live on their own. This is not always the case. When a child is ill or disabled, parents need to take on the role of advocate for their children, negotiating with the educational, social, and health care systems to obtain services that their children need. These parents have many difficult decisions to make. Blurring of responsibilities among health providers and family caregivers can place tremendous stress on families. Conflict may occur if family members and professionals disagree on what is best for the child (Hartman, DePoy, Francis, & Gilmer, 2000).

Children who are sick or disabled may require painful, invasive procedures, which stresses the parents before, during, and following them (LaMontagne, Wells, Hepworth, Johnson, & Manes, 1999). Parents want to protect their children from pain, but that is not always possible. Lack of control increases stress levels. Health providers can assist parents by showing them how they can be involved in treatments, such as describing procedures to children, instructing them in deep breathing and relaxation exercises, or even holding a hand during a procedure. Helping parents manage their own stress also has a positive impact on the child's care (LaMontagne et al., 1999).

While health care professionals take care of the needs of the children, the parents' needs are sometimes neglected. Parents of children with chronic illness or disability may experience emotional loss and feel responsible for their child's illness or disability. They mourn the loss of the child they expected and may experience chronic sorrow, described in Chapter 13. Their emotional adjustment can be lengthy and difficult. Sometimes they may perceive that they are in control. At other times, they may feel depression, anger, guilt, lack of control, powerlessness, and despair. Parents of children who are sick or disabled need to become expert caregivers and advocates in the often fragmented health care system. Stress may increase when developmental milestones are not met at anticipated times. Anxiety levels may be further exacerbated as a result of financial loss due to the expense of care and equipment and time away from work.

Career mobility may be limited as parents may choose to live in a geographical area where a child's health needs can be better met. They may be unable to change jobs, remaining in positions in order to retain their health care coverage and/or primary care physicians (Worthington, 1989). Financial resources can be even further strained if a parent must quit his or her job to stay home and care for a child who is ill.

Children with disabilities may not achieve independence. Parents may wonder who will care for their child when they are no longer able. They may feel angry, depressed, and envy families with more "typical" children. Parents often feel they should not leave the house and have fun while their child is at home ill or disabled (Cooper, 1996). Support systems that allow independent living away from the family are not always available (Hartman et al., 2000).

Health professionals can help by understanding that families may go through recurring periods of emotional crisis. At times they might be angry or hostile. Educating families about what to expect may help prevent or alleviate anger. Keeping the lines of communication open is also extremely important. Ask questions to help resolve issues and determine what a family needs or wants. You can then assist them in obtaining social and educational support.

Discussing a terminal illness is always difficult, particularly when it is a child who is dying. There is evidence that children know that they are dying but do not let others know that they know. Lack of communication among family members and between family and health care providers interferes with everyone's ability to cope with the situation. Health care providers can assist clients and families by empathetically listening and providing accurate and updated information on an ongoing basis (Black, 1998).

Sometimes decisions about whether to initiate or disconnect life-support systems must be made. These are difficult decisions, and family members need to be included. Values and spiritual beliefs influence one's definition of quality of life. The client's age and cognitive abilities, as well as the presence or absence of perceived pain levels, may be other considerations. Family relationships, including the existence of siblings, are additional factors. Finally, time is an important variable. In emergency situations, decisions need to be made immediately, with no time for lengthy deliberations. In the case of chronic illness, it is suggested that discussions regarding life support occur early, allowing time for planning and acceptance (Kirschbaum, 1996).

## Sibling Roles and Responsibilities

When a child is ill, parents and health providers focus on that child. What happens to the siblings living at home and experiencing the family stress? Siblings may experience guilt because they are healthy. They may become depressed, withdrawn, or use attention-seeking behavior. They may fear that they, too, will become sick (Murray, 1999; Sloper & While, 1996). Just as adult caregivers need adequate information regarding a client's diagnosis and prognosis, siblings also express a desire to understand more about the illness or disability their brother or sister is experiencing. Health providers can teach and support parents to communicate openly with all of the children in the family and invite siblings to be involved in the care plan. Sibling support groups may also be beneficial in helping children adjust (Murray, 1999).

The roles and responsibilities of a healthy child may change when a sibling becomes ill or disabled. Older children are often enlisted to care for younger siblings, while parents attend to the needs of the child who is ill or disabled. The older child may resent these changes in roles and responsibilities. This is especially true if parents overindulge an ill child or spend extended periods of time away from home visiting a child in the hospital (Sloper & While, 1996).

If a child has a physical or emotional disability, a sibling may experience feelings of embarrassment and not want to be seen with the child with problems. This may also lead to feelings of guilt and depression. Although educational information regarding illness or disability may be written for adults and not be suitable to share with children, they need to be informed. Providing appropriate educational interventions to siblings will help them understand what is happening, allay their fears, and reduce their sense of guilt or embarrassment.

Encourage siblings to talk about their feelings without fear of consequences. Answer questions honestly. While all members of the family may be required to take on additional responsibilities, adults need to assure children that they will be treated as children and not as adult caretakers (Fleitas, 2000). Parents should be encouraged to spend as much time with the healthy children as possible to decrease disruption in family life. Health providers need to help parents understand that their reaction to the child's illness will affect their other children's responses and behaviors (Sloper & While, 1996).

# Caregiver Burden

Following initial diagnoses, accidents, or injuries, there may be an abundance of family and friends to help both client and caregiver. However, as time progresses, people return to their own lives. Caregivers may be left alone to adjust to their altered lives. Caring for a friend or relative can be a positive experience. Some caregivers report developing a strong bond with their "clients" and feel good about themselves as a result of the experience (Findeis et al., 1994; Rabkin, Wagner, & DelBene, 2000; Walker, Martin, & Jones, 1992).

However, providing long-term care can lead to "caregiver burden" (Hoffman & Mitchell, 1998). Caregiver burden has been described in studies of clients with many diagnoses (Cooper, 1996; Freedman, Griffiths, Krauss, & Seltzer, 1999; Gulick, 1995; Harrington et al., 1996; Hendryx-Bendalov, 2000; Perlesz & O'Loughlan, 1998; Steketee, 1997; Thompson & Haran, 1985; Zwygart-Stauffacher et al., 2000). It encompasses both objective and subjective components. Objective burden refers to the tasks caregivers must perform and the changes that occur in their lives as a result of performing tasks, such as dressing, bathing, feeding, and transporting clients. Subjective burden results from the emotional factors stemming from caregiving responsibilities, such as fatigue, stress, anger, depression, social isolation, fear, and role adjustment. Lack of resources and financial strain can also affect caregiver burden (Hoffman & Mitchell, 1998; Montgomery & Borgatta, 1989).

When friends or family members become caregivers, their lives are disrupted. They must rearrange schedules to meet the needs of the client. While some people make this adjustment easily, others do not. Studies indicate that the quality of the relationship between the caregiver and the client has an impact on the perceived levels of burden and satisfaction with the caregiver role (Robinson, 1990; Snyder, 2000). If the premorbid relationship was characterized by open communication, shared interests, and a family orientation, perceived burden is low and satisfaction is high. This is true even when objective burden is high. Although health care providers cannot change family histories or relationships, they may assist burdened caregivers by referring them to family counselors or therapists who may be able to help.

Clients may require more assistance over time, especially if the illness or disability is progressive or chronic. When this occurs, caregivers have less time for themselves. Overload and burnout may occur. They may lose sleep if they are frequently interrupted during the night to provide assistance. Caregivers may lose contact with former friends and feel socially and emotionally isolated. They may also experience grief and chronic sorrow, as described in Chapter 13, as they watch their loved ones decline. At the same time, they may also experience anger, resentment, and frustration because their own lives have been disrupted. Some caregivers may resort to maladaptive practices, turning to prescription and nonprescription drugs or alcohol to help them face each day (Faison et al., 1999; Marsh, Kersel, Havill, & Sleigh, 1998). Others postpone taking care of their own health needs because they are so busy caring for someone else (Stein et al., 2000). However, failure to alleviate their stress and burden can ultimately lead to increased doctors' visits and medical expenses (O'Brien, 2000).

As discussed in Chapter 17, high caregiver burden, frustration, and inability to provide adequate care can increase risk for abuse (Lachs, Williams, O'Brien, Hurst, & Horwitz, 1996; Marshall, Benton, & Brazier, 2000). For example, it is estimated that over 2 million older adults are mistreated in the United States each year. Abuse can occur in the home or in a residential facility. The abuser may be a health provider or a family caregiver. Because of differing definitions of abuse and lack of reporting, the exact extent of this problem is not known at this time. It may include neglect and physical, emotional, and financial abuse (Gray-Vickrey, 2000; Swagerty, Takahashi, & Evans, 1999). Clients who depend on others for assistance with activities of daily living and/or who are cognitively impaired are at high risk for abuse (Lachs, Berkman, Fulmer, & Horwitz, 1994). Health care professionals play an important role in recognizing signs of abuse and taking appropriate steps to stop its occurrence. Those who are aware and educated about this issue are more likely to detect and report cases of abuse (Tilden et al., 1994).

Abuse may be difficult to detect. Individuals with cognitive impairment may have trouble defining the problem (Gray-Vickrey, 2000; Swagerty et al., 1999). People with physical impairments may have bruising caused by bumping into walls or falling. Care must be taken when making assumptions. Clients may be reluctant to discuss injuries with people outside of the family because they may be embarrassed or afraid of retaliation. Some individuals may fear that they will be moved out of their homes and institutionalized. Given the choice, they prefer to remain silent rather than be moved.

Although there are federal laws concerning child abuse, there is no federal law mandating reporting of domestic violence. The laws regarding the reporting of abuse differ from state to state. However, most states do require health professionals to report suspected abuse of children and people who are elderly, disabled, or institutionalized. In addition, most health care facilities have procedures for dealing with and reporting suspected abuse. It is important to know your state regulations and departmental policies. Students suspecting abuse should notify their immediate supervisors so they can take appropriate action. An attempt should be made to independently interview the client and caregiver, take notes, and compare the information. It is essential that discrepancies are documented using the exact words of the caregiver and the client. Health care providers can be found negligent if they fail to report suspected abuse of members of the mandated populations. Penalties may include fines, imprisonment, and loss of license (Barnett, Miller-Perrin, & Perrin, 1997; Bird et al., 1998; Swagerty et al., 1999).

# Caring for the Caregiver

A review of the literature indicates that well-informed caregivers who are confident in their abilities and have developed appropriate coping strategies exhibit lower stress levels and less caregiver burden. Health care professionals who suspect caregiver burden can help by educating them about common stresses associated with caregiving and by referring them to appropriate resources to assist them in developing strategies for coping with difficult situations (Parks & Novielli, 2000).

## Respite Care

Both the amount of care provided and the duration of the illness influence caregiver burden (Lemkin, 1995). It is important that the caregiver receive some relief from his or her duties. Respite care, as a social service, is designed to support family caregivers by providing temporary daytime or overnight relief. It was designed to assist with crisis intervention and avoid institutionalization (Lawton, Brody, & Saperstein, 1989). Eligibility is typically limited to families of clients with severe disabilities (Knoll et al., 1992). It is a beneficial system that supports both clients and family caregivers on an ongoing basis.

Health professionals can assist caregivers by helping them identify appropriate resources. Some local governments have volunteer "sitters" for short periods of time. Formal adult day care programs provide opportunities for caregivers to work, do errands, or just take a break from everyday duties. Bus services may be available to transport individuals to and from the day care facility. Other family members can be asked to provide care for short periods of time. While primary caregivers may be uncomfortable giving up "control," health providers can help them understand that it is in the best interest of the client and themselves.

## Support Groups

As discussed in Chapter 6, peer support groups can be an effective adjunct for both clients and caregivers. Caregivers may be reluctant to leave their loved one alone to attend a support group, but again, may be encouraged to do so for the benefit of the client. Some caregiver support groups are concurrently offered in the same facility as client support groups. This forum provides the opportunity for everyone to share ideas and strategies for handling problems.

Peer visitor support programs offer another alternative. For example, in one program, a group of caregivers with previous experience took part in a supervised peer support program. They underwent a training program and participated in a biweekly, twelve-week program in which they visited peers who had just begun to care for a family member. Peer visitors provided informational support, suggested potential coping strategies, and discussed problem-solving methods based on their own experiences. In addition, they listened to the concerns of the new caregivers and affirmed that they were doing a good job. All of the participants rated the experience as being extremely beneficial (Stewart, Doble, Hart, Langille, & MacPherson, 1998).

## Humor

As discussed in Chapter 2, humor has been shown to help people maintain balance in their lives. Developing and maintaining a sense of humor can assist caregivers in preventing or overcoming caregiver burden. The strategy can be as simple as reading a humorous book or watching funny movies to relieve stress. Although some caregivers might feel guilty devoting time to laughter, particularly if their loved one is in pain or uncomfortable, those who understand the importance of self-care are less likely to experience guilt. If they are unable to leave the client alone, encourage caregivers to seek respite care to allow some time for enjoyment (Pasquali, 1991).

While humor can reduce stress, it can also serve as a barrier to effective communication (Bethea, Travis, & Pecchioni, 2000). Careful judgment is needed. For example, caregivers may use humor to describe problems or situations to health providers. Anecdotal accounts and jokes may help alleviate uneasiness. Conversely, a caregiver may be using humor because he or she is unable to express a need. In those cases, the caregiver may actually be conveying a serious cry for help. Health providers need to ask probing questions to determine the extent of potential problems and offer appropriate assistance, when indicated.

# Relationships between Professional and Family Caregivers

Families involved in long-term caregiving stress the importance of having a good relationship with a competent and caring professional. The effective professional relates well to a family and demonstrates an appreciation for the caregiver's knowledge and skills (Nottingham, 1995). Nottingham (1995) stresses the importance of distinguishing between caring and caregiving: "The caring professional is concerned about another person's well-being and human development. Caregiving without caring involves going through the motions of doing a job that the professional has been hired to do. People know whether they are in the hands of a caring person who is caregiving or whether they are just having an encounter with a care provider" (p. 17).

Caring health providers understand and appreciate the needs of family caregivers and include them in treatment planning. Those who are uncaring want to be in control. Inexperienced health professionals sometimes make the mistake of maintaining too much control. Being able to relinquish control and decision making to clients and their families encourages them to take responsibility for their own care (Nottingham, Haigler, Smith, & Davis, 1993).

In the acute care setting, planning for home care needs to begin upon admission to the hospital, with communication between clients, family members, and health providers. Shared knowledge results in better treatment planning for both the clinical setting and upon discharge. Organizational policies and procedures may hamper effective communication, though (Ray & Miller, 1990). One study showed that the disagreement between family caregivers and staff nurses about health issues of older hospitalized clients was attributed to the limited time nurses had available to communicate with them (Rose, Bowman, & Kresevic, 2000). Although busy health providers have limited time to communicate with family members, it is well worth the time in terms of clients' health status, staffing needs, and health care dollars. Early involvement of family members in discharge planning results in fewer inpatient hospital days and fewer cases of readmissions (Naylor et al., 1994).

Communication between health providers and family caregivers affects clients' health following discharge from the hospital (Bull & Kane, 1996). In a study of clients hospitalized for heart failure, family caregivers who reported a high level of involvement in discharge planning were more satisfied with care than those who did not. In addition, these caregivers felt more prepared to take care of their family member and more accepting of their caregiver role (Bull, Hansen, & Gross, 2000). It is the responsibility of health care providers to ensure that caregivers feel competent in their roles, have realistic expectations, and know who to contact for post-discharge questions (Findeis et al., 1994).

When working with family caregivers in the home, health care professionals must remember that they are in the family's domain. Interventions need to reflect the family values and belief systems. Some families are comfortable with their homes being converted into miniature hospitals; others resist this, minimizing disruption of home and family life. It is important to actively listen to caregivers, view them as experts in the care of family members, and validate their strategies (Toth-Cohen, 2000).

For example, some clients might be comfortable having grab bars and a raised toilet seat installed in the bathroom, while others may find it embarrassing when they have visitors. Work with clients and family members to develop an acceptable solution that ensures safety. You might be able to try another approach, without making structural modifications. With your encouragement, they can contact you if there is a change in abilities and equipment is needed to be installed. Consider alternative solutions. Another possibility might be a portable commode that could be used in the bathroom on a daily basis and put away when there are visitors.

## Summary

This chapter addressed the effects of illness and disability on members of a family system. The role of the family in health care was discussed, and the importance of an interdependent relationship between professional and family caregivers was presented. Family caregivers are at risk for developing depression, caregiver burden, and burnout. Strategies to assist caregivers were explored.

## REFLECTIVE QUESTIONS

1. a. What comprises a "family" to you?
   b. Who comprises your family of origin?
   c. Who comprises your family of creation?
   d. What roles have been "assigned"?
2. Assume that one of your parents became seriously ill or disabled today.
   a. In your family, who would accept the primary caregiving role?
   b. What burdens would be imposed on this person?
   c. What kind of supports would be available?
   d. What health provider behaviors do you think would be most helpful?
3. a. What conflicts might occur in your family if a decision needed to be made regarding the care of someone who was ill or disabled?
   b. What conflicts might develop between your family and health care providers?
   c. How might these conflicts be resolved?
4. Imagine that you are 5 years old and your younger brother has just been born with a disability.
   a. What effects might this have on your family?
   b. How might the relationships change?
   c. What additional roles and responsibilities might you need to assume?
   d. How might this have changed your life as a 5-year-old? 10-year-old? 15-year-old?
5. How can you instill trust in clients and family caregivers in the current health care climate?

## CASE STUDY

Yvette is a third-year physical therapist student, who is living on the East Coast with her grand-parents while she attends college. Her parents and brother live on the West Coast, and her mother is the only child of the grandparents. Recently, Yvette's grandmother was hospitalized following a cerebrovascular accident (stroke). She is currently receiving home care services. As Yvette is the only one in the family to attend college, is majoring in a health care profession, and lives at the house with her grandparents, the family expects her to be their advocate.

The grandfather is not happy with the services that are being provided. Although the nurse comes once each week, he believes that she should be there daily. The grandmother is receiving physical therapy services three times each week for strengthening, conditioning, and ambulatory activities, but the grandfather thinks the therapist is "pushing" his wife too hard. A home health aide comes in every day to assist the grandmother with activities of daily living, but the grandfather feels that she is invading his wife's privacy.

The occupational therapist has suggested changes in the home environment, including removal of scatter rugs, installation of grab bars in the bathtub, and a commode and hospital bed for the bedroom.

Yvette thinks that although the clinicians are providing technically competent care, they are insensitive to the psychosocial needs of her family.

1. How are the family dynamics affected by the circumstances?
2. How are the roles and responsibilities of each family member altered?

3. What can be done to bridge the geographic distance that exists?
4. What steps can be taken to develop a trusting relationship with each family member?

## REFERENCES

Alzheimer's Association. (2001). *General statistics/demographics* [Online]. Available: http://www.alz .org/research/current/stats.htm. Date accessed: 6/6/05.

Arno, P., Levine, C., & Memmott, M. M. (1999). The economic value of informal caregiving. *Health Affairs, 1*(2), 182–188.

Banja, J. D. (1992). Tragedy and traumatic brain injury. *Journal of Head Trauma Rehabilitation, 7*(4), 112–114.

Barg, F. K., Pasacreta, J. V., Nuamah, I. F., Robinson, K. D., Angeletti, K., Yasko, J. M., & McCorkle, R. (1998). A description of a psychoeducational intervention for family caregivers of cancer patients. *Journal of Family Nursing, 4,* 394–413.

Barnett, O. W., Miller-Perrin, C. L., & Perrin, R. D. (1997). *Family violence across the lifespan: An introduction.* Newbury Park, CA: Sage.

Bethea, L. S., Travis, S. S., & Pecchioni, L. (2000). Family caregivers' use of humor in conveying information about caring for dependent older adults. *Health Communication, 12*(4), 361–376.

Biegel, D. E., Sales, E., & Schulz, R. (1991). *Family caregiving in chronic illness.* Newbury Park, CA: Sage.

Bird, P. E., Harrington, D. T., Barillo, D. J., McSweeney, A., Shirani, K. Z., & Goodwin, C. W. (1998). Elder abuse: A call to action. *Journal of Burn Care and Rehabilitation, 19,* 522–527.

Black, D. (1998). The dying child. *British Medical Journal, 316*(7141), 1376–1378.

Bull, M. J., Hansen, H. E., & Gross, C. R. (2000). Differences in family caregiver outcomes by their level of involvement in discharge-planning. *Applied Nursing Research, 13*(2), 76–82.

Bull, M. J., & Kane, R. L. (1996). Gaps in discharge-planning. *Journal of Applied Gerontology, 15,* 506–520.

Coberly, S., & Hunt, G. G. (1995). *The MetLife study of employer costs for working caregivers.* Washington, DC: Washington Business Group on Health.

Cooper, M. (1996). Obsessive–compulsive disorder: Effects on family members. *American Journal of Orthopsychiatry, 66*(2), 296–304.

Dunn, B. (1993). Growing up with a psychotic mother: A retrospective study. *American Journal of Orthopsychiatry, 63*(2), 177–188.

Faison, K. J., Faria, S. H., & Frank, D. (1999). Caregivers of chronically ill elderly: Perceived burden. *Journal of Community Health Nursing, 1*(4), 243–253.

Findeis, A., Larson, J. L., Gallo, A., & Shekleton, M. (1994). Caring for individuals using home ventilators: An appraisal by family caregivers. *Rehabilitation Nursing, 19*(1), 6–11.

Fleitas, J. (2000). When Jack fell down, Jill came tumbling after: Siblings in the web of illness and disability. *American Journal of Maternal Child Nursing, 25*(5), 267–273.

Folkman, S. (1997). Positive psychological states and coping with severe stress. *Social Science and Medicine, 45*(8), 1207–1221.

Freedman R. I., Griffiths, D., Krauss, M. W., & Seltzer, M. M. (1999). Patterns of respite use by aging mothers of adults with mental retardation. *Mental Retardation, 37*(2), 93–103.

Gray-Vickrey, P. (2000). Combating abuse: I. Protecting the older adult. *Nursing, 30*(7), 34–38.

Gulick, E. E. (1995). Coping among spouses or significant others of persons with multiple sclerosis. *Nursing Research, 44*(4), 220–225.

Hanson, E. C. (1995). Evaluating cognitive services for non-literate and visually impaired patients in community pharmacy rotation sites. *American Journal of Pharmaceutical Education, 59,* 48–55.

Harrington, V., Lackey, N. R., & Gates, M. F. (1996). Needs of caregivers of clinic and hospice cancer patients. *Cancer Nursing, 19*(2), 118–125.

Hartman, A., DePoy, E., Francis, C., & Gilmer, D. (2000). Adolescents with special health care needs in transition: Three life histories. *Social Work in Health Care, 31*(4), 43–57.

Hendryx-Bendalov, P. M., (2000). Alzheimer's dementia: Coping with communication decline. *Journal of Gerontological Nursing, 26*(8), 20–24.

Hoffman, R. L., & Mitchell, A. M. (1998). Caregiver burden: Historical development. *Nursing Forum, 33*(4), 5–10.

Kirsch, I. S., Jungeblut, A., Jenkins, L., & Kolstad, A. (1993). *Adult literacy in America: National adult literacy survey.* Washington, DC: U.S. Government Printing Office.

Kirschbaum, M. S. (1996). Life support decisions for children: What do parents value? *Advances in Nursing Science, 19*(1), 51–71.

Knoll, J., Covert, S., Osuch, R., O'Connor, S., Agosta, J., & Blaney, B. (1992). Supporting families: State family support efforts. In V. Bradley, J. Knoll, & J. Agosta (Eds.), *Emerging issues in family support* (pp. 57–97). Washington, DC: American Association on Mental Retardation.

Lachs, M. S., Berkman, L., Fulmer, T., & Horwitz, R. I. (1994). A prospective community-based pilot study of risk factors for the investigation of elder mistreatment. *Journal of American Geriatric Society, 42,* 169–173.

Lachs, M. S., Williams, C., O'Brien, S., Hurst, L., & Horwitz, R. I. (1996). Older adults: An 11 year longitudinal study of adult protective service use. *Archives of Internal Medicine, 156,* 449–453.

Laditka, J. N., & Laditka, S. B. (2000). Aging children and their older parents: The coming generation of caregiving. *Journal of Women and Aging, 12*(1/2), 189–204.

LaMontagne, L. L., Wells, N., Hepworth, J. T., Johnson, B. D., & Manes, R. (1999). Parent coping and child distress behaviors during invasive procedures for childhood cancer. *Journal of Pediatric Oncology Nursing, 16*(1), 3–12.

Lawton, M. P., Brody, E. M., & Saperstein, A. R. (1989). A controlled study of respite service for caregivers of Alzheimer's patients. *Gerontologist, 29,* 8–16.

Lemkin, P. (1995). How much can I give? The other side of caregiving. *Caring Magazine, 14*(4), 41–43.

Levine, C., & Zuckerman, C. (2000). Hands on/hands off: Why health care professionals depend on families but keep them at arm's length. *Journal of Law, Medicine and Ethics, 28*(1), 5–18.

Lindgren, C. L., Connelly, C. T., & Gaspar, H. L. (1999). Grief in spouse and children caregivers of dementia patients. *Western Journal of Nursing Research, 21*(4), 521–537.

Mace, N. L., & Rabins, P. V. (1991). *The 36-hour day* (2nd ed.). Baltimore: The Johns Hopkins University Press.

Marosy, P. (1997). Elder caregiving in the 21st century. *Caring Magazine, 16*(5) 18–21.

Marsh, N. V., Kersel, D. A., Havill, J. H., & Sleigh, J. W. (1998). Caregiver burden 1 year following severe traumatic brain injury. *Brain Injury, 12*(12), 1045–1059.

Marshall, C. E., Benton, D., & Brazier, J. M. (2000). Elder abuse: Using clinical tools to identify clues of mistreatment. *Geriatrics, 55*(2), 42–53.

Montgomery, R., & Borgatta, E. (1989). The effects of alternative support strategies on family caregiving. *The Gerontologist, 29,* 457–464.

Murray, J. S. (1999). Siblings of children with cancer: A review of the literature. *Journal of Pediatric Oncology Nursing, 16*(1), 25–34.

Nottingham, J. A. (1995). Navigating the seas of caregiving: Allies and ideas for success. *Caring Magazine, 14*(4), 16–20.

Nottingham, J., Haigler, D., Smith, D., & Davis, P. (1993). *Characteristics, concerns and concrete needs of formal and informal caregivers. Understanding and appreciating their marathon existence.* Americus: Georgia Southwestern College Publications.

O'Brien, J. (2000). Caring for caregivers. *American Family Physician, 62*(12), 2584–2587.

Ostwald, S. K., Hepburn, K. W., Caron, W., Burns, T. B., & Mantell, R. (1999). Reducing caregiver burden: A randomized psychoeducational intervention for caregivers of persons with dementia. *The Gerontologist, 39*(3), 299–309.

Parks, M. S., & Novielli, K. D. (2000). A practical guide to caring for caregivers. *American Family Physician, 62*(12), 2613–2619.

Pasacreta, J. V., Barg, F., Nuamah, I., & McCorkle, R. (2000). Participant characteristics before and 4 months after attendance at a family caregiver cancer education program. *Cancer Nursing, 23*(4), 295–303.

Pasquali, E. A. (1991). Humor: Preventive therapy for family caregivers. *Home Healthcare Nurse, 9*(13), 13–17.

Pearlin, L. I., & Aneshensel, C. S. (1994). Caregiving: The unexpected career. *Social Justice Research, 7,* 373–390.

Perlesz, A., & O'Loughlan, M. (1998). Changes in stress and burden in families seeking therapy following traumatic brain injury: A follow-up study. *International Journal of Rehabilitation Research, 21,* 339–354.

Phillips, L. (1995). On becoming a caregiver: Default or election—and does it matter? *Caring Magazine, 14*(4), 12–25.

Rabkin, J. G., Wagner, G. J., & DelBene, M. (2000). Resilience and distress among amyotrophic lateral sclerosis patients and caregivers. *Psychosomatic Medicine, 62,* 271–279.

Randall, A. D., & Boonyawiroj, E. B. (1999). Client education and family systems. *Physical Therapy, 13*(3), 18–22.

Ray, E. B., & Miller, K. I. (1990). Communication in the health care organization. In E. B. Ray & L. Donahew (Eds.), *Communication and health: Systems and application* (pp. 92–107). Hillsdale, NJ: Erlbaum.

Robinson, K. (1990). Predictors of burden among wife caregivers. *Scholarly Inquiry for Nursing Practice, 4,* 189–208.

Rose, H. R., Bowman, K. F., & Kresevic, D. (2000). Nurse versus family caregiver perspectives on hospitalized older patients: An exploratory study of agreement at admission and discharge. *Health Communication, 12*(1), 63–80.

Schumacher, K. L., Stewart, B. J., Archbold, P. G., Dodd, M. J., & Dibble, S. L. (2000). Family caregiving skill: Development of the concept. *Research in Nursing and Health, 23,* 191–203.

Sloper, P., & While, D. (1996). Risk factors in the adjustment of siblings of children with cancer. *Journal of Child Psychology, 37*(5), 597–607.

Smith, J. E., & Smith, D. L. (2000) No map, no guide: Family caregivers' perspectives on their journeys through the system. *Case Management Journal, 2*(1), 27–33.

Snyder, J. R. (2000). Impact of caregiver–receiver relationship quality on burden and satisfaction. *Journal of Women and Aging, 12*(1/2), 147–167.

Spillman, B. C., & Pezzin, L. E. (2000). Potential and active family caregivers: Changing networks and the "sandwich generation." *The Millbank Quarterly, 78*(3), 347–374.

Steele, R. G., Forehand, R., & Armistead, L. (1997). The role of family processes and coping strategies in the relationship between parental chronic illness and childhood internalizing problems. *Journal of Abnormal Child Psychology, 25*(2), 83–94.

Stein, M. D., Crystal, S., Cunningham, W. E., Ananthanarayanan, A., Andersen, R. M., Turner, B. J., Zierler, S., Morton, S., Katz, M. H., Bozzette, S. A., Shapiro, M. F., & Schuster, M. A. (2000). Delays in seeking HIV care due to competing caregiver responsibilities. *American Journal of Public Health, 90*(7), 1138–1140.

Steketee, G. (1997). Disability and family burden in obsessive–compulsive disorder. *Canadian Journal of Psychiatry, 42,* 919–927.

Stewart, M. J., Doble, S., Hart, G., Langille, L., & MacPherson, K. (1998). Peer visitor support for family caregivers of seniors with stroke. *Canadian Journal of Nursing Research, 30*(2), 87–117.

Swagerty, D. L., Takahashi, P. Y., & Evans, J. M. (1999). Elder mistreatment. *American Family Physician, 59*(10), 2804–2808.

Thompson, D. M., & Haran, D. (1985). Living with an amputation: The helper. *Social Science Medicine, 20*(4), 319–323.

Tilden, V. P., Schmidt, T. A., Limandri, B. J., Childo, G. T., Garland, M. J., & Loveless, P. A. (1994). Factors that influence clinicians' assessment and management of family violence. *American Journal of Public Health, 84,* 628–633.

Toth-Cohen, S. (2000). Role perceptions of occupational therapists providing support and education for caregivers of persons with dementia. *American Journal of Occupational Therapy, 54*(5), 509–515.

Walker, A. J., Martin, S. K., & Jones, L. J. (1992). The benefits and costs of caregiving and care receiving for daughters and mothers. *Journal of Gerontology, 3,* S130–S139.

Webster, G., Daisley, A., & King, N. (1999). Relationship and family breakdown following acquired brain injury: The role of the rehabilitation team. *Brain Injury, 13*(8), 593–603.

Wilson, F. L. (2000). Are patient information materials too difficult to read? *Home Healthcare Nurse, 18*(2), 107–115.

Worthington, R. C. (1989). The chronically ill child and recurring family grief. *Journal of Family Practice, 29*(4), 397–400.

Zwygart-Stauffacher, M., Lindquist, R., & Savik, K. (2000). Development of health care delivery systems that are sensitive to the needs of stroke survivors and their caregivers. *Nursing Administration Quarterly, 24*(3), 33–42.

# ADDITIONAL READINGS FOR PART I

Barnett, R. C., Biener, L., & Baruch, G. K. (Eds). (1987). *Gender and stress.* New York: Free Press.

Blenky, M. F., Clinchy, B. M., Goldberger, N. R., & Tarule, J. M. (1986). *Women's ways of knowing: The development of self, voice, and mind.* New York: Basic Books.

Braun, K. L., Pietsch, J. H., & Blanchette, P. (Eds.). (2000). *Cultural issues in end-of-life decision-making.* Newbury Park, CA: Sage.

Brownell, J. (1996). *Listening, attitudes, principles and skills.* Boston: Allyn and Bacon.

Cooke, R. (2001). *Dr. Folkman's war.* New York: Random House.

Doka, K., & Davidson, J. (1998). *Living with grief: Who we are, how we grieve.* Washington, DC: Hospice Foundation of America.

Faderman, L. (1998). *I begin my life all over again.* Boston: Beacon Press.

Fadiman, A (1997). *The spirit catches you and you fall down.* New York: Farrar, Strauss, & Giroux.

Fiser, R., & Ury, W. (1991). *Getting to yes: Negotiating agreement without giving in.* Boston: Houghton Mifflin.

Gray, J. (1992). *Men are from Mars, women are from Venus: A practical guide for improving communication and getting what you want in all your relationships.* New York: HarperCollins.

Groopman, J. (2000). *Second opinions.* New York: Viking Press.

Hogan, L. (2001). *The woman who watches over the world.* New York: Norton.

Kapleau, P. (1998). *The Zen of living and dying.* Boston: Shambhala Press.

Karp, D. (2001). *Burden of sympathy.* New York: Oxford Press.

Karrass, C. (1992). *How to get what you want: The negotiating game* (rev. ed.). New York: HarperCollins.

Keirsey, D., & Bates, M. (1984). *Please understand me: Character and temperament types.* Del Mar, CA: Prometheus Nemesis.

Levine, C. (Ed). (2000). *Always on call. When illness turns families into caregivers.* Edison, NJ: United Hospital Fund.

Lown, B. (1999). *The lost art of healing: Practicing compassion in medicine.* New York: Ballantine Books.

Mayer, B. S. (1995). Conflict resolution. In R. L. Edwards (Ed.), *Encyclopedia of social work* (19th ed., Vol. 1, pp. 613–622). Washington, DC: NASW Press.

McBride, J. (1996). *The color of water.* New York: Riverhead Books.

Nava, Y. (2000). *It's all in the frijoles.* New York: Simon & Schuster.

Osborne, H. (2000). *Overcoming communication barriers in patient education.* Gaithersburg, MD: Aspen.

Pruitt, G., & Rubin, J. Z. (1986). *Social conflict: Escalation, stalemate and settlement.* New York: Random House.

Renz, M. A., & Greg, J. B. (2000). *Effective small group communication in theory and practice.* Boston: Allyn and Bacon.

Schellenberg, J. (1996). *Conflict resolution theory, research, and practice.* Albany: State University of New York Press.

Shouse, D. (1996). *How to be a more effective group communicator.* Mission, KS: SkillPath.

Spector, R. E. (1996). *Cultural diversity in health and illness.* Stamford, CT: Appleton & Lange.

Spiro, H. M., Curnen, M. G. M., & Wandel, L. P. (Eds.). (1998). *Facing death: Where culture, religion, and medicine meet.* New Haven, CT: Yale University Press.

Stewart, J., & Logan, C. (1998). *Together, communicating interpersonally.* Boston: McGraw-Hill.

Tan, A. (1989). *The joy luck club.* New York: Raven Press.

Tan, A. (2001). *The bonesetter's daughter.* New York: Putnam.

Tannen, D. (1990). *You just don't understand: Women and men in conversation.* New York: Ballantine Books.

# Part II

# *Goal-Setting: Client–Professional Collaboration*

When illness or injury leads to disablement, financial, social, emotional, and other concerns can seriously impact each client's unique lifestyle and quality of life. Quality of life is a subjective concept that depends on each person's perception of wellness. Part II addresses the collaboration between the client and the health professional. Chapter 5 describes important considerations in the client–professional relationship, highlighting the fact that no two clients can be treated alike, even when they share the same illness or impairment. It discusses the role of ethical guidelines and their importance in establishing a client–provider relationship characterized by mutual trust and respect. Professional ethics are reviewed in both historical and clinical contexts to help illustrate contemporary challenges, as well as the importance of considering issues, such as self-determination, end-of-life concerns, and weighing any possible risks against the benefits of proposed interventions.

Chapter 6 presents important concepts related to motivation and adherence, such as locus of control, self-efficacy, self-esteem, and the role of social support systems. It stresses the importance of understanding and incorporating clients' perspectives when designing care plans in order to develop explicitly shared expectations for outcomes. This is a significant step toward empowering clients to become active in their own recovery.

Chapter 7 presents legislation and health care accreditation criteria that have been established to help safeguard important rights. Although these standards help ensure that clients are given the opportunity to participate in developing goals and plans for services, barriers to collaboration do exist. Therefore, strategies for overcoming these obstacles are also included in this section.

Successful collaboration requires sensitivity to all dimensions of the human experience, including the physical, psychological, and existential domains. Chapter 8 addresses the interdependence of the mind, body, and spirit. The science of psychoneuroimmunology is briefly reviewed because this area of study has provided important physiological explanations to help us understand these connections.

# 5

# *Client Rights and Provider Responsibilities*

I still can't get over the conversation I had with my client Paula today. Apparently, the orthopedic surgeon came by to discuss her surgery. What impressed her most was the amount of time that he spent with her. He perched himself on the edge of her bed, asked her about her concerns, and then actually listened and responded to them! First, she shared her fears about anesthesia and that the surgery might make things worse. She had expected him to be interested in that much. But then he asked her about her home life, what her duties would be upon discharge, and how she planned to deal with the fact that she would have to remain on bedrest for several days after the surgery. She felt that he really cared about her answers. He also took the time to draw a picture for her so that she would clearly understand just what would happen in the operating room. He assured her that everyone who touched her would be as gentle as possible. As if to prove his point, he gently touched her arm. Once she was fully comfortable with the explanation, he continued to chat for a few minutes longer, even getting her to laugh at a joke or two. Only then did he ask her to sign a consent form. She felt like she was this doctor's only patient.

—*From the journal of Antonella Molinari, nursing student*

This chapter describes the rights of clients and the responsibilities of providers in the health care relationship. The relationships that health care providers establish with their clients and their clients' significant others are among the most important factors that influence the success of treatment outcomes. Understanding clients as people, not just as illnesses, is imperative. Developing explicit trust, confidence, empathy, hope, and reduction of fear are critical to positive outcomes. As discussed in Chapter 2, effective communication builds a solid relationship between the client and care provider. This therapeutic relationship, with appropriate boundaries, is as important to the recovery process as selecting optimal interventions.

Developing an appropriate relationship within which to address the client's quality of life depends on the health care provider's ability to discern the type of relationship the client is seeking. This requires understanding the client's current and changing priorities and needs and adjusting the goals to facilitate progress toward recovery. As health care providers, we also bring our own attitudes, prejudices, cultures, histories, hurts, fears, and beliefs into relationships with our clients. A therapeutic relationship depends on our ability to set aside our personal issues in order to maintain a positive attitude and desire to meet the needs that are presented by the client.

Clients have important rights, such as the right to informed consent. The manner in which health care professionals honor these rights determines the tone of the relationship that develops between the client and the provider. Showing care and compassion, the physician described above not only satisfied his responsibility to honor this client's right to informed consent, but also established a wonderful relationship in the process. Why does this encounter seem so remarkable?

# The Health Care System

As illustrated in Figure 5–1, the health care system is a complex entity that is influenced by the community around it. Cultural and social values influence the nature of the community. This is evident in the fact that the health care system in the United States is like no other in the world. Our health care system is comprised of a variety of public and private organizations that employ individual health care providers from multiple health care professions who, in turn, offer services to clients.

The philosophy of our health care system has evolved from one dominated by paternalism to one currently dominated by bureaucracy. Siegler (1985) offers the framework in Figure 5–2 to discuss three major periods in medical history: the Age of Paternalism, the Age of Autonomy, and the Age of Bureaucracy.

## Age of Paternalism

This era was, by far, the longest in medical history, lasting thousands of years. It was rooted in the ethical principles of beneficence and nonmaleficence and emphasized healing rather than curing clients. Relationships between clients and providers were bonded in trust. Medical gains were modest during this era. However, this "traditional and relatively ineffective system of healing must have addressed and satisfied many basic human needs of patients [since it lasted] for millennia" (Siegler, 1985, p. 454).

Before 1850, few scientifically "proven" medical treatments existed. Medical care was primarily supportive, designed to keep the client as comfortable as possible. It depended on the placebo effect; that is, both client and provider believing treatments would be effective (Benson & Friedman, 1996). The physician's role was to identify and use all of the resources of the client, family, and community to bring about healing. Referral to other health care professionals was rare. The predominant legal and ethical principles that governed health care

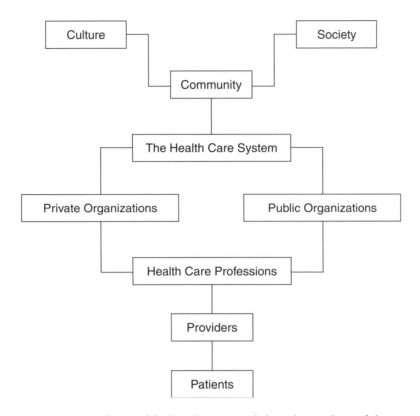

**FIGURE 5–1**    The Health Care System and the relationships of the entities Involved.

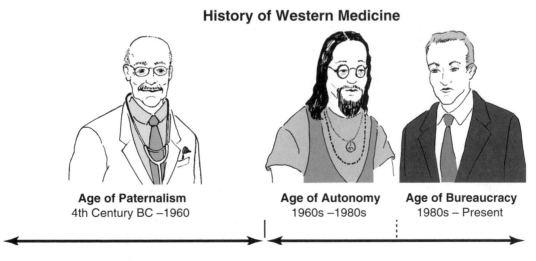

**FIGURE 5–2**    History of Western Medicine.

were essentially Judeo-Christian values. We had well-defined "God-given" rights that influenced all political, social, and legal concerns (Loewy, 1987).

In the late 1800s to early 1900s, the isolation of bacteria, and identification of the serious diseases they could cause, significantly changed medicine. The availability of vaccines meant that many serious illnesses could be prevented, and the discovery of penicillin brought new hope for cures (Benson & Friedman, 1996). Physicians began a transition from helpers to scientists. Unlike their clients, they understood the science of medicine and were held in the highest esteem by clients for the "miracles" they could perform. During this time, paternalism began to take on a negative connotation.

It was common for physicians to withhold information or treatment if they judged that it was in the "best interest" of the client. Most clients essentially did "whatever the doctor ordered" without question (Cassell, 2000). Although the ethical principles of beneficence and nonmaleficence still weighed most heavily in solutions of ethical questions, an uprising was brewing (Morris, 2000).

## Age of Autonomy

The civil rights movement of the 1960s gave way to postmodern philosophy and the Age of Autonomy (Bell, 1996). The philosophy of this time is perhaps best characterized by the phrase, "Whatever works for me," because everything was based on the needs and desires of the individual, with no generally accepted values. The "void of an outside, wholly objective, God's eye view of Truth" (Morris, 2000, p. 7) created the need to develop client rights to govern health care. The emphasis of these rights was to protect clients as consumers. The driving ethical principles shifted away from beneficence and nonmaleficence to autonomy with the overarching goal of creating a more equal relationship between the client and the provider. Ideally, this relationship would be based on mutual respect, mutual participation, and shared decision making. Clients would be provided with information to allow them to make their own decisions about care (Siegler, 2000).

This shift has significantly influenced client–provider relationships as health care continues to evolve. Although clients have become more equal in the health care relationship, malpractice lawsuits have become more common, highlighting the issue of "wronging clients." The waning ability to develop trust in the health care relationship has caused many providers to practice "defensive medicine" (Sulmasy, 1997). Complex regulatory codes and client rights laws have emerged, giving rise to the Age of Bureaucracy.

## Age of Bureaucracy

Prior generations understood health care to mean a visit to a physician or other health care professional and the administration of some form of intervention or prescription, followed by discharge from care. High technology diagnostics, replacement of organs, and other life-sustaining and extending measures did not exist. The cost of such care, therefore, was not what it is today (Loewy, 1987). The rapid advances in medicine have resulted in equally rapid increases in the cost of health care. However, the availability of new and costly interventions is only partly to blame for our current crisis. The shift from the Age of Paternalism to the Age of Autonomy was accompanied by "opinion shopping." Until the advent of managed care, clients who were not satisfied with the opinion of one health care professional could visit multiple care providers until they found the answers or services they were seeking.

Until the 1980s, health care professionals had little concern or training in cost containment—that was the job of health care administrators. To discuss matters of cost or insurance with clients was considered distasteful. Health care professionals, acting in ignorance, did nothing to contain the rapidly rising costs of health care. Naturally, cost containment grew out of "regulations" established by health care administrators, rather than the ethical criteria used to guide clinical practice. If we are to achieve a movement away from the detrimental effects of managed care, health care professionals must take responsibility for cost containment based on ethical principles. This requires honest communication with clients, who trust their care providers. When intervention is futile, and not expected to make any difference in clients' quality or quantity of life, it is the responsibility of health care providers to guide clients toward acceptance of reality (Helft, Siegler, & Lantos, 2000; Low & Kaufman, 1999).

During this Age of Bureaucracy, providers are now accountable to many entities aside from their clients, including hospitals, health maintenance organizations, insurance companies, and government agencies. We now must balance the welfare of clients against the interests of the health care system (Minogue, 2000). Decision making is no longer in the exclusive realm of the client–provider relationship. Efficiency and expediency, based primarily on concerns related to cost, have emerged as major forces in the provision of health care. The provider's obligation to honor the ethical principles of beneficence, nonmaleficence, self-determination, and justice has become a major challenge. Patients (now commonly referred to as clients or consumers) must have strong advocates or exceptional self-advocacy skills to receive acceptable levels of care.

Confidentiality, which has been a basic tenet of the client–provider relationship since the time of Hippocrates, is at great risk because of the volume of written data generated today. Information technology has been both a help and a hindrance in maintaining confidentiality of the medical record. Once a sacred document shared only by the client and physician, the medical record is now of interest to third parties, including payers, quality care assurance reviewers, and researchers. Yet, health care professionals are still solely responsible for maintaining the confidentiality of medical records. Any breach of this responsibility could seriously undermine trust and may invite litigation (Dierks, 1993).

This responsibility also applies to verbal information. Providers have the legal and ethical duty to share information only on a need-to-know basis. Other health care professionals involved in the client's care meet the need-to-know criteria, but family members, payers, and lawyers do not. Clients must explicitly give consent to share medical information. The only exceptions to this rule are legal mandates, such as subpoenas and mandated reporting. Health care professionals are mandated reporters, in some circumstances, which means that if they believe that the safety of clients or others is at risk, they must share otherwise-confidential information to obtain appropriate legal or medical assistance.

The first ever federal guidelines to protect confidentiality took effect on April 14, 2003. As part of the Health Insurance Portability and Accountability Act of 1996 (HIPAA), Congress charged the Department of Health and Human Services to establish guidelines to ensure client privacy. The regulations apply to covered entities, including health care providers, hospitals, and third party payers. HIPAA dictates appropriate use of clients' personal medical information for all forms of communication, including verbal, written, and electronic media.

Covered entities that misuse client information are subject to criminal and/or civil penalties (U.S. Department of Health and Human Services, 2003).

## Age of Justice

Many health care professionals believe that we are now moving toward a health care system based on distributive and rights-based justice (Cassell, 2000; Weber, 1993). Weber (1993) believes a common-good, community-based approach is needed in the interest of cost containment and as an appropriate balance for autonomy. Although self-determination is a "good" that deserves preservation, it should be balanced with other "goods." A justice-based model would emphasize clients as "citizens."

The argument in favor of a system based on justice is to provide everyone with equal access to basic care. On the surface, beneficence and nonmaleficence seem to be honored under such a system. However, treatment beyond the basic level, such as experimental medication, would be accommodated only if it would not undermine the ability to meet the basic health care needs of all. Although this approach may seem extreme, it already exists in the United States government subsidy programs of Medicare and Medicaid. These programs distribute health care benefits based primarily on demonstrated medical necessity, and nothing considered experimental or potentially futile is covered, except in rare instances when benefit for an individual client can be clearly demonstrated.

Opponents of a justice-based system worry about who will determine the value or futility of proposed treatments. Currently, health care payers understandably oppose costly treatments if they are of questionable benefit, but offer the option of filing an appeal to such decisions. It is still possible to secure coverage on a case-by-case basis if a strong and effective argument is made. Appeals of this nature require a significant amount of time, interest, and knowledge on the part of the health care provider, who must prepare and often present the argument. Bureaucrats, who are able to "decipher" the elements of successful appeals, employ professional consultants to counterargue on their behalf. Since professional consultants are paid for the time involved in preparing and presenting arguments and clinical practitioners are not, the payer has an unfair advantage in this system. Could a justice-based system resolve this problem?

Our society has had a disposition toward excessive individualism. It is widely recognized that we need greater emphasis on public health and preventive measures, as well as more opportunity for the public to help shape the health care system (Dougherty, 1997). Health care reform has been "the great debate" for nearly a decade now. The controversy lies in how to accomplish health care reform in a way that ensures equal access and coverage for all. It is clear that the employer-based system in place today is not effective. Employers cannot represent employees' health interests well because they have a conflict of interest. While they do have an interest in the health of their employees, they also have an interest in keeping health care insurance premiums as low as possible, in order to keep profits high. A second problem is that not all people are employed. The result is that people who are less advantaged become disenfranchised. As members of our community, they are entitled to receive care that compensates for their disadvantages (Angell, 2000; Dougherty, 1997).

Many believe that we can achieve a single payer, universal health care plan by extending Medicare to all ages. The insurance industry argues that this would simply lead to bigger government, more bureaucracy, and ineffective health care. Does the best solution lie in investor-owned managed care companies? Probably not. They have obligations to their investors as well as to their enrollees (employers). This is evident in the many ways that medical services are limited, while high profits are maintained. Once again, care of the client suffers. As the debate continues, the need is greater than ever. Health care costs and the number of people with inadequate or no insurance coverage continue to rise (Angell, 2000).

The insurance company wanted to discharge my client Mrs. Jeffrey today. She recently had a stroke. Even though she is able to transfer and use the toilet safely, she is still unable to feed herself or take care of her hygiene needs. How can an insurance company send someone home who is still so dependent? Fortunately, my supervisor has a lot of experience working with case managers. She was able to contact the insurance company, explain the client's needs, and negotiate for another week of inpatient care. It's really frightening to think that doing this kind of work will be essential when I become a licensed health care provider.
—*From the journal of Mary Beth Newton, occupational therapy student*

In today's health care system, we can become easily frustrated by the paperwork, bureaucracy, and need to advocate for clients. It helps to remain focused on our primary concern: what is best for the client. But this is not enough. As members of the health care system, we also have the responsibility to work toward changing our methods of service delivery. This requires keeping informed of pending legislation that affects health care, including changes in health care finance and insurance regulations. Besides expressing concern about our current system to our sympathetic colleagues, legislators, insurance executives, and others who affect the health care system must understand our perceptions of the problems. Power comes in numbers. Being actively involved in professional organizations, such as the American Medical Association, American Physical Therapy Association, American Occupational Therapy Association, American Nursing Association, National Social Work Association, and American Speech-Language-Hearing Association, is more effective than trying to accomplish this on our own. Clients should be encouraged to contact their legislators to share their own experiences and frustrations. Feedback from the "grassroots" level is important to ensure effective health care reform.

# Health and Quality of Life

The World Health Organization (2000a) defines health as a "state of complete physical, social, and mental well-being, and not merely the absence of disease or infirmity." This broad-based definition implies that health depends on a multitude of factors, ranging from physical abilities to social and personal resources (World Health Organization, 2000b). When illness or injury disrupts clients' lives, financial, social, emotional, and other resources may be significantly altered. Immediate concerns arise. Will I live or die? What will be my family's source of income? Who will care for my aging parent or young child? All of these concerns can seriously impact quality of life.

Quality of life is a subjective concept that depends primarily on how we perceive the world and ourselves in it. Our quality of life is good when we (and our significant others) are mentally, emotionally, and physically well, particularly if we feel understood and supported. Quality of life also depends on how fully our basic human needs are being met, and whether we have the opportunity to pursue and achieve goals that are important to us (Dennis, Williams, Giangreco, & Cloninger, 1993). Many events can interrupt this state of well-being, however. The onset of an illness or injury causing impairment of function is one example. When someone becomes ill or disabled, nothing is the same any more. All aspects of life are affected: physical, social, psychological, and spiritual. Quality of life is closely related to one's own perception of health (Cunningham, Burton, Hawes-Dawson, Kington, & Hays, 2000). Even in the presence of illness or injury, quality of life can be considered "good," depending on one's perception. Health-related quality of life specifically addresses the impact health has on the overall quality of life.

# Quality of Life Assessment

The assessment of quality of life involves evaluating a number of subjective concepts. Clients' personal needs, strengths, and talents contribute to form a unique experience. In addition, there are concerns related to specific illnesses or injuries. For example, there may be a need for technology to establish functional communication, environmental control, or mobility. Clients will have their own experiences of prejudice that may cause them to feel stereotyped or stigmatized. Fears, or perhaps realities, of being segregated and having a very limited social network will also affect health-related quality of life and general sense of well-being (Dennis et al., 1993).

It is important to recognize that quality of life is affected by cultural influences. As discussed in Chapter 3, values and beliefs that are expressed in customs, languages, and traditions are important concepts to consider. Our own cultural values influence our perception of what may be important to our clients, but we must remain cognizant of the fact that there is significant variation in values among groups, families, and individuals with different life experiences. Men and women, children and adults, people with disabilities and those without, are just a few examples of contrasting groups that experience life differently from each other (Dennis et al., 1993).

Quality of life is quite complex. It can only be discussed relative to each person's individual experience. Our sense of well-being is influenced by the passage of time, changes in our relationships, and changes in circumstances. Never is this experienced more than during a life-altering event, such as receiving a diagnosis of a serious illness.

There is no single definition of quality of life that can address what is important to everyone. The objective measures included in quality of life indices are certainly correlated with quality of life perceptions, but it is important to remember that quality of life is essentially a subjective concept. With this in mind, let us look at some of the quality of life indices that are being used in health care research to determine treatment outcomes.

Clients' perceptions are the best indicators of whether treatment goals have been reached. Therefore, quality of life indices are designed to measure clients' perceived sense of well-being. They provide objective measures of psychological, physical, and social functions that are important to the client (Jette & Downing, 1994). Keep in mind that these instruments provide an objective "snapshot" of quality of life; they do not reflect the subjective and fluid nature of it. These tools are primarily used for research and help us determine the effectiveness of generalized approaches to treatment. It is critical to establish evidence-based practice. However, these tools can be of some value in individualized treatment planning because they remind us to include comprehensive measures of health in our examinations and interventions.

The Medical Outcomes Study (MOS) Short Form, SF-36 (Ware & Sherbourne, 1992), and its subset version, SF-12 (Ware, Kosinski, & Keller, 1996), are among the most popular and useful quality of life indices. Many recent studies have utilized these instruments, helping to validate them across different populations (Damiano et al., 2000; Finkelstein, 2000; Holtzman, Caldwell, Walvatne, & Kane, 1999; Hultling et al., 2000; Jette & Downing, 1994; Sherbourne, Sturm, & Wells, 1999). These tools are norm-referenced and assess health-related quality of life. They include important factors related to physical, psychological, emotional, and social health. The longer survey (SF-36) is reportedly less acceptable to clients because of the time it takes to complete (Andresen, Fouts, Romeis, & Brownson, 1999).

The SF-36 and SF-12 are generic instruments designed to be relevant to quality of life for everyone. However, Cunningham and coworkers (2000) found that not all MOS items were particularly relevant to elderly African Americans. This group did not rate items, such as social isolation, physical function, and role limitations, as highly relevant. However, spirituality and weight-related health were of particular concern. This means that health-related quality of life instruments that do not measure spiritual health may not be particularly useful for this population. These instruments have a finite number of items. If the health concepts that are important to our clients are not included, a specific tool may be of limited use.

A number of disability-specific tools have been used in recent studies (Abetz, Jacoby, Baker, & McNulty 2000; Andresen et al., 1999; Damiano et al., 2000; Holtzman et al., 1999; Wilkinson et al., 2000). They were developed to evaluate changes in the specific characteristics of the disability for which they have been designed. These tools are generally used in conjunction with the generic quality of life instruments in order to capture the full range of variables being studied. As mentioned earlier, there is evidence that objective quality of life indices can be useful in treatment planning. The quality of life themes they measure offer significant value and should be included in some way in our client examinations and interventions. Interviewing the client and significant others to gather information about what is truly important to them is an essential step to developing goals that address all of the client's needs.

# Disablement

The term *disablement* envelops all of the events that impact health-related quality of life. Disablement is the process precipitated by the onset of illness or injury. The study of disablement and its impact on quality of life, survival, health status, and functional ability has been a priority for some time. The concept of disablement is far reaching and represents "the various impact(s) of chronic and acute conditions on the functioning of specific body systems, on basic human performance, and on people's functioning in necessary, usual, expected, and personally desired roles in society" (Verbrugge & Jette, 1994, p. 1).

One of the most significant problems in this area of study has been the use of conflicting terminology to represent disability-related concepts. Work to establish a comprehensive disablement model and associated terminology has yielded two major disablement schemas. It is critical to both research and clinical practice that all health care providers involved in the rehabilitation process speak the same "language." This will ensure that our written and verbal communication will be appropriately interpreted (Jette, 1994). The two major conceptual models found in the rehabilitation literature are discussed below.

## Disablement Models

### NAGI MODEL

The first comprehensive disablement model appeared in the literature in the 1960s. Developed by sociologist Saad Nagi, this model follows the disablement process from the onset of an active pathology (illness or injury), to impairment (anatomical, physiological, mental, or emotional dysfunction), to functional limitation (limitation in performance at a personal level), and finally, disability (limitation of performance in society) (Nagi, 1965). Consider John, who has a diagnosis of diabetes mellitus. The active pathology, diabetes, may progress to the level of impairment if circulation becomes so compromised that a lower extremity amputation is necessary. The amputation will then result in functional limitations. The most common is the inability to ambulate without assistive devices. Our society was not specifically designed to accommodate the needs of individuals with lower extremity amputations, so it is also likely that John will be disabled. This means that he will encounter barriers when trying to assume the role in society he enjoyed prior to the amputation.

The Nagi model has been modified since its inception. Pope and Tarlov (1991) introduced the concept of quality of life into the schema, a concept that has been most helpful and widely used. Quality of life refers to the total well-being of the client, including physical, psychological, social, cultural, and spiritual factors. Most importantly, quality of life is based on the clients' own values, expressed individually as their state of well-being.

Verbrugge and Jette (1994) have further expanded the Nagi model. Termed the "disablement process," this approach is appealing because it describes how acute and chronic conditions affect physical functions and how personal, social, or environmental factors influence disablement. This creates a conceptual model for linking bodily functions, social and environmental demands, and the available support systems.

Current disablement models often consider only three areas of function when measuring the effects of impairment: activities of daily living (ADLs), instrumental activities of daily living (IADLs), and paid employment. These concepts are critical factors in achieving physical independence and self-sufficiency. ADLs allow clients to take care of their personal needs. IADLs move the client further along the autonomy scale to include activities, such as housekeeping, managing money, and shopping, and employment provides the ultimate level of independence—financial self-sufficiency.

However, there is more to living a meaningful life than being able to manage these tasks. The disablement process model that was proposed by Verbrugge and Jette (1994) adds factors that are important for determining the client's satisfaction with life, such as hobbies, sports, and participation in religious activities. It also factors in external supports, such as personal care attendants and environmental adaptations, including access to home or office, as well as lifestyle and behavioral aspects, psychosocial attributes, and social connections.

Research has indicated that there is never a straight path from pathology to impairment, functional limitations, and disability (Hermann & Reese, 2001; Jette, 1994). Each client is unique, and multiple factors impact the ultimate effect of diseases and impairments. We need to look beyond the client's physical status and focus on the human side of health care: addressing the values of each client (Rothstein, 2001).

### INTERNATIONAL CLASSIFICATION

An alternative model was introduced in 1980 by the World Health Organization (1980). Known as the International Classification of Impairments, Disabilities, and Handicaps (ICIDH), this model is similar to the Nagi model in the first two concepts (active pathology and impairment) but significantly differs in the latter two concepts (functional limitation and disability). The ICIDH failed to make a distinction between limitation in social performance and the cause of limitation (Guccione, 1991; Jette, 1994; Nagi, 1991). In the ICIDH, the term "disability" described the inability to perform any activity in a "normal" manner, and "handicap" defined the social disadvantages that result from having a disability. The weak link between cause and effect in the ICIDH has made the Nagi model the preferred schema.

In May 2001, the World Health Assembly approved a new system of classification. Entitled the International Classification of Functioning, Disability, and Health (ICF), this classification system is structured around three broad components: body functions and structure; activities and participation; and additional information on severity and environmental factors (Centers for Disease Control, 2001). Now that the international system incorporates social factors, it may well become preferred over the Nagi model because of its international recognition.

## Variations in Response to Disablement

It is common to see different responses to disablement among clients who have acquired the same impairment. Responses depend on the physical, psychological, social, and spiritual concepts that make clients who they are. Immature coping strategies, pain, substance abuse, anger, manipulation, and noncompliance are among a number of difficult factors that can negatively impact progress toward recovery (Brown, King, Butow, Dunn, & Coates, 2000; Morrison, Ramsey, & Synder, 2000). In contrast, effective coping strategies, presence of social and emotional support, and limited family or financial worries can positively influence the recovery process.

The ability to cope with major life changes depends on one's ability to adapt. Several factors influence this. If the client has never experienced a challenge of this magnitude before, the onset of illness or injury can cause a temporary loss of adaptability. Consider the differences in adaptability between Carla and Mary. Both are in their 30s and have just been diagnosed with cancer. Carla has never encountered any adversity in her life. Her parents are still alive and well. She is happily married with two young, healthy children. In contrast, Mary experienced the death of both parents when she was a teenager, then survived the physical abuse by the uncle who took care of her after her parents' death. Assuming that she has "recovered successfully" from these two traumatic histories, and has developed effective coping strategies, Mary may be better able to adapt to the changes that are likely to occur over the next several months.

Age is also a factor. There is a significant decline in the ability to adapt and accept change with advancing age (Collins, 1999). Consider Martha Jones, a 78-year-old woman who frequently falls. Her most recent fall resulted in a fracture of her right hip. Her family is concerned about her ability to continue to live alone. They want her to sell her home of 57 years and move in with one of them. She's very angry and resentful. She believes that she has everything she needs in the house and doesn't need anybody's help. Surrounded by all that is familiar, she likes her comfortable and predictable daily routine and is unwilling to move.

Health care providers can help clients improve their ability to adapt through effective client education, psychological intervention, and spiritual support (Sawyer, 2000). Darrow, Speyer, Marcus, Ter Maat, and Krome (1998) report that education makes it easier for clients and their significant others to adapt to illness (or injury). Effective education, intervention, and support depends on careful identification of the various issues that have the potential to impact quality of life.

# The Client–Provider Relationship

A good relationship between a client and a health care provider depends on effective communication, mutual respect, and mutual trust. The client has a relatively dependent and vulnerable role in the relationship, placing the primary responsibility for the relationship's success on the provider. Clients do have the responsibility to communicate as honestly and effectively as possible and do what they can to promote mutual trust and respect, but the legal and ethical burden is always on the provider.

## Boundaries

There are significant differences between personal and professional relationships. Personal relationships are mutual in nature and serve the needs of all participants equally. There is a reciprocal give-and-take between the parties, with each expecting to give and receive support and attention.

Unlike family or friends, clients pay money to spend time with us. They are entitled to receive health care services, empathy, and compassion but should never feel the need to return the same. Developing and honoring professional boundaries works to ensure that the helping nature of the health care relationship stays directed toward the client.

It is the responsibility of the health professional to establish and maintain financial, emotional, and physical boundaries (Simon, 1992). Financial expectations should be clearly defined. If an insurance company is to be billed, the client must agree to this in advance. If the client is to provide a copayment at the time of the visit, this should be made clear, too.

At times, clients wish to express their gratitude by giving health care providers small gifts. Many employers have formal policies about employees accepting gifts, and these policies must be observed. It is generally felt to be ethical to accept small gifts, such as a batch of home-baked cookies, a box of candy, or flowers, but there are some gifts that are clearly inappropriate. These include money, gifts of a personal nature, such as clothing or jewelry, and expensive gifts, such as theater tickets. It is helpful to let clients know at the beginning of the relationship what these boundaries are. Some clinics post discreet signs or include this with other relevant information in brochures that are distributed to clients. This can help to prevent embarrassment or hurt feelings.

Touch is another important element in the healing relationship. Since touch is also an important element of personal relationships, it is critical that the touch we use in health care not be confused with personal touch. As highlighted in Chapter 3, comforting touch and other physical boundaries are culturally sensitive. It is important to acknowledge and respect the client's personal space and enter into this only when necessary, and then only with permission. This can be accomplished by asking questions, such as, "May I take a look at that shoulder now?" just prior to touching and moving the client's upper extremity.

Emotional boundaries are complex and difficult. Compassion must be felt for the client, which requires emotional involvement, but only to a certain point. The clinician must maintain enough emotional distance to preserve professional judgment and objectivity. It is important to avoid establishing friendships or romantic relationships with clients, because these relationships require an equal exchange of give-and-take. This is in direct conflict with maintaining the professional distance required in the health care relationship.

We must also be careful about disclosing personal information to clients. While we want to invite the client into a warm and engaging professional relationship, we should avoid a close and familiar personal relationship. An essential concept to remember is that the relationship is always for the benefit of the client, never for the provider. Before making decisions or taking any action, ask yourself, "What are the client's needs?" and "How will this help him (or her)?"

The medical examination involves taking a history, asking about personal and social circumstances, even about spiritual beliefs and values (see Chapter 8). When collecting this information, it is important to honor the client's right to privacy and do whatever possible to help preserve his or her dignity. Be certain that what is being asked is needed to establish or clarify treatment goals, rather than as a means to get to know the client on a personal basis. There is a fine line between maintaining a personal distance and achieving professional closeness (Purtilo, 1984). Clients generally seek a feeling of security in the health care relationship, which can be established only if there is mutual trust and respect, and the client's dignity is preserved.

## Preservation of Dignity

A client's dignity is threatened in the presence of illness or impairment because the self-image of the past may be inconsistent with the present one. The threat to dignity may be the primary source of the client's anxiety. By doing everything possible to preserve the client's dignity, the provider can minimize the client's anxiety (Purtilo, 1984). This can be as simple as observing common courtesies, such as apologizing to clients if they are hurt or offended by something we have said or done. Clients deserve to feel that they are genuinely respected. As outlined in Chapter 2, this is accomplished through effective communication, such as active listening, appropriate education, and answering questions with thoughtful answers.

The role of health care providers is to serve clients. This means that goals must be client-centered. Providers must plan treatments carefully, thinking critically about choices and reviewing any information about which they feel uncertain. An important goal of client interactions is to achieve mutual respect. Even when providers are personally offended or flustered, composure needs to be maintained, putting their own needs aside in favor of clients' needs (White, 1999).

## Trust, Respect, and Compassion

While we cannot always cure clients (eliminate health concerns), we can always facilitate healing (making whole). No matter how sophisticated the technology of health care becomes, healing relies on three simple human elements: compassion, touch, and conversation (Sulmasy, 1997). The physician described in the journal entry at the beginning of the chapter displayed each of these important elements. In doing so, he invited the patient to enter into a trusting relationship. Just because the invitation is extended, though, does not ensure that the client will accept it. Trust does not come easily in today's health care environment. By definition, trust involves risk and uncertainty, which can create anxiety (Sulmasy, 1997). Some people will do almost anything to avoid this.

Consider the case of Rob Jones, a 42-year-old lawyer, who sought medical care for frequent headaches. He had avoided seeing a doctor, assuming his headaches were stress-related and that nothing could be done. However, he became frightened when a relative, who was about his age, experienced a serious stroke and died. Although his doctor had little reason to believe that Rob was at risk for a stroke, the client demanded a magnetic resonance imaging (MRI) to avoid the anxiety of uncertainty. Because of his own need to avoid uncertainty and risk, the physician agreed. He feared that a malpractice lawsuit would be likely if it turned out that his judgment was in error. As expected, the MRI was negative, and so was the nature of the relationship between this client and provider.

There are many barriers to developing a trusting health care relationship. One barrier is that many clients feel rushed during medical encounters. The ability to understand and absorb information can be seriously hampered by this, especially when coupled with the stress that clients report when discussing matters of failing health.

Specialization of care creates another barrier (Dougherty, 1990). Clients frequently have multiple health professionals involved in their care. Unfortunately, conflicting information is not uncommon, and the client is left to sort it out. This can be a challenge, even for a bright, attentive, and assertive client.

The involvement of third-party payers is another barrier to developing trust. Trust between clients and health care professionals can be affected by clients' knowledge that other people will view their medical records. As a result, they may be reluctant to share certain information, such as drug or alcohol problems, abuse, sexual function, or incontinence.

Growing commercialism in medicine is another source of mistrust. Commercial advertising, for-profit ownership of hospitals, and other commercial aspects of health care have led to a perception of decreasing professionalism. Medicine, as a commercial enterprise, relegates clients to the role of consumers, who are empowered by lawsuits when they fail to get their "money's worth" (Dougherty, 1990).

As a client and practitioner get to know each other, a sense of security, trust, and respect will either grow or diminish. An effective practitioner does whatever he or she is able to establish a relationship based on these virtues, but it is not always possible. Whenever a provider does not feel compassion for a particular client, or believes that he or she cannot trust a client, then that provider has a responsibility to refer the client elsewhere for care.

Renate Justin, a Jewish physician, reported an experience influenced by prejudice and strong emotional overtones. A patient was referred to her because she spoke German. Unaware that her new physician was Jewish, the patient spoke freely during her initial visit, revealing that she was involved in the Nazi party and had been assigned to supervise Jewish slave labor during World War II. Her story was riddled with slanderous remarks about the Jewish slaves under her watch. Dr. Justin was able to contain her emotional response in the presence of the patient. After serious personal deliberation and soul-searching, she decided that, although she felt capable of providing basic medical care to this patient, she also had a duty to let the patient know that she was Jewish. She experienced significant relief when the patient opted to change providers (Justin, 2000).

A discussion about the client's values is essential to help the provider determine if there seems to be compatibility concerning many of the important issues that arise in health care. Opinions related to the sanctity of human life are of particular importance when counseling clients at the end of life. If conflicting views exist, it may not be possible to develop a relationship based on trust, respect, and compassion.

Dr. Justin, the physician mentioned in the above story, believed that she could feel compassion for her patient because of her medical illness but doubted that she could establish trust and respect for the patient. In spite of this, she believed that it would be possible to treat the patient (Justin, 2000). Health care professionals have a duty to put the client's needs first and to examine ethical conflicts from the client's point of view.

## Advocacy

Providers are always obligated to place clients' interests above their own. This includes avoiding conflicts of interest, such as owning stock in drug companies, health maintenance organizations, and medical equipment companies. Providers are frequently called upon to advocate for their clients, particularly when third-party payers have denied health care benefits. In the best interest of clients, providers should remain free from conflicts of interest to ensure availability to act as advocates whenever and wherever required.

# Provider Responsibilities

The Hippocratic Oath (Figure 5–3), long accepted as the "fundamental expression of medical ethics," extends to all health care professionals who work together with physicians to bring about benefit to the client (Bulger & Barbato, 2000, p. S7). There have been many modifications to this original oath. In fact, physicians have a choice about which oath they take today.

Bulger and Barbato (2000) note that taking any oath is an act of commitment. Many of the ideals expressed in the Hippocratic Oath still apply today. These include the commitment to remain competent, based on continued learning, caring for clients in a way that always seeks what is best for clients, respecting and keeping clients' personal information confidential, and avoiding any behavior that takes advantage of the clients' dependence and vulnerability. Because of a significant increase in diagnostic and treatment options, we now also have the obligation to provide care in a way that reflects responsible utilization of services in the interest of all clients and the health care system (Minogue, 2000).

"I will look upon him who shall have taught me this art even as one of my parents. I will share my substance with him, and will supply his necessities, if he be in need. I will regard his offspring even as my own brethren, and I will teach them this art, if they would learn it, without fee or covenant. I will impart this art by precept, by lecture, and by every mode of teaching, not only to my own sons but to sons of him who has taught me, and to disciples bound by covenant and oath, according to the law of medicine.

The regimen I adopt shall be for the benefit of my patients according to my ability and judgment, and not for their hurt or for any wrong. I will give no deadly drug to any, though it be asked of me, nor will I counsel such, and especially will I not aid a woman to procure abortion. Whatsoever house I enter, there will I go for the benefit of the sick, refraining from all wrongdoing or corruption, and especially from an act of seduction of male or female, of bond or free. Whatsoever things I see or hear concerning the life of men, in my attendance upon the sick or even apart therefrom, which ought not to be noised abroad, I will keep silence thereon, counting such things to be as sacred secrets."

FIGURE 5–3　The Original Hippocratic Oath.　*(Bulger & Barbato, 2000, p. S6).*

Providers' responsibilities to both clients and the health care system are often divergent, causing daily ethical dilemmas in health care. A dilemma is conflict that requires careful consideration of all possible solutions to identify the one that balances the interests of all involved. The guidelines for solving health care dilemmas lie in the legal and ethical parameters defined specifically for each health care profession. The first determination is always to ensure that the proposed solutions are legal. If not, they are immediately ruled out. If they are legal, ethical principles are then applied to ensure that the interests of all parties are observed and balanced.

## Legal and Ethical Guidelines

Client rights stem from federal, state, and local laws, case law, and contemporary values. Federal legislation governs the "big picture," known as the health care system, guiding the practices of insurance companies, health maintenance organizations, and government subsidies, including Medicare. Each state then governs the activities of its own hospitals, Medicaid programs, and the medical professionals who practice within its borders. The professional practice acts, established within each state, outline the guidelines that medical practitioners must agree to follow to become and remain licensed. Case law provides an historical collection of legal decisions that help to interpret medical questions that are brought to the courts.

Ethics complement and balance legal guidelines. Ethics are a set of moral principles that serve as a guiding philosophy for behavior. Most professional practice acts adopt the related profession's Code of Ethics within their legal guidelines. However, medical ethics can also be examined by using general approaches that offer culturally neutral frameworks and provide a common, basic language.

Beauchamp and Childress (1989) discuss an approach that relies on the four basic ethical principles of autonomy, beneficence, nonmaleficence, and justice. Others endorse this model (Darr, 1997; Gillon, 1994; Nosse, Friberg, & Kovacek, 1999). This is a simple system that involves examining all possible solutions to an ethical dilemma with respect to these ethical principles in order to identify the one best solution that balances the interests of everyone involved in the dilemma.

In the case described above, Rob insisted on having a MRI to rule out the risk of a stroke. The physician might have chosen another route if he had employed this approach to solving his dilemma. In the interest of autonomy, clients have the right to request any diagnostic or treatment option that they believe might be helpful. Rob felt that the MRI was needed to rule out the possibility of stroke and to reduce his stress. Beneficence requires health care practitioners to do whatever is in the best interest of their clients. Because the MRI would probably reduce the client's stress and rule out certain differential diagnoses, it could be considered to be in Rob's best interest. Nonmaleficence requires the provider to do no harm. The known risks of MRI are minimal and, therefore, probably not an issue. Justice, however, was not upheld in this case. Justice requires that resources be distributed responsibly. The physician in this case did not honor this ethical principle. By choosing lower cost diagnostics prior to proceeding with a more expensive test, he may have been able to honor all four ethical principles.

## AUTONOMY

Autonomy, or self-determination, demands a client–provider relationship based on trust, respect, truthfulness, information sharing, and confidentiality. The right to informed consent is rooted in this principle. Most clients exercise their right to autonomy by requesting full disclosure of their medical condition and options for treatment. However, others prefer to leave the decision making to the provider. Either option is an appropriate expression of autonomy and must be honored.

The legal doctrine of informed consent stems from the right to self-determination; that is, adults who are of sound mind have the right to make their own decisions about proposed medical care. While verbal consent may have been enough in the early days of this mandate, written consent in clients' records is required for legal protection today. Several issues must be addressed in the process: (1) Clients must be informed in a language that they can understand (lay terms and in their primary language); (2) all risks and benefits must be outlined; (3) any and all reasonable alternatives must be discussed; and (4) clients must sign a statement that indicates their understanding and acceptance of the treatment. This right can be waived in certain emergency situations or if treatment is legally mandated (Yale-New Haven Hospital and Yale University School of Medicine, 2000).

Clients faced with death have a heightened need and legal right to self-determination. Any ethical dilemmas in end-of-life care must be based on clients' own beliefs and values. The role of health care providers is to support clients, offering palliative care and the relief of suffering, enhancement of autonomy and individual sense of control, and assistance in achieving spiritual comfort during the process of dying (Carney & Meier, 2000; Jennings, 1997). Health care providers must exercise caution when acting as advocates to clients near the end of life. There is a fine line between advocacy and paternalism when clients are this vulnerable (Gadow, 1980).

The availability of experimental therapies, life-sustaining technologies, and active life-ending options (euthanasia) has complicated end-of-life decisions. If experimental therapies seem appropriate, informed consent, with accurate information and documentation regarding known risks and possible benefits, must be clearly presented to the client for consideration. Regarding termination of life-sustaining treatment, health care providers are obligated to comply with client wishes, even if this hastens death (Emanuel, 1996).

Technological mechanisms, developed in the interest of organ transplantation, are capable of indefinitely sustaining the function of many body systems. This has complicated the legal definition of death and caused dilemmas for families and health care practitioners alike (Smith, 1990). Advanced directives and legislative efforts to define "legal death" are intended to clarify the issues involved, but uncertainty over the withdrawal of life-sustaining treatment still occurs. Many hospitals today employ clinical ethicists to review cases marked by ethical uncertainty to help in making "right and good decisions in individual cases" (Siegler, 2000, p. S19). The emotional toll on family members and health care providers involved in such cases can be overwhelming.

Advanced directives allow competent adults to express their wishes regarding life-sustaining treatment should they become unable to make such decisions later. These directives seek to realize the basic values of human dignity, respect for self-determination, and the right to refuse treatment. Common directives include the living will and the durable power of attorney. The living will provides an opportunity to outline specific wishes regarding life-sustaining measures. The durable power of attorney names a successor to make these decisions, if the client becomes unable to do so (Hamel, 1988).

Although advanced directives may protect a client's right to self-determination, any ambiguity in the language may complicate decisions made on behalf of the client. Consider Caitlin, an infant who was born with anencephaly, rendering her prognosis for survival limited. Her parents directed the hospital staff to provide only palliative treatment. Over the weekend, Caitlin developed an apparently painful ear infection. This presented a clinical dilemma. The staff agonized over the decision to order antibiotics, wondering whether this would violate the parents' wishes. Ultimately, they administered the medication.

Nurses involved in critical care are often faced with moral dilemmas regarding resuscitation and withdrawal of treatment (Wurzbach, 1990). This is particularly true in the absence or ambiguity of advanced directives (Jones, 1994). If the decision is made to provide life-sustaining treatment, such as mechanical ventilation, the family and health care team may later be faced with the dilemma of whether to continue or discontinue use in the absence of improvement.

Euthanasia is a particularly controversial topic. While some people believe that it is simply a matter of clients exercising their right to autonomy by hastening death and "dying with dignity," others consider it to be an act of suicide and believe it is morally and legally wrong. Euthanasia could be viewed as the ultimate example of avoiding risk and uncertainty. Clients who are near death seek relief of symptoms that could include pain, depression, fear, and anxiety, especially if they expect their condition will only worsen. Most people would not voluntarily choose to experience pain and adversity, but numerous personal accounts support the idea that adversity can be a positive experience, even at the end of life (Bauby, 1997; Coughlin, 1993; Galli, 2000).

If euthanasia becomes a right, how long will it take to become an obligation in the interest of justice and cost containment? Will people who are elderly or catastrophically disabled feel obligated to make this choice to avoid being a burden on their families? We will see that under the principles of beneficence and nonmaleficence, every person deserves to feel loved, welcomed, and protected. Each is entitled to end-of-life care, not expedient elimination.

To date, Oregon is the only state in the United States that recognizes physician-assisted suicide as a legal option. However, the Assisted Suicide Consensus Panel of the Finding Common Ground Project, at the University of Pennsylvania Center for Bioethics, reported that other states will likely follow Oregon's lead unless negative issues arise (Tulsky, Ciampa, & Rosen, 2000). Physicians probably will not be ethically bound to provide this intervention if it is in direct contrast to their own beliefs and values (Emanuel, 1996). However, there is always an ethical obligation to provide information in a value-neutral manner. If client and provider beliefs are incongruent, the client should be referred elsewhere. The provider's ethical obligation to avoid either emotional or physical abandonment, when values are conflicting, is of utmost importance (Tulsky et al., 2000).

## BENEFICENCE AND NONMALEFICENCE

Medicine is a form of humanitarianism. Its purpose is to help clients through benevolence and concern (Bell, 1996). The motivation for most people who choose a medical career is the simple desire to help others. However, scientific and technological advances sometimes cloud our vision. What is "helpful" may not always be immediately obvious.

The ethical principle of beneficence requires providers to "do good" or "provide benefit," while nonmaleficence means to "do no harm." These two principles should be considered simultaneously because there is always a risk of harm when doing something to help a client (Gillon, 1994). When harm is unavoidable, everything possible should be done to minimize it. The benefit(s) must clearly outweigh the risk(s) of harm. Consider the benefits and potential risks involved in immunization. The potential benefit, immunization against infectious disease, probably outweighs the risk of pain from the injection and possible side effects, such as mild flu-like symptoms.

To honor beneficence and nonmaleficence, we must also honor autonomy, because clients' perceptions of benefit will vary. Consider Joan and Marie. Both required radical mastectomy for breast cancer. In Joan's opinion, the potential benefit of eliminating cancer overwhelmingly outweighed the harm of disfigurement. Conversely, benefit would outweigh harm for Marie only if she could receive reconstructive surgery at the same time as the mastectomy.

## JUSTICE

Justice or "fairness" requires that distribution of resources be done according to need, merit, and valid claims. This is the ethical obligation to "act on the basis of fair adjudication between competing claims" (Gillon, 1994, p. 185).

Three types of justice are involved in health care. Rights-based justice applies to the obligation providers have to respect client rights. As mentioned above, these rights stem from legal, as well as ethical, principles. Legal justice requires providers to honor morally acceptable laws. This means that licensed clinicians must observe all legal guidelines for practice, with the exception of laws that entitle clients to services that are morally objectionable to the provider. The most obvious examples are abortion and euthanasia. Clinicians have no legal obligation to provide these services if the services are in conflict with their own personal values, but, as indicated above, they do have an ethical obligation to assist the client in finding an appropriate alternative provider.

Distributive justice refers to the distribution of scarce resources. No nation can afford to provide *all* health care options to *all* citizens, so a fair and equitable formula for distribution is needed (Cassell, 2000). Simple equality is not the answer. From the time of Aristotle, it has been argued that "equals" should be treated "equally" and "unequals" should be treated proportionally "unequally" (Gillon, 1994). This means that society has a responsibility to provide care for the poor, less educated, and those racial or ethnic minorities who may bear disproportional burdens of morbidity and mortality (Dougherty, 1997). While medical professionals and politicians agree on this concept in health care, a solution has yet to be identified within the complex American health care system.

## SUMMARY

This chapter addressed client rights and provider responsibilities. A brief historical overview was provided, following the evolution of the health care system from the Age of Paternalism to the Age of Autonomy and finally to the Age of Bureaucracy. The Age of Justice is proposed as the age of the future. Legal and ethical principles that guide provider responsibilities were outlined, and contemporary medical concerns were discussed within a quality-of-life framework.

## REFLECTIVE QUESTIONS

1. Consider the journal entry at the beginning of this chapter. What makes this encounter seem so remarkable?
2. Think about a health care provider with whom you have a good relationship.
   a. What makes the relationship a good one?
   b. What does he or she do that demonstrates compassion?
   c. What does he or she do to earn your trust and respect?
   d. How does he or she encourage effective communication?
3. Boundaries are relative to the situation. Consider the following:
   • Receiving a gift
   • Disclosing personal information
   • Physical contact
   a. Contrast the boundaries that exist for each of these situations with respect to a personal relationship and professional relationship.
   b. Explain what circumstances would help you decide whether a boundary has been crossed in a professional relationship.
4. At times, clients cross the boundaries we have established. Without embarrassing the client, how could you reestablish boundaries in the following situations:
   a. A client asks you on a date
   b. A client gives you an expensive gift
   c. A client makes an offensive remark
   d. A client asks you a personal question
   e. A client touches you inappropriately
5. A client reveals to you that he or she is taking nonprescription medications. You suspect these medications are interfering with his or her medical condition. Considering the issue of confidentiality, could you share this information with others?
   a. If so, whom could you tell? Why?
   b. If not, why not?

# CASE STUDY

Your patient, Mary Cunningham, has a diagnosis of multiple sclerosis. In the time that you have been treating her, Mrs. Cunningham has experienced two exacerbations that have resulted in marked losses in function. She is in the midst of a remission at this time, but, given the typical course of progression of her illness, you believe that her condition is likely to deteriorate quickly if you withdraw skilled treatment. You realize that Mrs. Cunningham's insurance company will only pay for treatment as long as progress is being documented. You also know that Mrs. Cunningham is unable to pay privately for the cost of your services. At this time, the only "progress" you observe is that Mrs. Cunningham's condition is not getting any worse. You fear that your request to continue treatment is likely to be denied for lack of documented progress. Consider the ethical principles of autonomy, beneficence, nonmaleficence, and justice in the following exercises:

1. Discuss each of the four ethical principles relative to Mrs. Cunningham's case. Consider all stakeholders.
2. What is the best possible response, considering the specific issues involved in Mrs. Cunningham's case?
3. What factors contributed to your decision?
4. How will you express your decision to Mrs. Cunningham and to her insurance company?

# REFERENCES

Abetz, L., Jacoby, A., Baker, G. A., & McNulty, P. (2000). Patient-based assessments of quality of life in newly diagnosed epilepsy patients: Validation of the NEWQOL. *Epilepsia, 41*(9), 1119–1128.

Andresen, E. M., Fouts, B. S., Romeis, J. C., & Brownson, C. A. (1999). Performance of health-related quality-of-life instruments in a spinal cord-injured population. *Archives of Physical Medicine and Rehabilitation, 80*(8), 877–884.

Angell, M. (2000). Patients' rights bills and other futile gestures. *New England Journal of Medicine, 342*(22), 1663–1664.

Bauby, J. D. (1997). *The diving bell and the butterfly.* New York: Vintage.

Beauchamp, T. L., & Childress, J. F. (1989). *Principles of biomedical ethics* (3rd ed.). New York: Oxford University Press.

Bell, N. K. (1996). Responsibilities and rights in the promotion of health: Differing positions of the individual and the state. *Social Science and Medicine, 43*(5), 775–782.

Benson, H., & Friedman, R. (1996). Harnessing the power of the placebo effect and renaming it "remembered wellness." *Annual Review of Medicine, 47,* 193–199.

Brown, J. E., King, M. T., Butow, P. N., Dunn, S. M., & Coates, A. S. (2000). Patterns over time in quality of life, coping and psychological adjustment in late stage melanoma patients: An application of multilevel models. *Quality of Life Research, 9*(1), 75–85.

Bulger, R. J., & Barbato, A. L. (2000). On the Hippocratic sources of western medical practice. *Hastings Center Report, 30*(4), S4–S7.

Carney, M. T., & Meier, D. E. (2000). Palliative care and end-of-life issues. *Anesthesiology Clinics of North America, 18*(1), 183–209.

Cassell, E. J. (2000). The principles of the Belmont Report revisited: How have respect for persons, beneficence and justice been applied to clinical medicine? *Hastings Center Report, 30*(4), 12–21.

Centers for Disease Control. (2001). International classification of functioning, disability, and health (ICF). In *Classification of diseases, functioning, and disability* (10th rev.) [Online]. Available: http://www.cdc.gov/nchs/about/otheract/icd9/icfhome.htm. Date accessed: 6/6/05.

Collins, K. J. (1999). Physiological variation and adaptability in human populations. *Annals of Human Biology, 26*(1), 19–38.

Coughlin, R. (1993). *Grieving: A love story.* New York: Random House.

Cunningham, W. E., Burton, T. M., Hawes-Dawson, J., Kington, R. S., & Hays, R. D. (2000). Use of relevancy ratings by target respondents to develop health-related quality of life measures: An example with African-American elderly. *Quality of Life Research, 8,* 749–768.

Damiano, A. M., McGrath, M. M., Willain, M. K., Snyder, C. F., LeWitt, P. A., Reyes, P. F., Richter, R. R., & Means, E. D. (2000). Evaluation of a measurement strategy for Parkinson's disease: Assessing patient health-related quality of life. *Quality of Life Research, 9*(1), 87–100.

Darr, K. J. (1997). *Ethics in health services management* (3rd ed.). Baltimore: Health Professions Press.

Darrow, S. L., Speyer, J., Marcus, A. C., Ter Maat, J., & Krome, D. (1998). Coping with cancer: The impact of the Cancer Information Service on patients and significant others. *Journal of Health Communication, 3*(Suppl. Pt. 6), 86–96.

Dennis, R., E., Williams, W., Giangreco, M. F., & Cloninger, C. J. (1993). Quality of life as context for planning and evaluation of services for people with disabilities. *Exceptional Children, 59*(6), 499–512.

Dierks, C. (1993). Medical confidentiality and data protection as influenced by modern technology. *Medicine and Law, 12*(6–8), 547–551.

Dougherty, C. J. (1990). The costs of commercial medicine. *Theoretical Medicine, 11*(4), 275–286.

Dougherty, C. J. (1997). How to avoid flying blind: To truly improve U.S. healthcare, leaders must consider seven moral values. *Health Progress, 78*(2), 20–22.

Emanuel, E. J. (1996). Pain and symptom control: Patient rights and physician responsibilities. *Hematology/Oncology Clinics of North America, 10*(1), 41–56.

Finkelstein, M. M. (2000). Body mass index and quality of life in a survey of primary care patients. *Journal of Family Practice, 49*(8), 734–737.

Gadow, S. (1980). Caring for the dying: Advocacy or paternalism. *Death Education, 3*(4), 387–398.

Galli, R. (2000). *Rescuing Jeffrey.* Chapel Hill, NC: Algonquin Books.

Gillon, R. (1994). Medical ethics: Four principles plus attention to scope. *British Medical Journal, 309*(6948), 184–188.

Guccione, A. A. (1991). Physical therapy diagnosis and the relationship between impairment and function. *Physical Therapy, 71,* 499–504.

Hamel, R. P. (1988). Advanced directives compatible with Catholic moral principles. *Health Progress, 6*(3), 36–40, 88.

Helft, P. R., Siegler, M., & Lantos, J. (2000). The rise and fall of the futility movement. *New England Journal of Medicine, 343,* 293–296.

Hermann, K. M., & Reese, C. S. (2001). Relationships among selected measures of impairment, functional limitation, and disability in patients with cervical spine disorders. *Physical Therapy, 81*(3), 903–914.

Holtzman, J., Caldwell, M., Walvatne, C., & Kane, R. (1999). Long-term functional status and quality of life after lower extremity revascularization. *Journal of Vascular Surgery, 29*(3), 395–402.

Hultling, C., Giuliano, F., Quirk, F., Pena, B., Mishra, A., & Smith, M. D. (2000). Quality of life in patients with spinal cord injury receiving Viagra (sildenafil citrate) for the treatment of erectile dysfunction. *Spinal Cord, 38*(6), 363–370.

Jennings, B. (1997). Individual rights and the human good in hospice. *Hospice Journal, 12*(2), 1–7.

Jette, A. M. (1994). Physical disablement concepts for physical therapy research and practice. *Physical Therapy, 74*(5), 380–386.

Jette, D. U., & Downing, J. (1994). Health status of individuals entering a cardiac rehabilitation program as measured by the Medical Outcomes Study 36-Item Short-Form Survey (SF-36). *Physical Therapy, 74*(6), 521–527.

Jones, L. C. (1994). A right to die? *Intensive Critical Care Nursing, 10*(4), 278–288.

Justin, R. G. (2000). Can a physician always be compassionate? *Hastings Center Report, 30*(4), 26–27.

Loewy, E. H. (1987). Communities, obligations and health-care. *Social Science Medicine, 25*(7), 783–791.

Low, L. L., & Kaufman, L. J. (1999). Medical futility and the critically ill patient. *Hawaii Medical Journal, 58*(3), 58–62.

Minogue, B. (2000). The two fundamental duties of the physician. *Academic Medicine, 75*(5), 431–442.

Morris, D. B. (2000). How to speak postmodern: Medicine, illness, and cultural change. *Hastings Center Report, 30*(6), 7–16.

Morrison, E. F., Ramsey, A., & Synder, B. A. (2000). Managing the care of complex, difficult patients in the medical-surgical setting. *Medsurg Nursing, 9*(1), 21–26.

Nagi, S. (1965). Some conceptual issues in disability and rehabilitation. In M. Sussman (Ed.), *Sociology and rehabilitation* (pp. 100–113). Washington, DC: American Sociological Association.

Nagi, S. (1991). Disability concepts revisited: Implication for prevention. In A. Pope & A. Tarlov (Eds.), *Disability in America: Toward a national agenda for prevention* (pp. 309–327). Washington, DC: National Academy Press.

Nosse, L. J., Friberg, D. G., & Kovacek, P. R. (1999). *Managerial and supervisory principles for physical therapists.* Baltimore: Williams & Wilkins.

Pope, A., & Tarlov, A. (Eds.). (1991). *Disability in America: Toward a national agenda for prevention.* Washington, DC: National Academy Press.

Purtilo, R. (1984). *Health professional/patient interaction.* Philadelphia: W. B. Saunders.

Rothstein, J. M. (2001). Impairments: Always linked to meaningful disability? *Physical Therapy, 81*(3), 886–887.

Sawyer, H. (2000). Meeting the information needs of cancer patients. *Professional Nurse, 15*(4), 244–247.

Sherbourne, C. D., Sturm, R., & Wells, K. B. (1999). What outcomes matter to patients? *Journal of General Internal Medicine, 14*(6), 357–363.

Siegler, M. A. (1985). Who should decide? Paternalism in healthcare by James F. Childress. *Perspectives in Biology and Medicine, 28*(3), 453–456.

Siegler, M. A. (2000). Professional values in modern clinical practice. *Hastings Center Report, 30*(4), S19–S22.

Simon, R. I. (1992). Treatment boundary violations: Clinical, ethical, and legal considerations. *Bulletin of the American Academy of Psychiatry and Law, 20*(3), 269–288.

Smith, G. P., Jr. (1990). Recognizing personhood and the right to die with dignity. *Journal of Palliative Care, 6*(2), 24–32.

Sulmasy, D. P. (1997). *The healer's calling.* Mahwah, NJ: Paulist Press.

Tulsky, J. A., Ciampa, R., & Rosen, E. J. (2000). Responding to legal requests for physician-assisted suicide. *Annals of Internal Medicine, 132*(6), 494–499.

U.S. Department of Health and Human Services. (2003). *Fact sheet: Protecting the privacy of patients' health information.* Washington, DC: United States Department of Health and Human Services. [Online]. Available: http://www.hhs.gov/facts/privacy.html

Verbrugge, L. M., & Jette, A. M. (1994). The disablement process. *Social Science and Medicine, 38,* 1–14.

Ware, J. E., Kosinski, M., & Keller, S. D. (1996). A 12-item short-form health survey: Construction of scales and preliminary tests of reliability and validity. *Medical Care, 34*(3), 220–233.

Ware, J. E., & Sherbourne, C. D. (1992). The MOS 36-Item Short Form health survey (SF-36): I. Conceptual framework and item selection. *Medical Care, 30*(6), 473–483.

Weber L. J. (1993). The patient as citizen: A common-good approach to medical treatment decisions balances the emphasis on patient desires. *Health Progress, 74*(5), 12–15.

White, A. A., III. (1999). Compassionate patient care and personal survival in orthopaedics: A 35-year perspective. *Clinical Orthopaedics and Related Research, 361*, 250–260.

Wilkinson, G., Hesdon, B., Wild, D., Cookson, R., Farina, C., Sharma, V., Fitzpatrick, R., & Jenkinson, C. (2000). Self-report quality of life measure for people with schizophrenia: The SQLS. *British Journal of Psychiatry, 177*, 42–46.

World Health Organization. (1980). *International classification of impairments, disabilities, and handicaps.* Geneva, Switzerland: Author.

World Health Organization. (2000a). About WHO: Definition of health. In *World Health Organization.* [Online]. Available: http://www.who.int/aboutwho/en/definition.html

World Health Organization. (2000b). *The world health report 2000. Health systems: Improving performance.* Geneva, Switzerland: Author.

Wurzbach, M. E. (1990). The dilemma of withholding or withdrawing nutrition. *Image: The Journal of Nursing Scholarship, 22*(4), 226–230.

Yale-New Haven Hospital and Yale University School of Medicine. (2000). Patient's rights. In *Risk management handbook* [Online]. Available: http://info.med.yale.edu/caim/risk/patient_rights/patient_rights_2.html

# <u>6</u>

# *Motivation and Adherence*

I'm finding that when I begin each treatment by asking the clients how things are going and how they're handling everything, I see an enormous improvement in therapy results.

Just today, I encouraged Mr. Jorgensen to "go the extra mile." Because I was fully attentive and listened with my whole heart and soul, I was able to understand his psychosocial needs and found the words to encourage him to persevere. Although he was reluctant to ambulate further because of his pain, he responded to me and doubled the distance that he walked.

*—From the journal of Denise Motley, nursing student*

Most clients are highly motivated to get well. However, many of us have had the experience of working with clients who feel sorry for themselves, feel the world is against them, and want to spend the rest of their lives moping around or staying in bed. In addition, some clients are unwilling to make changes. Why do clients with the same diagnosis, age, gender, and socioeconomic status act so differently? Ideally, motivation is a two-part phenomenon. The client first has to possess a desire to achieve a goal and then commit to an action to accomplish that goal. This chapter discusses the theoretical concepts that influence client motivation and adherence and suggests strategies that health care practitioners can use to motivate them.

# Factors Affecting Motivation

## Locus of Control

Psychologists and other health care providers have long been interested in determining why individuals behave the way they do. Why do some people practice "wellness" behaviors, eating a balanced diet and exercising regularly, while others smoke and overindulge in food and alcohol, even though they know it is detrimental to their health? Why do some clients with chronic pain manage well, while others develop maladaptive behaviors?

One of the early researchers to study behavior was Julian Rotter. He described a theory that he called "locus of control," which is based upon life experiences and influenced by one's culture and family. According to Rotter's (1966) theory, people develop preconceived expectations about what will happen to them in the future. Those who believe they can influence what will happen to them are described as having an internal locus of control. They tend to be self-motivated and follow suggested treatment protocols because they believe they can make a difference in their lives. Other individuals have an external locus of control, believing that what happens to them is a result of outside influences or events. They may be less compliant with treatment protocols because they believe that their efforts will not make a difference.

Many studies have examined the relationship between locus of control and health-related behaviors. Hussey and Gilliland (1989) report that individuals with an internal locus of control are more health-oriented and more likely to follow suggested health care plans than those whose locus of control is external. In reviewing the nursing literature, Oberle (1991) found that some studies support Hussey and Gilliland's findings, while others contradict them. This may be due to the fact that locus of control is a dynamic concept with many points on its continuum. It can range from strongly internal to strongly external. In addition, the measures of locus of control assess tendencies that can vary and even change (Wallston, 1992).

Clients with chronic pain who have a strong internal locus of control are better able to deal with their pain than those with a strong external locus of control (Crisson & Keefe, 1988; Toomey, Mann, Abashian, & Thompson-Pope, 1991). However, because of its dynamic nature, locus of control can shift. Clients with chronic pain, treated in multidisciplinary pain management clinics, were able to increase their internal locus of control and, as a result, better manage their pain (Coughlin, Bandura, Fleischer, & Guck, 2000).

Wallston (1992) suggests that health-related behavior also depends on the value that people place on their health. People who perceive they can control their illness may place a higher value on health and comply with treatments in order to improve. In contrast, those who believe they have no control over their illness may place less emphasis on their health. They may be noncompliant with treatment, believing that their actions will not positively influence their health.

The good news for clients and health care providers is that locus of control is a fluid concept. Even clients with a strong external locus of control can learn to take control of their situations. While it is important for health care providers to understand locus of control, we must recognize that other factors also influence motivation and adherence.

## Self-Efficacy

The concept of self-efficacy was first introduced by Bandura (1977). This sense of competence and ability is related to how successful people believe they can be in accomplishing a task. Some people avoid a task if they do not believe they can adequately participate or complete it. In contrast, those who believe they will ultimately succeed continue their efforts, even if they are having difficulty. People judge their own abilities, and this, in turn, affects their behavior, level of motivation, and adherence with health care. This self-judgment can also determine how long someone persists with a difficult task. It is important to note that these personal judgments are not always accurate.

When people misjudge their abilities, they may become angry, frustrated, and lose their focus on the task. They believe things are more difficult than they really are. However, people with a strong sense of self-efficacy may see a difficult situation as more of a challenge, causing them to try even harder (Bandura, 1982). This may partly explain why clients may react differently to the same circumstances.

Individuals with a strong sense of self-efficacy are better able to cope following a disability or illness (Maciejewski, Prigerson, & Mazure, 2000; Robinson-Smith, Johnston, & Allen, 2000). For instance, one study noted that self-efficacy positively affected the functional outcomes for women with osteoarthritis of the knee (Harrison, 2004). Strong self-efficacy is also related to better physical and mental health and exercise compliance (Resnick & Jenkins, 2000; Resnick, Palmer, Jenkins, & Spellbring, 2000). Women who survived breast cancer and participated in a strength/weight training program for six months demonstrated a high degree of self-efficacy and were very adherent to the program (Ott et al., 2004). Fortunately, like locus of control, self-efficacy is a dynamic concept. People can improve their sense of competence by observing others accomplishing tasks and by learning to successfully complete tasks themselves (Bandura, 1997; Resnick et al., 2000).

This is important information for health care professionals. We can assist our clients by introducing them to clients with similar diagnoses who have functionally integrated their illness or disability into their lives. These clients can serve as role models for those who have recently been diagnosed or injured. In addition, we can assist our clients by establishing reasonable short-term goals. Clients develop a sense of accomplishment, improve their sense of self-efficacy, and become motivated to comply with future treatments as they successfully achieve goals.

## Self-Esteem

Self-esteem describes how individuals feel about themselves. Do they accurately assess their self-worth in comparison to others? Do they have pride in their abilities? A person with strong self-esteem is more likely to feel in control of his or her life and be more motivated to be an active participant in health care than a person with low self-esteem (Turner, 1999).

Many factors affect self-esteem. For example, clients in a rehabilitation setting or skilled nursing facility may feel better if they are able to wear their own clothing rather than hospital attire. A woman who uses a wheelchair may feel better about herself if a hairdresser is available to cut, color, and style her hair. Someone with burns might improve his self-esteem if he learns to apply cosmetics to mask his injuries. It may also help to have personal items nearby to remind them of their homes and families. A simple compliment from a health care provider can help boost a client's self-esteem, too. What may appear to be insignificant to us might be extremely important to a client.

## Social Support

In addition to locus of control, self-efficacy, and self-esteem, social support plays a significant role in determining a client's motivation. It involves interaction between at least two people, which can enhance well-being. Social support shows people that they are loved, cared about, and valued (Schumaker & Brownell, 1984). Lack of social support has been associated with low levels of motivation and may lead to nonadherence; therefore, it is beneficial to consider social support mechanisms when developing plans of care.

When obtaining clients' histories, it is important for health providers to ask about support systems. People with illness or injury may find that they are unable to perform many of their activities of daily living. Frustration, anger, and lack of motivation may follow. A social support system can make it easier for clients to function. For example, people may be able to keep medical appointments if they have transportation. Members of a social support system may encourage a client to comply with treatment plans, such as reminding a client to take medication, eat healthy meals, and exercise. This support can motivate a client to keep trying and forge ahead, even in difficult times.

In a study of caregivers for clients discharged from an outpatient geriatric assessment center, it was found that those caregivers who agreed with health provider recommendations had greater adherence to treatment protocols and were more likely to help the clients reach the goals (Bogardus et al., 2004). In a broader sense, when caregivers and health providers work together and caregivers believe in the efficacy of recommendations, client care is the winner.

Adherence to medical treatment is 1.7 times higher for clients with close family ties and 1.53 times lower in those experiencing conflict. Clients who live with a spouse or another adult have somewhat greater adherence to medical treatment than adults who live alone (DiMatteo, 2004).

Stress of caregivers can significantly impact adherence. In a study of caregivers of children with disabilities, as major problems arose for the children, i.e., loss of functional skills, accommodations needed for adaptive equipment to achieve mobility, transition to school, and terminal stages of disease, family stress levels increased and adherence to home exercise programs diminished (Rone-Adams, Stern, & Walker, 2004). Health care professionals need to be aware of these factors affecting motivation and adherence so that they can refer caregivers to applicable sources of assistance, such as support groups, other health disciplines, stress and time management programs, and respite care.

If clients do not have support systems in place, they can be referred to appropriate community resources. For example, Meals on Wheels can provide adequate nourishment. Transportation may be provided by local town governments. A home health aide might assist with activities of daily living. It is the responsibility of health care providers to be knowledgeable about the programs and resources in the client's community, so they can inform them about these services.

In addition to locus of control, self-efficacy, self-esteem, and social support, there are other factors that affect a client's motivation and ability to participate with health care. These factors include:

- depression
- anxiety

- denial
- fear
- illness variables, such as fatigue and pain
- incongruent client–provider goals
- culture
- health care history
- practical logistical arrangements

These additional factors are explored in other chapters and are mentioned here to highlight their impact on client/family motivation and adherence.

Motivation and adherence go hand-in-hand. In a study investigating why children do not take their asthma medication (that is to say lack of adherence to the treatment regimen), the children gave reasons of lack of motivation, difficulty remembering to do so, and social barriers. This occurs even in the face of their perceived consequences of not self-medicating, i.e., feeling sick and not being able to participate in peer activities (Penza-Clyve, Mansell, & McQuaid, 2004).

# Role of Health Care Providers in Promoting Motivation and Adherence

Mrs. Menendez is at home recuperating from total hip replacement surgery. She fractured her hip when she fell on the ice in front of her home. Recently discharged from the hospital, she will receive services from the Visiting Nurses Association.

My supervisor and I visited Mrs. Menendez to evaluate her home to eliminate falling hazards. I was appalled! She had numerous scatter rugs throughout her home. I suggested she remove them immediately so that she wouldn't trip on them. She was reluctant to move them. The rugs had belonged to her mother, and she enjoys having them in her home; they make her feel comfortable and connected to her family. In addition, she has a 20-pound Boston Terrier. Although the dog is 4 years old, he has a habit of jumping on people. I was concerned that he would knock her over. I really thought she should put him in a kennel while she recuperated. She said, "No way! I love my dog and missed him when I was in the hospital." She likes to have him sit on her lap in the evening because he helps her "relax and calm down."

Her husband is another problem. While I was trying to encourage Mrs. Menendez to do things for herself, he wanted to wait on her "hand-and-foot." He didn't want her to move from her comfortable chair in the living room. I tried to explain that she needed to walk to become stronger, to improve her balance, and increase her endurance. He didn't want to listen to me. He was afraid that she might fall again, and he didn't want to "lose her." They've been married for over 50 years. What was I to do?

—*From the journal of Samantha Marino, physical therapist student*

The interaction between Samantha and the Menendez family illustrates the importance of the health provider in motivating clients to comply with care. Health providers need to recognize clients' values and priorities and incorporate them into a care plan to establish reasonable and effective outcomes. For example, Mrs. Menendez might have considered removing the scatter rugs, if she knew she could replace them once she was more stable on her feet. Samantha could suggest that the dog be put into a closed room while Mrs. Menendez is walking and be present when she is seated. In addition, Samantha could also work with Mr. Menendez to establish goals to increase his wife's strength and endurance. With these strategies, she would include him as a valued team member. Perhaps he could record his wife's daily progress. Samantha needs to understand and respect that Mr. Menendez, the dog, and the scatter rugs are all part of Mrs. Menendez's frame of reference. She can utilize these resources to motivate her client to comply with treatments.

# Strategies to Enhance Motivation and Adherence

## Goal-Setting

"Goal-setting has long been regarded as a cornerstone of effective rehabilitation" (Lawler, Dowswell, Hearn, Forster, & Young, 1999, p. 402). Studies indicate that including clients in goal-setting is critical to their treatment success (Bohannon, Andrews, & Smith, 1988; Cott & Finch, 1991; Wressle, Oberg, & Henriksson, 1999). Goals must be established to meet clients' needs, not those of health providers. When clients are involved in establishing goals, they become partners in their care (Playford, Dawson, Limbert, Smith, Ward, & Wells, 2000; Skinner, 2004). Because the goals have relevancy in their lives, they tend to be more committed to them. We will further discuss this concept in Chapter 7, when we explore meaningful outcomes through shared goal setting.

Once goals have been established, it can be helpful for clients to write out their goals in their own words. They may record them in a journal or calendar so that they can regularly review them. You can help clients establish realistic timeframes for completing these goals. It is important to note, though, that goals do not always indicate forward progress. Some goals may be to maintain function or to slow the rate of decline that occurs with some long-term illnesses (Cott & Finch, 1991). In addition, having clients sign personal contracts stating they will adhere to treatment plans has also been shown to improve motivation and adherence (Becker, 1985; Jones & Kovalcik, 1988).

Clients are most successful in achieving treatment outcomes when their goals are specific, challenging, and achievable, and they have the opportunity to successfully practice the skills (Bandura, 1977, 1995; Locke, Shaw, Saari, & Latham, 1981). Therefore, we must be careful to agree upon goals that are neither too high or too low. If a goal is set too high, clients will be unable to achieve success. If a goal is too low, clients may achieve success, but will lack a sense of accomplishment. In either case, this may lead to frustration and nonadherence.

Health care professionals and clients need to recognize that most people will not adhere to treatment programs 100 percent of the time. For example, clients occasionally forget to take medications or follow dietary recommendations. These minor lapses are considered normal. According to Barsa del Alcazar (1998), clients who are "moderately adherent" are demonstrating adaptive behavior. This is especially true of clients who are undergoing long-term treatments such as dialysis. Health care professionals need to recognize and accept this adaptive behavior because it allows clients to continue to have control of their own lives. They can also help clients' family members understand this behavior so they will continue to be supportive, rather than critical, of the behavior of their loved ones over time.

When presented with a list of potential motivators, children favored using rewards as positive reinforcement. Interestingly, although they found prompting by their parents to be aggravating, they did recognize that this cueing fostered greater adherence (Penza-Clyve et al., 2004).

Following illness or injury, clients' goals frequently include returning immediately to their previous state of health. Health care professionals need to discuss prognosis and anticipated timeframes for recovery. Educating clients about the importance of short-term goals, and their relationship to long-term goals, is critical (Bradley, Bogardus, Tinetti, & Inouye, 1999).

Many clients need to make long-term lifestyle changes, such as proper nutrition and physical exercise. In an investigation of promoting adherence to lifestyle changes in people with diabetes, several techniques were recognized:

- progressively prepare individuals to be ready to change
- explore their determination to change and confidence in their ability to do so
- help them establish very specific short- and long-term goals
- establish goals that are congruent with their interests and progress
- provide feedback to build confidence
- progress activities incrementally
- monitor client's progress toward goals
- "coach" the client so that he or she may make positive and independent choices and find solutions to obstacles
- create a team approach (Koenigsberg, Bartlett, & Cramer, 2004).

Clients need to understand that improvement and, hopefully, recovery takes time and effort. Consider Annette Springfield, who required maximum assistance with all activities of daily living (ADLs) following a spinal cord injury. Initially, she was depressed and refused treatments from both physical and occupational therapists, but she did want to resume her life as it had been prior to her injury. When attempting to perform her ADLs, Mrs. Springfield became frustrated and angry. Trying to use assistive devices took too much time and energy, and she just wanted the nurses to dress and bathe her. She did not see value in doing anything that she could not easily accomplish.

The rehabilitation staff helped Mrs. Springfield understand that she needed to master simple activities before she could progress to more complex ones. Many treatment sessions were scheduled in an open clinic space, where she had the opportunity to interact with and observe other clients who had also sustained spinal cord injuries and were able to accomplish what she believed she could not. Over time, Mrs. Springfield began to realize she was making progress and becoming more independent. She then became more motivated. Observation of people who are overcoming or who have successfully overcome similar challenges can promote motivation (Bandura, 1977, 1995).

When clients understand and appreciate the link between short- and long-term goals, they may be more motivated to adhere to programs. In addition, early and continued involvement in goal-setting promotes active participation and responsibility in their own care.

## Education

Client education is an important component of health care (Becker, 1985; Jensen, Gwyer, Shepard, & Hack, 2000; Mostrom & Shepard, 1999; Vanderhoff, 2005). Studies have shown that educated clients practice wellness behaviors and, if ill or injured, remain motivated and adhere to treatment programs (Sluijs, 1991). Client education needs to be culturally sensitive, a topic that is described in Chapter 3, and utilize the components of effective communication discussed in Chapter 2, such as speaking clearly and providing pictures whenever possible. Ask clients if they will be able to adhere to the program that you have both agreed upon. If not, ask why and make appropriate modifications. Attempt to eliminate any barriers that might interfere with adherence.

According to Treichler (1967), classroom students remember:

- 10 percent of what they read
- 20 percent of what they hear
- 30 percent of what they see
- 50 percent of what they see and hear
- 70 percent of what they discuss with people whose opinions they value
- 80 percent of what they personally experience
- 90 percent of what they teach to others

In the clinical setting, clients and families are also learners. Providing clients with written directions, pictures, and time to discuss instructions and ask questions will help them remember prescribed treatment programs. Have clients repeat directions or demonstrate tasks to ensure they understand. In addition, according to Treichler's model, learners retain 90 percent of what they teach to others. Therefore, giving clients the opportunity to teach their program to significant others, under your guidance, may aid in their retention.

Sluijs (1991) noted that the more information clients are given at one time, the more likely they are to forget. They will forget even more if they are worried, concerned, or in pain when they receive information. When possible, try to mitigate anxiety and discomfort at the outset. Yet, how often do we overload clients with information during our first encounter? Ideally, provide clients with basic information during the initial meeting, emphasizing the most important components of the instruction. More complex information can be given at a later time. During subsequent sessions, determine whether clients correctly remember instructions. However, the client may only have one treatment session. In that case, communicate only the most essential information. Encourage clients to contact you with questions or concerns.

People have different teaching and learning styles. Most people tend to teach the way they prefer to learn (Brock & Allen, 2000; Mostrom & Shepard, 1999). However, this may not always be effective. Our teaching approach may not match the client's learning style. While some individuals prefer to hear only the facts, others prefer a more personable approach. Allow time for clients to tell you how they feel and to ask questions. This strategy may instill comfort and prepare clients to absorb the information you are prepared to communicate. While some people learn best by watching a demonstration and listening to instructions, others prefer trying things immediately. Recognizing and making adjustments for individual learning styles can make health care professionals more effective teachers and clinicians (Lawrence, 1997; Vanderhoff, 2005).

Today, a great deal of information on health care is available. Clients can open a newspaper, watch television, or listen to the radio to hear about the latest medical research. In addition, more people have access to the Internet, at home or through local libraries and schools. Clients need to be educated on how to evaluate all sources of information, since some are unreliable (Vanderhoff, 2005). As health care professionals, we need to be well informed so that we can answer questions appropriately and ensure that clients receive accurate information. Motivation and adherence can be enhanced if clients are well educated regarding their diagnosis and prognosis.

## Feedback

Positive feedback has been shown to improve self-esteem, enhance individuals' perceptions of their own competency, and improve motivation and adherence (Bandura, 1977, 1995; Goudas, Minardou, & Kotis, 2000; Jones & Kovalcik, 1988; Locke et al., 1981). Health care professionals track clients' progress in medical records, but do we adequately share this information with clients? Understanding the progress they have made can give clients a sense of control and motivate them to continue (Lawler et al., 1999). It is important to give feedback in a timely manner. Positive feedback may be provided whenever clients follow through with program guidelines or make progress toward their goals.

Clients can also give positive self-feedback. For example, they may track their own progress in journals or calendars. Reviewing this information can be a motivator. Consider Mrs. Thompson, who was trying to lose weight and increase her endurance following cardiac surgery. She had been in a cardiac rehabilitation program for several months and had become discouraged. As a result, she started "forgetting" about her exercise and walking program and no longer made time to adhere to other aspects of her treatment plan. Her exercise physiologist suggested she review the progress she had recorded in her journal. Reading the entries, Mrs. Thompson was surprised at how far she had come. When she began the program, she was barely able to walk the length of her driveway. She recognized that she had increased her endurance, by small increments, and was now able to walk more than 1 mile in 30 minutes. In addition, she had lost 12 pounds. Identifying these accomplishments enhanced her self-esteem and motivated her to return to her program with renewed energy.

## Peer Support Groups

Peer group participation has been shown to help people clarify values, improve self-esteem, increase knowledge, develop coping strategies, maintain healthy lifestyle habits, and reduce or eliminate addictions (Bernard, 1991; Horowitz, 1985). In fact, groups are so beneficial and popular, it seems as though they exist for almost any problem, condition, or diagnosis. Interacting with others who have gone through or are going through similar experiences may assist clients in understanding their own limitations or impairments and give them greater confidence in their ability to succeed (Resnick et al., 2000; Turner, 1999). Groups offer social support and provide a forum for sharing stories and strategies for success. Support groups also benefit family members who are learning to live with an individual who has been diagnosed with an illness or who has sustained an injury.

Peer support groups can be especially effective in promoting positive health and wellness behaviors. For example, Turner (1999) described peer-led initiatives as a social support system for adolescents. Teens often feel more comfortable talking to one another rather than discussing their concerns with adults. Turner cautions, however, that when teen peer groups are developed, peer leaders need extensive training in listening and basic counseling skills in order to be effective. He emphasizes the need for adequate training, adult support, and the availability of appropriate referral resources. There must also be a trained adult available whom they can contact immediately if the need arises. Developing effective peer support programs can be quite time-consuming, but the results are worth the effort.

While health care professionals direct some peer support groups, group members direct others, as in the teen group noted above. Such programs can be a positive adjunct to professional health care services. However, when developing these programs, health care providers must remember that peer leaders have the same concerns and problems as group members. Therefore, it is important to provide professional social support mechanisms for all peer leaders if their problems begin to overwhelm them (Sherman, Sanders, & Yearde, 1998).

Information regarding peer group meetings is often available from local newspapers, hospitals, libraries, or churches. National resources, such as the Muscular Dystrophy Association and the United Cerebral Palsy Association, can be found on the Internet. Practitioners may consider developing peer support groups at their own facilities if none are available in the community.

## Functional Programs

Following illness or injury, many clients are concerned with their ability to be independent. Studies have shown that clients are more motivated to adhere to treatment programs that are functionally related (Bohannon et al., 1988; Brody, 1999; Cott & Finch, 1991; Pollock, 1993). In addition, clients are more likely to comply with programs that cause the least disruption in their lifestyles. Finding ways to fit treatment plans into a client's normal routine helps ensure long-term adherence (Becker, 1985; Brody, 1999).

Keep programs realistic and avoid complex instructions. Provide variety and choice when possible to prevent clients from becoming disinterested. Develop functional programs based on daily routines. For example, if a client needs to follow a complicated medication schedule, suggest the client purchase a weekly medication dispenser. Guide the client to identify the best time each week to fill the dispenser and establish a realistic strategy for remembering to take the medication on time. If the medication needs to be taken with food, he or she may want to leave the dispenser on the table where meals are eaten.

Be sure that home programs are functional in nature. Consider Mrs. Farrari. She slipped in the supermarket and fractured her shoulder. The therapist first suggested a nonfunctional exercise program. Mrs. Farrari stated the exercises were "boring" and did not interest her. After careful questioning about her home environment, where she lived alone, the therapist suggested that Mrs. Farrari move frequently used items to higher shelves. The client relocated teacups and glasses in the kitchen cabinets and towels and facecloths in the bathroom closet. As a result, as her day progressed so did her accomplishments of her treatment goals.

While a more structured exercise program might have accelerated her progress, she would not have made any progress if she did not adhere to the therapeutic program.

It is especially beneficial for families with children who have disabilities to integrate home exercise programs with a functional routine, such as bathing, dressing, and playing. It is incumbent upon the health provider to collaborate with caregivers to simplify activities so that stress is minimized and limited time and energy are used most effectively (Rone-Adams et al., 2004).

## Primary and Secondary Control-Enhancing Strategies

Some clients start out motivated but lose their impetus over time. This is especially true for clients dealing with chronic impairment or terminal illness. No matter how hard they work, their condition is not likely to significantly change. Maintaining motivation can also be difficult for elderly people. Even healthy people experience decreased hearing acuity and loss of muscle tone, strength, flexibility, and, sometimes, memory as they age. They cannot participate in activities the way they could when they were younger.

How can we help these clients sustain their motivation to adhere to programs and achieve therapeutic outcomes? Studies have shown that a two-step approach, involving primary and secondary control-enhancing strategies, can be very effective (Chipperfield, Perry, & Menec, 1999; Rothbaum, Weisz, & Snyder, 1982). These strategies allow clients to feel in control of their lives, maintain their self-esteem, and remain motivated.

Primary control-enhancing strategies allow people to accomplish desired goals in new ways by modifying the environment. Consider Mrs. McKenzie, who loved to walk to the corner store to get her daily newspaper. As her rheumatoid arthritis progressed, she purchased a motorized scooter that allowed her to continue her routine. When primary control-enhancing strategies no longer achieve the goals, secondary strategies can be utilized to retain a form of personal control. Instead of modifying the environment, clients who use secondary control-enhancing strategies modify their internal environment by altering their expectations. As her condition worsened, Mrs. McKenzie found that she could not control the scooter and began to have her newspaper delivered to her home.

## SUMMARY

This chapter discussed the theoretical concepts related to motivation and adherence, including locus of control, self-efficacy, self-esteem, and the importance of social support systems. Strategies to enhance motivation and adherence involved understanding the importance of shared goal-setting, developing realistic and functional goals, ensuring that clients understand instructions, developing and adjusting educational programs to meet clients' learning styles, and providing clients with positive feedback. In addition, methods to help clients adjust goals to effectively deal with chronic illness and impairments were presented. Barriers to motivation, such as depression, anxiety, fatigue, pain, and denial, will be discussed in other chapters.

Identifying realistic, achievable goals that are relevant, meaningful, and mutually valued by both the clients and the health provider is a critical motivational tool.

When working with clients, we need to remember that many feel a loss of control as a result of illness or injury. We can empower them by facilitating a move toward independent management of their care. Even if complete independence of a task is not possible, many people are able to direct aides, nurses, therapists, and others to assist in a way that is comfortable for the clients. Regaining control of even small tasks can provide motivation to adhere to established programs so that long-range goals can be realized.

## REFLECTIVE QUESTIONS

1. Think about a person you know who is highly motivated. What factors do you think help keep that person motivated?
2. Think about a person you know who lacks motivation and has difficulty following through with most things.
   a. What factors do you believe contribute to his or her lack of motivation?
   b. Describe three strategies that might help the person become or stay motivated.
3. a. When do you feel challenged?
   b. What motivates you to keep trying?
   c. What barriers interfere with your motivation?
4. What are some important attitudes and beliefs that you can use to elicit clients' motivation?
5. What skills do you need to develop and/or improve to become a more effective motivator?

## CASE STUDY

Russell Lewis is a 14-year-old boy who sustained multiple trauma in a motor vehicle accident. He is quite depressed and refuses to cooperate with treatments.

His parents, grandparents, and younger sister are very concerned about his prognosis and make sure that someone is always with him, the grandparents all day and the parents and sister during the evening following work and school. Although the physician informed them that Russell may never walk again, they believe that he will. They are very active in their local church, and the entire congregation is praying for Russell's speedy recovery.

1. Consider the earlier discussion about locus of control.
   a. Where might Russell be at this point in time on the continuum from internal to external locus of control?
   b. What factors form your rationale?
2. Given the dynamic nature of locus of control and self-efficacy, as well as the specifics of this case, what kinds of interventions might help shift Russell's locus of control in a more positive direction?
3. Bandura and others found that clients are most successful in achieving treatment outcomes when goals are specific, challenging, and achievable, and they are afforded the opportunity to practice specific skills.
   a. Develop at least three goals for Russell that meet these criteria.
   b. How will you include Russell in establishing these goals?
4. a. What do you think might motivate Russell?
   b. What might be barriers to his adherence?

# REFERENCES

Bandura, A. (1977). Self-efficacy: Toward a unifying theory of behavioral change. *Psychological Review, 84*(2), 191–215.

Bandura, A. (1982). Self-efficacy mechanism in human agency. *American Psychologist, 37*(2), 122–147.

Bandura, A. (1995). *Self-efficacy in changing societies.* New York: Cambridge University Press.

Bandura, A. (1997). *Self-efficacy: The exercise of control.* New York: W. H. Freeman.

Barsa del Alcazar, C. (1998). Spectrum of adherence among hemodialysis patients. *Journal of Nephrology Social Work, 18,* 53–65.

Becker, M. H. (1985). Client adherence to prescribed therapies. *Medical Care, 23*(5), 539–554.

Bernard, B. (1991). The case for peers. *The Peer Facilitator Quarterly, 8,* 20–27.

Bogardus, S. T., Bradley, E. H., Williams, C. S., Maciejewski, P. K., Gallo, W. T., & Inouye, S. K. (2004). Achieving goals in geriatric assessment: Role of caregiver agreement and adherence to recommendations. *Journal of the American Geriatric Society, 52*(1), 99–105.

Bohannon, R., Andrews, A., & Smith, M. (1988). Rehabilitation goals of patients with hemiplegia. *International Journal of Rehabilitation Research, 11*(2), 181–183.

Bradley, E., Bogardus, Jr., S., Tinetti, M., & Inouye, S. (1999). Goal-setting in clinical medicine. *Social Science and Medicine, 49,* 267–278.

Brock, S., & Allen, J. (2000). Working with type in health care: Same words, different meanings? *Journal of Psychological Type, 53,* 4–10.

Brody, L. (1999). Principles of self-management and exercise instruction. In C. M. Hall & L. T. Brody (Eds.), *Therapeutic exercise: Moving toward function* (pp. 33–42). Philadelphia: Lippincott Williams & Wilkins.

Chipperfield, J. G., Perry, R. P., & Menec, V. H. (1999). Primary and secondary control-enhancing strategies: Implications for health in later life. *Journal of Aging and Health, 11*(4), 517–539.

Cott, C., & Finch, E. (1991). Goal-setting in physical therapy practice. *Physiotherapy Canada, 43*(1), 19–22.

Coughlin, A. M., Bandura, A. S., Fleischer, T. D., & Guck, T. P. (2000). Multidisciplinary treatment of chronic pain patients: Its efficacy in changing patient locus of control. *Archives of Physical Medicine and Rehabilitation, 81,* 739–740.

Crisson, J. F., & Keefe, F. J. (1988). The relationship of locus of control of pain coping strategies and psychological distress in chronic pain patients. *Pain, 35,* 147–154.

DiMatteo, M. R. (2004). Social support and patient adherence to medical treatment: A meta-analysis. *Health Psychology, 23*(2), 207–218.

Goudas, M., Minardou, K., & Kotis, J. (2000). Feedback regarding goal achievement and intrinsic motivation. *Perceptual and Motor Skills, 90,* 810–812.

Harrison, A. L. (2004). The influence of pathology, pain, balance, and self-efficacy on function in women with osteoarthritis of the knee. *Physical Therapy, 84*(9), 822–831.

Horowitz, L. (1985). The self-care motivation model: Theory and practice in healthy human development. *Journal of School Health, 55*(2), 57–61.

Hussey, L. C., & Gilliland, K. (1989). Compliance, low literacy, and locus of control. *Nursing Clinics of North America, 24,* 605–611.

Jensen, G. M., Gwyer, J., Shepard, K. F., & Hack, L. M. (2000). Expert practice in physical therapy. *Physical Therapy, 80*(1), 28–43.

Jones, J., & Kovalcik, E. (1988). Goal-setting: A method to help clients escape the negative effects of stress. *Stress Reduction, 83*(1), 257–261.

Koenigsberg, M. R., Bartlett, D., & Cramer, J. S. (2004). Facilitating treatment adherence with lifestyle changes in diabetes. *Journal of American Family Physicians, 69*(2), 309–316.

Lawler, J., Dowswell, G., Hearn, J., Forster, A., & Young, J. (1999). Recovering from stroke: A qualitative investigation of the role of goal-setting in late stroke recovery. *Journal of Advanced Nursing, 30*(2), 401–409.

Lawrence, G. (1997). *Looking at type and learning styles.* Gainesville, FL: Center for Applications of Psychological Type.

Locke, E. A., Shaw, K. N., Saari, L. M., & Latham, G. P. (1981). Goal-setting and task performance. *Psychological Bulletin, 90*(1), 125–152.

Maciejewski, P. K., Prigerson, H. G., & Mazure, C. (2000). Self-efficacy as a mediator between stressful life events and depressive symptoms. *British Journal of Psychiatry, 176,* 373–378.

Mostrom, E., & Shepard, K. F. (1999). Teaching and learning about patient education in physical therapy professional preparation: Academic and clinical considerations. *Journal of Physical Therapy Education, 13*(3), 8–17.

Oberle, K. (1991). A decade of research in locus of control: What have we learned? *Journal of Advanced Nursing, 16,* 800–806.

Ott, C. D., Lindsey, A. M., Waltman, N. L., Gross, G. J., Twiss, J. J., Berg, K., Brisco, P. L., & Henricksen, S. (2004). Facilitative strategies, psychological factors, and strength/weight training behaviors in breast cancer survivors who are at risk for osteoporosis. *Orthopedic Nursing, 23*(1), 45–52.

Penza-Clyve, S. M., Mansell, C., & McQuaid, E. L. (2004). Why don't children take their asthma medications? A qualitative analysis of children's perspectives on adherence. *Journal of Asthma, 41*(2), 189–197.

Playford, E. D., Dawson, L., Limbert, V., Smith, M., Ward, C. D., & Wells, R. (2000). Goal-setting in rehabilitation: Report of a workshop to explore professionals' perceptions of goal-setting. *Clinical Rehabilitation, 14*(5), 491–496.

Pollock, N. (1993). Client-centered assessment. *American Journal of Occupational Therapy, 47*(4), 298–301.

Resnick, B., & Jenkins, L. S. (2000). Testing the reliability and validity of the Self-Efficacy for Exercise Scale. *Nursing Research, 49*(3), 154–159.

Resnick, B., Palmer, M. H., Jenkins, L. S., & Spellbring, A. M. (2000). Path analysis of efficacy expectations and exercise behavior in older adults. *Journal of Advanced Nursing, 31*(6), 1309–1315.

Robinson-Smith, G., Johnston, M. V., & Allen, J. (2000). Self-care, self-efficacy, quality of life and depression after stroke. *Archives of Physical Medicine and Rehabilitation, 81,* 460–464.

Rone-Adams, S. A., Stern, D. F., & Walker, V. (2004). Stress and compliance with a home exercise program among caregivers of children with disabilities. *Pediatric Physical Therapy, 16,* 140–148.

Rothbaum, F., Weisz, J. R., & Snyder, S. S. (1982). Changing the world and changing the self: A two-process model of perceived control. *Journal of Personality and Social Psychology, 42,* 5–37.

Rotter, J. B. (1966). Generalized expectancies for internal versus external control of reinforcement. *Psychological Monographs, General and Applied, 80,* 1–28.

Schumaker, S. A., & Brownell, A. (1984). Toward a theory of social support: Closing conceptual gaps. *Journal of Social Issues, 40*(4), 11–36.

Sherman, B. R., Sanders, L. M., & Yearde, J. (1998). Role-modeling healthy behavior: Peer counseling for pregnant and post-partum women in recovery. *Women's Health Issues, 8*(4), 230–238.

Skinner, T. C. (2004). Psychological barriers. *European Journal of Endocrinology, 151* (Suppl. 2), T13–17.

Sluijs, E. (1991). *Patient education in physical therapy.* Utrecht, Netherlands: Nederlands Instituut voor Onderzoek Van de Eerstel I jnsgezondheidszorg NIVEL.

Toomey, T. C., Mann, J. D., Abashian, S., & Thompson-Pope, S. (1991). Relationship between perceived self-control of pain, pain description, and functioning. *Pain, 45,* 129–133.

Treichler, D. G. (1967). Are you missing the boat in training aids? In *Audiovisual communications.* New York: United Business Publications.

Turner, G. (1999). Peer support and young people's health. *Journal of Adolescence, 22,* 567–572.

Vanderhoff, M. (2005). Patient education and health literacy. *PT–Magazine of Physical Therapy, 13*(9), 42–46.

Wallston, K. A. (1992). Hocus-pocus, the focus isn't strictly on locus: Rotter's social learning theory modified for health. *Cognitive Therapy and Research, 16*(2), 182–199.

Wressle, E., Oberg, B., & Henriksson, C. (1999). The rehabilitation process for the geriatric stroke patient: An exploratory study of goal-setting and interventions. *Disability and Rehabilitation, 21*(2), 80–87.

# 7

# *Collaborative Treatment Planning*

I had a terrible experience in the clinic today. I was working in the gym with Mrs. Swanson, a woman who had her left leg amputated above the knee because of complications related to her diabetes. Just as she was finishing her exercises, one of the medical residents came by. Apparently, Mrs. Swanson agreed to participate in a study that was designed to examine how well clinicians at our hospital collaborate with patients on establishing goals and treatment plans. I asked for permission to sit in on the interview. What a mistake! This is how the interview went:

*Interviewer:* Who decides what you are going to do in physical therapy?

*Mrs. Swanson:* Well, Suzy does, of course! She's so smart. I don't know how I would have gotten this far without everything she has taught me.

*Interviewer:* Do you ever suggest to Suzy that you would like to try a different exercise or work on something specific that you need to be able to do at home?

*Mrs. Swanson:* Oh, no. She really knows just what I need to learn. After all the schooling she's had, how would I know anything more?

At first, I felt touched and kind of proud, but as the interview continued, I became embarrassed. The questioning continued about Mrs. Swanson's home situation. She mentioned how sad she was that she probably wouldn't be able to participate in her weekly line dancing class now that she was missing a leg. She started sobbing and talking about how she would be no good to anyone any more. I really thought that I had done a good job of incorporating her goals into my treatment plan. Today, I realized that I had not.

—*From the journal of Suzanne Ballis, physical therapist student*

In Chapter 6, we discussed the importance of establishing collaborative relationships with our clients that are based on genuine concern and mutual respect and trust. A healthy client–provider relationship involves understanding clients' perspectives and leads to explicitly shared expectations for outcomes. In this chapter, we describe collaborative relationships, identify common barriers, and discuss strategies that can be used to enhance collaboration. Approaches to modifying health beliefs, values, and behaviors are included because they may be underlying factors in the development of an effective collaborative treatment plan.

# Collaboration

As we discussed in Chapter 6, collaborative goal setting is an important step toward empowering clients to take responsibility for their own recovery. Providing opportunities to make real choices in treatment goals and planning stimulates clients to utilize their own skills and resources to achieve positive outcomes. Goals that are important in clients' lives tend to be functional, meaningful, and motivating (Chinman et al., 1999; Randall & McEwen, 2000; von Korff, Gruman, Schaefer, Curry, & Wagner, 1997). They lead to more positive outcomes because the client is more invested in the treatment plan, and there is a better sense of achievement (Ridgway, 1988). In addition, client satisfaction is positively associated with the degree of client and family involvement in the collaborative design and implementation of health care plans (Massey & Wu, 1993).

All health care providers agree, at least conceptually, that plans of care should be client-centered and established and managed in collaboration with clients and all of their care providers (Baker, Marshak, Rice, & Zimmerman, 2001; Commission on Accreditation of Rehabilitation Facilities, 1998; Joint Commission on Accreditation of Healthcare Organizations, 1999; Lamorey & Ryan, 1998; Nelson & Payton, 1997; Randall & McEwen, 2000; Smith, Smith, King, Frieden, & Richards, 1993). While effective collaboration may be the single most significant factor in determining client outcomes, it continues to pose significant challenges to health care professionals (Backlar, 1998; Chinman et al., 1999; Neistadt, 1995; Nelson & Payton, 1997; Woodend, Nair, & Tang, 1997). On the public front, legislators have developed a number of initiatives to help solve this problem.

Legislation has been enacted to identify important rights of individuals with disabilities and their families, including the right to participate in developing goals and plans for services. See Table 7–1 for a summary of these laws. Those having most significant impact include the Rehabilitation Act of 1973 (Public Law 93-112); the Rehabilitation, Comprehensive Services and Developmental Disabilities Amendment of 1978 (Public Law 95-602); the Individuals with Disabilities Education Act of 1997 (IDEA), and this act's predecessors, the Education for All Handicapped Children Act (Public Law 94-142) and the Education of the Handicapped Amendments of 1986 (Public Law 99-457). These legislative changes carry a mandate to use a team process to identify the most appropriate plans to meet the needs of individuals receiving federally funded services (McGonigel & Garland, 1988).

In pediatric care, the transdisciplinary model emerged to meet this demand. Transdisciplinary teams consist of the child's parents, along with professionals from a variety of disciplines (Lamorey & Ryan, 1998). Ideas and expertise are shared among team members to evaluate and meet the needs of the child being served. Once the collaborative plan is established, team

**TABLE 7–1**    Disability Rights Legislation

| Legislation | Population Served | Summary |
| --- | --- | --- |
| Rehabilitation Act of 1973 | Any person with a disability receiving federally funded services | • First "rights" legislation to prohibit discrimination against people with disabilities.<br>• Established the Rehabilitation Service Administration to oversee grants to assist in meeting the current and future needs of people with disabilities. |
| Comprehensive Services and Developmental Disabilities Amendment of 1978 | Any person with a disability receiving federally funded services | • Amended the Rehabilitation Act of 1973.<br>• Established state vocational rehabilitation services.<br>• Called for information and referral programs so that people needing these services would be aware of the federal and state programs available. |
| Education for All Handicapped Children Act of 1975 | Children ages 3–21 | • Recognized that the education needs of disabled children were not being fully met<br>• Ensured that all children with disabilities would have available to them special education and related services designed to meet their unique needs as identified by an Individualized Education Plan (IEP). |
| Education of the Handicapped Amendments of 1986 | Children ages birth through age 2 | • Expanded the services enabled by the Education of the Handicapped Act to children under the age of 3.<br>• Required that each eligible child and family receive a written Individualized Family Service Plan (IFSP) based on a multidisciplinary assessment and identification of services to meet needs. |
| Individuals with Disabilities Education Act of 1997 | Children ages 3–21 | • Reauthorized and strengthened the Education for All Handicapped Children Act of 1975.<br>• Strengthened the academic expectations and accountability.<br>• Bridged the gap between what children with disabilities learn and what is required in regular curriculum. |

members train each other to provide hands-on interventions. For example, a special education teacher may train the child's parents in behavioral techniques to obtain their child's attention and cooperation. An occupational therapist may instruct a special educator in the principles of positioning to facilitate the child's involvement in classroom activities that require upright sitting. Professional members of the team assume a consultative role, providing assistance to bring about changes in the care plan as needed. Active family involvement is central to the process, and this helps to ensure that a holistic approach is maintained.

Fortunately, funding outside of the medical system is available for this population. Through early intervention and public education, federal and state funds cover some of the costs of meeting the ever-changing needs of children with developmental disabilities. This allows health care professionals to be involved over time, providing more opportunity for trusting relationships to develop.

Early intervention programs cover services for children from birth to age 3. The family establishes goals and a plan with guidance from the early intervention team. The child is seen primarily in the home setting, where important aspects of his or her life are more naturally incorporated into the goals and treatment program. As the child's third birthday approaches, this team of health care professionals assists in the transition to a school program that may provide services through age 21.

Consider the case of Lisa Marie, a 2-year-old girl with a diagnosis of cerebral palsy. She has been treated by the same physical therapist (PT), occupational therapist (OT), and speech/language pathologist (SLP) since she came home from the neonatal intensive care unit. The individualized family service plan (IFSP) was coordinated by a case manager and involved Lisa Marie's parents and all health care professionals who would be involved in her care. Although only one member of the health care team can visit each month, collaborative planning occurs, involving all team members, especially the family. Occasional tension does exist between the practitioners and Lisa Marie's parents regarding what is "right" for her care, but this tension forces periodic reexamination of the goals and the progress being made.

Because family involvement is essential, team members have established bonds with Lisa Marie and her mother, father, and two older siblings. All family members have learned how they can help to facilitate Lisa Marie's development. Her parents use effective handling skills, which were taught by the PT and OT. Her older brother, Eric, helps to position Lisa Marie in the seating system she uses for eating meals and participating in family activities. The SLP has taught Eric to position Lisa Marie in a way that minimizes the risk of aspiration when she is eating. Lindsay, Lisa Marie's older sister, enjoys playing video games with her. These games are prerequisites for power-mobility training, which Lisa will begin once she makes the transition to her new school-based program next year.

Lisa Marie will soon be 3 years old, and the therapists have been helping to prepare everyone for the transition to a public preschool program in the fall. She will be entering an innovative program, in which children with special needs are integrated with neighborhood children who have no identified special needs. Each of Lisa Marie's therapists has participated in the development of her individualized education plan (IEP). In addition to submitting written reports of all aspects of Lisa Marie's life, they also participated in a team meeting with the family and school-based personnel. Her services must be linked to educational goals, so part of the work of both teams of professionals has been to help the family understand which services would be "appropriate."

Through this example, one can see that the programs that evolved out of IDEA legislation have significantly helped to formalize collaborative goal setting. Within the early intervention and special education systems, IFSPs and IEPs are established through a process that involves rehabilitation professionals, parents, teachers, and any other personnel who work with the child. It is the responsibility of the child's advocates to carve out a program that meets the identified needs most fully. For the child receiving services in a public school setting, functional goals, such as achieving independence in communication, toileting, and feeding, can be included, but sophisticated negotiation skills may be required on the part of the family to achieve successful inclusion in the educational plan.

Home care for adults with long-term illnesses or disabilities could probably offer the same benefits, but funding is significantly more limited for adult rehabilitation services. Obtained primarily through medical reimbursement programs, coverage is approved only to meet needs that are determined to be medically necessary. Although pediatric services provided through early intervention and public schools are federally mandated programs for which all eligible children are entitled, medical insurance does not provide this long-term guarantee of service. Lack of funding seriously limits the time that health care professionals can be involved. Not only does this restrict the clients' recovery potential, but also the collaborative relationship that might have developed between the client and provider.

# Barriers to Collaboration

Chinman and colleagues (1999) conducted a needs assessment in a large mental health clinic to determine the levels of interest and willingness of both clients and providers to participate in collaborative treatment planning. They found that (1) patients believed that providers were more interested in collaborative treatment planning than the providers actually reported they were, (2) patients had significantly more interest in collaborative treatment planning than providers thought they did, and (3) clients perceived themselves to be more capable of collaborative treatment planning than providers thought the clients were.

The providers in this study identified the most significant barriers to collaboration as clients' disabilities, noncompliance, and clients' lack of interest in collaboration. Conversely, clients perceived the main barriers as providers' lack of time, uncertainty that treatment goals would be helpful, and inadequate knowledge about how to collaborate in treatment planning.

The findings of Chinman and coworkers (1999) suggest that providers underestimate the willingness of clients to participate in collaborative management. Providers and clients differed significantly in their perceptions of how interested clients were in collaborating on treatment-planning. Sixty percent of the providers rated lack of client interest as a barrier, while only 15 percent of clients actually reported a lack of interest. In fact, most clients are motivated to participate in all aspects of their care. The researchers suggested two additional reasons why some practitioners fail to provide this opportunity. First, they must relinquish some power in the relationship if they are going to empower clients. Second, they feel that *they* know what is best for their clients. For collaborative treatment planning to be successful, practitioners need to provide clients with opportunities for participation and may need to educate them in the actual techniques of collaborative planning.

Nelson and Payton (1997) found that clients being treated by occupational therapists believed that they had some involvement in setting goals. However, upon questioning, the evidence to support this opinion was very weak. In fact, it was clear that clients allowed their occupational therapists to set goals for treatment because they assumed that the therapists would have a better understanding of what would be needed for a successful return to home or work. Although provider-identified goals generally meet some of the clients' needs, the needs that make each person unique might not be identified. This is significant because identifying these needs may result in the development of the most motivating goals (Neistadt, 1995; Nelson & Payton, 1997; Northen, Rust, Nelson, & Watts, 1995).

Clients expect therapists to know what questions to ask to retrieve important information regarding concerns, goals, resources, treatment ideas, and outcomes. While this may occur in long-term care, professionals working in fast-paced environments may have only one opportunity to ask clients to identify their goals. Asking one question about goals during the initial examination is not enough. For example, Nelson and Payton (1997) noted that one of the subjects in their study mentioned that he had a 4-month-old baby at home. He had not reported this to his occupational therapist, nor had he identified taking care of the baby as one of his goals. This certainly was a missed opportunity for developing motivation, a therapeutic relationship, and appropriate goals.

Clients' main concerns may not be identified at all during the initial examination, probably because a comfortable relationship has not yet been established. According to Thorne (1993), clients will progress through three stages of development in their relationships with health care providers. The first stage is characterized by naïve trust. During this phase of the relationship, clients rely on the knowledge of health care professionals to establish goals and plans. They assume that health care providers will know what is best to help them return to their premorbid lifestyles. This stage is generally followed by disenchantment, which occurs because personal goals that may have been highly motivating to the client were not included. Finally, a stage of guarded alliance emerges. This stage offers the best opportunity for collaborative goal setting. In short, clients' main concerns are usually identified later in the course of treatment rather than during the initial examination. Unfortunately, many clients may never have the opportunity to reach this stage in today's health care environment. The number of encounters with health care professionals is quite limited, and clients move quickly from one or more treatment environments to discharge.

Clients may rely on health care professionals to share established goals with other members of the team (Morgan, 1997). This is unlikely to happen. Even clients who are ill enough to require care in an intensive care unit may move from that setting to transitional care, and finally, to outpatient or home care, sometimes after only a few days in each setting. Transfers of service are likely to be accompanied by a complete change in the members of the health care team, with little or no continuity other than what is provided by written reports. These reports often fail to relay details that are important to consider.

Another potential barrier to collaboration is failure to take clients' premorbid lifestyle and history into account, except in a very superficial way. Clients may feel "stripped" of their previous identity. Their former lifestyle may seem somewhat irrelevant in light of significantly altered physical or cognitive function. On the other hand, when important aspects of the premorbid lifestyle are considered, motivating factors can be identified and used to develop an effective treatment plan.

Consider the case of Jenny, whose story of successful recovery from traumatic brain injury was summarized by Price-Lackey and Cashman (1996). Hers was actually a story of self-recovery. When the therapists involved in her rehabilitation failed to capture and incorporate Jenny's life history, she became frustrated, discharged herself from her residential treatment program, and struggled to develop her own, eventually successful program.

Had the therapists fully examined Jenny's history, they would have discovered that, throughout her life, she had been remarkably independent and self-disciplined. She sought out progressively more challenging experiences, which were unusually demanding and somewhat dangerous, and worked diligently until she mastered them. An important theme that continually emerged was that Jenny had effectively used cognitive restructuring to reframe adverse situations (see Chapter 14). This enabled her to view potentially negative experiences as opportunities for change and growth and strive for completion in the face of adversity.

In the narrative histories taken after her recovery, it became clear that Jenny eventually used these cognitive restructuring skills, learned in childhood and adolescence, to achieve recovery after her head injury. Unfortunately, she was not able to call upon this special talent until after she had discharged herself from therapy. She described her self-directed therapy as a long and lonely process. Counseling that emphasized cognitive restructuring would have been extremely helpful to Jenny in the early stages of recovery, but failure to identify this important aspect of her history prevented this from happening.

Failure to incorporate clients' life histories is indicative of a larger problem. Providers tend to conceptualize clients in terms of diagnoses, symptoms, and needs that must be matched with appropriate treatment options. Conversely, clients conceptualize their needs in terms of the functional abilities and resources needed to help them return to their premorbid lifestyles. Coordination and integration of both perspectives through effective collaboration is needed. Both providers and clients have important contributions to make in the treatment process (Chinman et al., 1999; von Korff et al., 1997).

# Strategies for Improving Collaboration

Asking clients to identify the biggest problems they are facing in managing their illness may provide the basis for improved collaboration. Consider the following example:

> I tried something new with my patients this month. About one week prior to each client's appointment, I sent out a brief questionnaire. Clients were asked to answer a few basic, open-ended questions before coming in for their visits. The questions addressed concerns or problems they might be experiencing with their health or lifestyle. I was amazed at the results. I had expected the majority would respond, but every one of my clients did! The other expectation I had was that this simple reflection would help focus our sessions. It did, but other benefits occurred, too. Patients reported feeling more relaxed during the visit because they knew all of their concerns would be addressed. One of my clients suggested that I add a section to record my answers to concerns discussed during the visit. They'll be given a copy of this to take home.
>
> *—From the journal of Cathy Smith-Peterson, nurse practitioner student*

In addition to asking clients to identify questions or problems, it may be helpful to ask them other pointed questions at various intervals in the treatment process. For example, they could be asked to define their own role in maintaining and improving their health, how they perceive the role of the health care professional, and how they define concepts, such as help, therapy, rehabilitation, goals, and outcomes. This type of discussion not only provides baseline information about client beliefs, it can also provide an opportunity to clarify any confusion the client may be experiencing (von Korff et al., 1997).

As discussed in Chapter 6, client education is an essential element of health care. In addition to information about a specific illness or disability, some clients may have to learn how to be more active participants. This might require instruction in helpful concepts and terminology. By modeling the process of evaluation and task analysis and communicating in terms that clients can easily understand, health providers can facilitate their clients' learning how to independently solve functional problems. For example, if a client tends to identify problems in broad-based terms such as, "I want to be able to provide for my family," you may need to help him or her reframe the problem in terms of specific functions. This will facilitate achievement of the ultimate goal of every health plan—independent health care management.

If clients are included in planning, their involvement should be active enough that they realize their collaborative role. This means that if clients are asked to identify their goals for treatment, responses should mirror the goals recorded in their health care records. Incorporating clients' goals into the plan of care requires active listening to ensure that we fully understand what clients are conveying. Their ideas then need to be developed into attainable and measurable goals that not only meet the criteria for standards of professional documentation but also maximize the chance of health insurance reimbursement (Chinman et al., 1999).

It is important for providers to identify clients' health beliefs, values, and practices because these can be key determinants of motivation and behavior. For example, if a client believes that herbal supplements offer more benefit than the insulin that has been prescribed as a treatment for diabetes, a change in this belief must be encouraged before a successful outcome can be achieved.

Forms designed to guide treatment planning tend to include information required by payers but may be relatively void of prompts to record client beliefs, strengths, resources, hopes, dreams, and practical needs. Including this information on these forms can enhance collaborative care by providing data of value to the entire health care team (Gage, 1994).

# Modifying Health Behaviors

Various approaches to changing or modifying health behaviors are documented in the medical literature. Treatment interventions based on behavior theory seem most likely to have positive outcomes, particularly when clients and providers work together toward shared goals (Brown, 1992; Hirano, Laurent, & Lorig, 1994; Lorish & Gale, 1999, 2002; Meyer & Mark, 1995; Sikkema & Kelly, 1996; von Korff et al., 1997).

To effectively design and implement treatment interventions and promote motivation and adherence to protocols and wellness programs, health care professionals need to understand basic theories of behavior and change. Three such theories are the Health Belief Model, the Transtheoretical Model for Health Behavior Change, and the Five As Behavioral Intervention Protocol.

## Health Belief Model

The Health Belief Model, developed by Hochbaum, Leventhal, Kegeles, and Rosenstock, utilizes psychological theories of decision making to determine what actions individuals might choose when presented with several options of health care choices (Maiman & Becker,

1974; Rosenstock, 1966). This model is based upon the earlier seminal work of Lewin and colleagues, who believed that health behaviors and choices are influenced by the value people place on a potential outcome and their belief that a certain course of action would result in that desired outcome (Lewin, Dembo, Festinger, & Sears, 1944). According to the Health Belief Model, in order for people to change behavior, they must be ready to make a change, believe that the value of making the change is stronger than the consequences of not making the change, and believe that they have the ability to be successful in achieving their goal. In addition, there must be some incentive, either internal or external, that spurs them to action.

## Transtheoretical Model for Health Behavior Change

Change in health behavior is a process that takes time. According to Prochaska and Velicer (1997), even when progress toward change occurs, clients are likely to relapse into earlier stages. In fact, relapse appears to be a necessary element in the process. Clients are likely to pass through six nonlinear stages on their way to change, including:

- Precontemplation–No thought of change
- Contemplation–Considering change
- Preparation–Preparing to change
- Action–Implementing change
- Maintenance–Maintaining change
- Termination–Change is integrated

During precontemplation, clients are not expecting to make any changes within the next six months. At this stage, people may be uninformed as to the consequences of their behaviors or may have given up, having been unsuccessful at earlier attempts to change. These clients tend to refuse to discuss or consider consequences of their actions. Although they may be perceived and labeled as unmotivated, they may not be ready to change. Providing them with additional information regarding the positive aspects of change can help them progress to the next stage, known as contemplation.

In the contemplation stage, clients are aware of the need to change and are considering doing so within the next six months. They have "done their homework" and have learned the pros and cons of their situation. However, these clients can sometimes feel overwhelmed with information and become stuck in this stage for months. They are not ready for action, but encouraging them, providing additional resources, and reducing their barriers to change may help them move to the next stage, known as preparation.

During the preparation stage, people plan to take action in the near future. They know what they need to do and have a plan as to how they will achieve their goals. In addition, they recognize that the positive aspects of change outweigh the negative elements. They are prepared and tend to quickly move to the action stage where observable changes can be measured.

Health professionals perceive clients in the action stage as highly motivated. When clients adhere to home programs, lose weight, and join gyms or health clubs, the health providers feel a sense of satisfaction for having helped them achieve their goals.

Once people achieve their goals, they progress to the maintenance stage and can remain there for six months to five years. During this period, they continue to develop self-confidence and are less tempted to relapse to their former behavior. However, clients often do relapse and may return to any of the earlier stages.

The final stage, termination, occurs when clients have reached their goals, incorporated positive lifestyle changes, and are confident that they will not return to their "old ways."

Health care professionals who understand where clients are in the process of change can better provide appropriate support and help them move forward. Attempting to force a person who is in the precontemplation stage to the action phase can be frustrating for both the client and the health provider and will usually result in only short-term success and a high dropout or relapse rate.

## Five A's Behavioral Intervention Protocol

Lorish and Gale (2002) built upon the theoretical components of the models discussed above and developed the Five A's Behavioral Intervention Protocol. The five steps are easy to follow, take little time to complete, and have been shown to be more successful in promoting client motivation and adherence than information and advice alone.

The steps of the Five A's include:

- Address the issue: Present the need for intervention and determine what clients are willing to do.
- Assess the clients: Determine previous attempts to change behavior, assess willingness to change at this time, and evaluate the current level of motivation.
- Advise the clients: Help the clients understand the benefits of change and the consequences of not changing, by using professional knowledge and demeanor.
- Assist the clients: Negotiate an agreeable plan of care.
- Arrange follow-up: Schedule another appointment to review progress, address barriers, and renegotiate the protocol.

In order for clients to change, they must be knowledgeable about their situation, motivated to change, and have the resources to change. The Five A's address all of these issues and involve a dialogue between the health care provider and the clients to reduce barriers and negotiate positive behavioral changes.

Numerous behavioral techniques have been found to improve health management among clients who have chronic illnesses (Baum & Creer, 1986; Beresford et al., 1992; Curry & McBride, 1994; Haynes, Taylor, & Sackett, 1979; Ignacio-Garcia & Gonzalez-Santos, 1995). As described in Chapter 6, these include the following:

- Collaborative goal setting
- Assessing readiness for new behaviors
- Teaching new behaviors in small, manageable steps
- Providing personalized feedback
- Encouraging self-monitoring of changes and symptoms
- Counseling in techniques to obtain appropriate social support

Incorporating these behavior techniques may facilitate clients' independence of important health management skills.

Further, von Korff and coworkers (1997) identified four key behavioral principles for consideration:

*Principle 1. Illness management skills are learned, and behavior is self-directed.* Most clients grow and develop without concerns related to illness or disability. Until a need arises, these illness management skills cannot be practiced. Clients who have survived previous hardships will adapt to illness or disability more readily. Those who have not will benefit from additional counseling and education. However, until clients value the information as necessary for their own health, independent management is not likely to occur. Patience is needed with those learning these skills for the first time.

*Principle 2. Motivation and self-confidence are important determinants of behavior.* As discussed in Chapter 6, clients must be motivated to make changes in their health behaviors. They also must believe that they are capable of being successful. It is critical to identify what is most important in their lives, what they enjoy doing, and what they find easy to do. Goals established with these elements in mind are more likely to be motivating and achievable. For example, if the goal is to quit smoking, it might be motivating to focus the client's attention on a child or spouse who would be left alone should he or she die from lung disease.

*Principle 3. Social factors influence health behaviors.* The social environments at home, work, and in the health care system can support or impede health behaviors. Changes in these environments may be necessary to promote optimal health. Consider Jon, a college sophomore who has been diagnosed with Hepatitis C. His liver biopsy shows early signs of cirrhosis. He lives near campus with a group of friends who host "keg" parties nearly every weekend night. Since he finds it impossible to avoid drinking in this environment, his health care provider might help him to see that moving into a new setting would be a healthy choice.

*Principle 4. The process of monitoring and responding to changes, symptoms, emotions, and functions improves adaptation to illness.* Learning to adapt to an illness or disability requires the acquisition of many new skills. The process of monitoring and responding to changes related to the illness or disability provides a natural and incremental method for learning to deal with all that is entailed. Sebastian is a 22-year-old man who sustained a cervical 7 spinal cord injury approximately fourteen months ago. His initial recovery was hampered by the involvement of his well-meaning, but overprotective, mother. Over time, family counseling has helped both Sebastian and his mother understand the importance of separation. Recently, he has assumed full responsibility for managing his new life.

Education and persuasion can be used to help motivate clients, but strategies to overcome barriers toward progress must be continually refined. Rewards, such as recognition and praise, may be helpful in encouraging the maintenance of positive changes.

## SUMMARY

This chapter emphasized the importance of establishing goals and treatment plans in collaboration with clients in order to maximize motivation, adherence, and positive outcomes. The concept of collaboration was discussed from both client and provider perspectives, and common barriers to collaborative planning were identified. Principles of behavior theory, which may be helpful in modifying health behaviors, were reviewed.

# REFLECTIVE QUESTIONS

1. If you became disabled, what elements of your life story would you want your health care provider to identify and understand?
   a. What gives your life meaning?
   b. How would this information be important to establishing treatment goals for you?
2. Think about a health care encounter experienced by you, a friend, or family member that was not client-centered.
   a. How might collaboration have improved the experience?
   b. How might the outcome have been different?
3. How do you feel about sharing decision-making power with clients?
4. How might you empower clients to become partners with you in their care?
5. How will you respond if a client disagrees with your recommendations?

# CASE STUDY

Mrs. Johnson is being seen at the Diabetes Clinic at her local hospital. A special diet has been recommended because of her diabetes. It has been one month since she was last in, and she has gained four pounds. Her blood sugar levels are very high, and she admitted that she's been eating ice cream and candy. She also stated that she hasn't been walking like she was advised to do. She told her nutritionist, Andrea, "I'm 75 years old, and I've been eating like this all my life. It's what I do for enjoyment. If God decides he wants to take me, then so be it."

1. What can Andrea do to ensure that Mrs. Johnson's plan of care is client-centered and managed in collaboration with other care providers?
2. What barriers exist for successful collaboration between Mrs. Johnson and the health care team?
3. What strategies can you develop to overcome these barriers?
4. a. What behavioral techniques could be used with Mrs. Johnson to improve her health management?
   b. What principles support your response?

# REFERENCES

Backlar, P. (1998). Can we bridge the gap between the actual lives of persons with serious mental disorders and the therapeutic goals of their providers? *Community Mental Health Journal, 33,* 465–471.

Baker, S. M., Marshak, H. H., Rice, G. T., & Zimmerman, G. J. (2001). Patient participation in physical therapy goal setting. *Physical Therapy, 81*(5), 1118–1126.

Baum, D., & Creer, T. L. (1986). Medication compliance in children with asthma. *Journal of Asthma, 23,* 49–59.

Beresford, S. A., Farmer, E. M., Feingold, L., Graves, K. L., Sumner, S. K., & Baker, R. M. (1992). Evaluation of a self-help dietary intervention in a primary care setting. *American Journal of Public Health, 82,* 79–84.

Brown, S. A. (1992). Meta-analysis of diabetes patient education research: Variations in intervention effects across studies. *Research in Nursing and Health, 15*(6), 409–419.

Chinman, M. J., Allende, M., Weingarten, R., Steiner, J., Tworkowski, S., & Davidson, L. (1999). On the road to collaborative treatment planning: Consumer and provider perspectives. *The Journal of Behavioral Health Services and Research, 26*(2), 211–218.

Commission on Accreditation of Rehabilitation Facilities. (1998). *1998 medical rehabilitation standards manual.* Tucson, AZ: Author.

Curry, S. J., & McBride, C. M. (1994). Relapse prevention for smoking cessation: Review and evaluation of concepts and interventions. In G. S. Omenn, J. E. Fielding, & L. B. Lave (Eds.), *Annual review of public health* (pp. 345–366). Palo Alto, CA: Annual Reviews.

Education of the Handicapped Act Amendments of 1986, Pub. L. No. 99–457, 20 *U.S. Code* § 1401 (1986).

Education for All Handicapped Children Act of 1975, Pub. L. No. 94–142, 20 *U.S. Code* § 1401 (1975).

Gage, M. (1994). The patient-driven interdisciplinary care plan. *Journal of Nursing Administration, 24,* 26–35.

Haynes, R. B., Taylor, D. W., & Sackett, D. L. (Eds.). (1979). *Compliance in health care.* Baltimore: Johns Hopkins University Press.

Hirano, P. C., Laurent, D. D., & Lorig, K. (1994). Arthritis patient education studies, 1987–1991: A review of the literature. *Patient Education Counseling, 24,* 9–54.

Ignacio-Garcia, J. M., & Gonzalez-Santos, P. (1995). Asthma self-management education program by home monitoring of peak expiratory flow. *American Journal of Respiratory and Critical Care Medicine, 151*(2), 353–359.

Individuals with Disabilities Education Act Amendments of 1997, Pub. L. No. 105–17, 20 *U.S. Code* § 1401 (1997).

Joint Commission on Accreditation of Healthcare Organizations. (1999). *The 1999 comprehensive accreditation manual for hospitals: The official handbook.* Oakbrook Terrace, IL: Author.

Lamorey, S., & Ryan, S. (1998). From contention to implementation: A comparison of team practices and recommended practices across service delivery models. *Infant-Toddler Intervention, 8*(4), 309–331.

Lewin, K., Dembo, T., Festinger, L., & Sears, P. S. (1944). Level of aspiration. In J. M. Hunt (Ed.), *Personality and the behavior disorders: A handbook based on experimental and clinical research* (pp. 333–378).New York: The Ronald Press.

Lorish, C. D., & Gale, J. R. (1999). Facilitating behavior change: Strategies for education and practice. *Journal of Physical Therapy Education, 13*(3), 31–37.

Lorish, C. D., & Gale, J. R. (2002). Facilitating adherence to healthy lifestyle behavior changes in patients. In K. F. Shepard & G. M. Jensen (Eds.), *Handbook of teaching for physical therapists* (2nd ed.; pp. 351–385). Boston: Butterworth-Heinemann.

Maiman, L. A., & Becker, M. H. (1974). The health belief model: Origins and correlates in psychological theory. In M. H. Becker (Ed.), *The health belief model and personal health behavior* (pp. 9–26). Thorofare, NJ: Charles B. Slack.

Massey, O. T., & Wu, L. (1993). Service delivery and community housing: Perspectives of consumers, family members, and case managers. *Innovations and Research, 2,* 9–15.

McGonigel, M. J., & Garland, C. W. (1988). The individualized family service plan and the early intervention team: Team and family issues and recommended practices. *Infants and Young Children, 1*(1), 10–21.

Meyer, T. J., & Mark, M. M. (1995). Effects of psychosocial interventions with adult cancer patients: A meta-analysis of randomized experiments. *Health Psychology, 14,* 101–108.

Morgan, U. (1997). The introduction of collaborative care plans. *Professional Nurse, 12*(8), 556–558.

Neistadt, M. E. (1995). Methods of assessing clients' priorities: A survey of adult physical dysfunction settings. *American Journal of Occupational Therapy, 49*, 428–436.

Nelson, C. E., & Payton, O. D. (1997). The planning process in occupational therapy: Perceptions of adult rehabilitation patients. *American Journal of Occupational Therapy, 51*(7), 576–583.

Northen, J. G., Rust, D. M., Nelson, C. E., & Watts, J. (1995). Involvement of adult rehabilitation patients in setting occupational therapy goals. *American Journal of Occupational Therapy, 49*(3), 214–220.

Price-Lackey, P., & Cashman, J. (1996). Jenny's story: Reinventing oneself through occupation and narrative configuration. *American Journal of Occupational Therapy, 50*(4), 306–314.

Prochaska, J. O., & Velicer, W. F. (1997). The transtheoretical model of health behavior change. *American Journal of Health Promotion, 12*(1), 38–48.

Randall, K. E., & McEwen, I. R. (2000). Writing patient-centered functional goals. *Physical Therapy, 80*(12), 1197–1203.

Rehabilitation Act of 1973, Pub. L. No. 93–112, § 102.1, Vocational Rehabilitation Services (1973).

Rehabilitation, Comprehensive Services, and Developmental Disabilities Amendments of 1978, Pub. L. No. 95–602, § 705.4, Comprehensive Services for Independent Living (1978).

Ridgway, P. (1988). *The voice of consumers in mental health systems: A call for change.* Washington, DC: National Institute of Mental Health.

Rosenstock, I. M. (1966). Why people use health services. *Milbank Memorial Fund Quarterly, 44*, 94–127.

Sikkema, K. J., & Kelly, J. A. (1996). Behavioral medicine interventions can improve the quality of life and health of persons with HIV disease. *Annals of Behavioral Medicine, 18*, 40–48.

Smith, Q., Smith, L., King, K., Frieden, L., & Richards, L. (1993). *Health care reform, independent living, and people with disabilities.* Houston, TX: Independent Living Research Utilization Program.

Thorne, S. (1993). *Negotiating health care: The social context of chronic illness.* Newbury Park, CA: Sage.

von Korff, M., Gruman, J., Schaefer, J., Curry, S. J., & Wagner, E. H. (1997). Collaborative management of chronic illness. *Annals of Internal Medicine, 127*(12), 1097–1102.

Woodend, A. K., Nair, R. C., & Tang, A. S-L. (1997). Definition of life quality from a patient versus health care professional perspective. *International Journal of Rehabilitation Research 20*(1), 71–80.

# 8

# *The Mind-Body-Spirit Connection*

I had a really amazing experience today. If I hadn't seen it for myself, I would have thought somebody was making this stuff up—or at least really exaggerating. As part of my clinical rotation, I am assigned to the Wellness Clinic, affiliated with the hospital. I have been attending the Stress Management class, which met once a week for seven weeks. The clients learned many different techniques: meditation, mindfulness, exercises, diet, etc. There was even some discussion about the role of prayer.

Last night was the last session of the class, and the clients were talking about what changes they had made since they started attending. It was incredible. One woman had lowered her blood pressure 10 points. Another had decreased her neck pain from 8 down to 2, on a scale of 1 to 10. Someone else is now able to fall asleep without using medication. I guess this stuff really works! I'd really like to know how. It seems like the activities are so simple, but the effects are so powerful.

—*From the journal of Fred Morris, nursing student*

Although physical dysfunction is the most common reason that people seek health care services, it is impossible to treat the body without consideration of the mind and spirit as well. This chapter describes the interrelatedness of the mind, body, and spirit, explores the historical basis for a holistic approach to health care, and provides some concrete strategies for addressing the client as a whole in health care practice.

# Holism

The biomedical model of health care places the emphasis on curing rather than on healing. When clients do not get "well," health providers may feel as though they have failed, while clients may feel abandoned and unsupported. In contrast, a holistic approach, based on a biopsychosocial model of health care, considers social, cultural, and emotional histories and beliefs about illness and health care (Engel, 1977). The holistic approach recognizes that each person is unique and requires care that encompasses mind, body, spirit, culture, and family and social support systems. Halstead (2001) has termed this "humanistic care" because it requires the skills of personal interaction, caring, and compassion.

When clients entrust us with their care, it is important to view each one individually and to include each dimension of the human experience—physical, psychological, and spiritual—in our examination and plan of care. There is a significant body of research to support this holistic approach to health care. Kenneth Pelletier has done extensive work in behavioral medicine, clinical biofeedback, and neurophysiology. He notes that a holistic approach to client care helps us to more fully understand the needs of our clients. As health care providers, we cannot limit ourselves to the client's physical dimension. Each client's world includes family, friends, coworkers, job and living situations, early background, self-concept, and role in the environment (Pelletier, 1977). When the mind or spirit is in a state of distress, the body is also affected. Conversely, when the body is unhealthy, the mind and spirit may be negatively affected.

Interest in holistic medicine has increased steadily over the past decade. Clients are anxious to learn about and try anything that might improve their health. A growing body of scientific literature supports the benefits of client education, meaningful involvement, and empowerment. However, clients often lack the discernment needed to evaluate the wide range of alternative and complementary interventions for which information is readily available.

Health care providers may need to assist clients in choosing appropriate options. There are several published guides that providers may find useful in evaluating the appropriateness of various practices or techniques (Cohen, 1998; Jonas & Levin, 1999; Novey, 2000; O'Mathuna & Larimore, 2001; Reisser, Mabe, & Velarde, 2001; Spencer & Jacobs, 1999). Novey (2000) recommends careful examination of the following evidence before recommending any type of alternative or complementary practice, such as acupuncture, herbal remedies, or yoga, to ensure that the recommendations fit client needs:

- Origin
- Indication for use
- Evidence of efficacy
- Mechanism for action
- Required training for practitioner
- Safety
- Contraindications

The role of spirituality has received particular attention (Koenig, 1999; Matthews, 1998; McBride, 1999), largely due to the support of the International Center for the Integration of Health and Spirituality (ICIHS). By providing funding for research in this area, ICIHS hopes to supply both professionals and the public with information that promotes a comprehensive understanding of how the interaction of spirituality and health influences our lives (International Center for the Integration of Health and Spirituality, 2002).

Scientists and clinicians who are skeptical about the value of spirituality in health care claim that there is inadequate scientific evidence to support the claims made. In part, this is due to the presiding culture in Western medicine. Mental and physical health care have long been considered separate and isolated systems. However, the structural and financial constraints of the current health care system have fragmented physical health care even further. For example, the cardiovascular system is treated and studied independently of the immune system, unrelated to the brain and nervous system. Fortunately, this trend has been changing because of the work supported by ICIHS and others.

# Spirituality

Spirituality can be broadly defined as the life force in each of us (Craigie & Hobbs, 1999). The spirit, or soul, is an immaterial entity that motivates and inspires. Like the mind and body, the spirit requires adequate "nourishment" and "exercise" to remain healthy. That is, spiritual energy must be replenished on a regular basis. Clients who are hospitalized due to illness or disability can lose access to support systems, spiritual resources, and spiritual practices. A healthy spirit may positively influence the body and mind, so the care plan must address clients' spiritual needs. This does not mean that all health care providers should be equipped to meet the spiritual needs of clients, but we all have a responsibility to provide guidance and/or referral to appropriate resources. There can be great value in simply reminding our clients to access their preexisting spiritual strength in difficult times (McColl et al., 2000).

Spirituality takes the form of religious faith for the majority of people in the United States. Based on 1999 Gallup polls, 86 percent of the population believes in God, and another 8 percent believes in a "universal spirit/higher power" (Gallup Poll, 1999). Others achieve spiritual fulfillment by alternative means, but an unmistakable energy or power is central to all spiritual practices. Meditation, yoga, tai chi, and even simple altruism can all be considered spiritual. A general awareness of the scope of spiritual expression is important if we are to understand our clients' spiritual health and needs.

# Ancient Insights and Modern Practices

The body of knowledge that supports holistic care has an early foundation. In medieval times, health care providers understood that the mind, body, and spirit were inseparable (Chopra, 1993; Newman, 1998). Hildegard of Bingen, a twelfth-century nun and health care practitioner, was a proponent of a low-fat diet, rich in fresh fruits and vegetables, whole grains, and seafood, no sugar, and minimal salt and alcohol. Prescribed treatment regimens consisted of fasting, herbal remedies, and other detoxifying techniques. Meditation, introspection, and prayer were essential components of treatment (Newman, 1998).

The techniques of St. Hildegard were not unlike those that formed the basis of Ayurveda, the ancient Indian medical science. Ayurveda stems from the Vedas, India's ancient books of knowledge. The literal translation of the term *Ayurveda* is life (Ayu) science (Veda) (Chauhan, 1998). Control of one's own physiology is gained through the use of herbs, diet, massage, exercise, music, and meditation. These ancient traditions form the basis of the practice of Deepak Chopra, an endocrinologist who directs The Chopra Center for Well-Being in LaJolla, California. The Center boasts an exceptionally high rate of spontaneous cancer remission. Critics of the practice are quick to point out that this high rate may simply be due to the fact that the Center is looking for and measuring this phenomenon, while other practices do not necessarily collect this information (Chopra, 1993). Clients often visit Chopra's Center as a last resort. When they learn that a cure may be possible, it comes into the realm of believable. The belief and expectations generated by the relationship between client and care provider are intended to influence the outcome, and apparently, they do. Chopra believes that success in the program depends on the client's ability to activate the internal "pharmacy" and natural defenses of the body. By achieving a balance in and awareness of the mind, body, and spirit connection, a person can help control bodily functions. Among the many reported benefits of his program are control of heart rate, blood pressure, gastric acid secretion, and bowel motility.

Herbert Benson, of the Mind/Body Institute at the Beth Israel Deaconess Medical Center and Harvard Medical School in Boston, Massachusetts, has been teaching the relaxation response to his clients for many years (Benson, 1996). He incorporates several of the same concepts that Chopra uses in his practice. Benson describes his model of care as a three-legged stool. One leg is based on the use of medications. The second relies on the use of medical procedures, including surgery, to correct physical problems. The third leg of the stool represents self-care practices. Clients are taught the importance of managing their stress, eating well, and exercising (Benson & Stuart, 1992). An important aspect of Benson's self-care program is the client's inner belief system and its ability to promote healing.

Benson and Chopra agree that the *placebo effect* may play an important role in clients' responses. The placebo effect is based on the expectations of both the client and the health care provider that the treatment will actually help. There is significant scientific evidence to support the relevance of client and practitioner belief systems in the overall care of clients. The placebo effect is one of the most powerful techniques available to us. When the placebo effect takes place, it is an indication that the client has been able to activate his or her own internal "pharmacy," a source that is much more accurate and effective than externally administered drugs (Benson & Stuart, 1992; Chopra, 1993; Stefano, Fricchione, Slingsby, & Benson, 2001).

One important component of practicing self-care is daily stress management. Benson teaches clients to meditate once or twice daily for 20 minutes. Kabat-Zinn (1990) also incorporates daily meditation at the Stress Management Clinic at the University of Massachusetts Medical Center in Worcester, Massachusetts. Dean Ornish (1990), who has done pioneering work in reversing heart disease, is also a proponent of meditation. Although practices vary, three essential features are common to the techniques of meditation (Benson, 1996). First, the person must sit or lie in a quiet and comfortable place. Second, the person must clear his or her mind of all thoughts, ideas, worries, and distractions. Finally, the individual uses a focal point, such as a word, sound, or phrase. Another technique is to focus on the breath (Kabat-Zinn, 1990). Yoga, tai chi, karate, and chi qong have all been described as moving meditation and are believed to have the same beneficial effects (Chen & Snyder, 1999; Ross, Bohannon, Davis, & Gurchiek, 1999).

The common denominator in all these practices is clearing the mind of all stresses. Hans Selye, often referred to as the "father of stress," was a pioneer in psychosomatic medicine. He described stress as an integral element in any living being (Selye, 1974). Responding to stress may be part of our biological makeup, but it is also healthy to keep it balanced. Clearing the mind of stressful thoughts elicits the relaxation response (Benson, 1996), which turns off the arousing effects of the sympathetic nervous system. The body returns to a calmer state, improving immune system function and cardiovascular health, and diminishing anxiety and depression (Benson, 1996; Kabat-Zinn, 1990; Koenig, 1999; Ornish, 1990).

Researchers have demonstrated that the active practice of prayer, along with a positive attitude, healthy lifestyle, and substantial physical and emotional support of the community, significantly improves medical outcomes (Benson, 1996; Koenig, 1999; Matthews, 1998; McCullough & Larson, 1999; Meyers, 1999). Although the studies are too numerous for our discussion, the following list highlights the wide range of documented health benefits that have been found among adults who practice their spiritual beliefs on a regular basis:

- Significantly reduced blood pressure
- Stronger immune systems
- Fewer health problems
- Fewer hospitalizations
- Shorter lengths of stay when hospitalized
- Stronger social support systems
- Stronger family ties
- Stronger and healthier marriages
- Stronger sense of well-being and acceptance
- Lower rates of depression

The mental health benefits of regular spiritual practices are not limited to adults. Adolescents who practice their spirituality are significantly less likely to consider suicide, use drugs or alcohol, or engage in delinquent behaviors or in early sexual activity (Donahue & Benson, 1995).

While many clients believe positive outcomes are the result of divine intervention, scientists offer alternative explanations. According to Koenig (1999), deep spiritual belief and regular attendance at religious services are generally accompanied by positive health habits, including healthy eating, regular wellness care, compliance with medical advice, and abstinence from drinking, smoking, and unsafe sexual practices. In addition, the social support offered by a religious community prevents isolation and may even provide physical or financial support for those in need.

Some researchers argue that it is the healthy lifestyle that is responsible for all of the measured health benefits. Certainly, a healthy lifestyle can strengthen the immune system, lower stress levels, decrease the sympathetic nervous system response, and promote early detection of illness. Whether the positive benefits can be explained in scientific or spiritual terms, it is clear that the inner peace of a deep, personal faith is beneficial to many of our clients (Koenig, 1999; Matthews, 1998).

# Mind-Body-Spirit

The essential connection between the mind, body, and spirit exists in the limbic system, which lies deep in the brain at the level of the midbrain and brainstem. The limbic system is the emotional center of the body, and it is responsible for regulation of the autonomic nervous system (ANS). Table 8–1 provides a summary of the limbic system functions. The ANS has two complementary subsystems, the sympathetic nervous system (SNS) and the parasympathetic nervous system (PNS). In a healthy person, these two systems act collaboratively to maintain a steady state, as well as to ensure the efficiency of our automatic survival skills (Umphred, 1995).

The SNS responds to rapid or unexpected change. Fear, anger, or arousal of any kind will stimulate the SNS to become active. All systems of our body are affected. This generalized response has been described as a "fight-or-flight response." Identified by Walter Cannon of Harvard Medical School in the early 1900s, this response involves involuntary physiological changes. When an individual perceives a situation as challenging, the sympathetic response occurs automatically (Cannon, 1929).

Once activated, the SNS causes constriction of blood vessels and an increase in blood pressure, heart rate, and respiratory rate. The pupils dilate, and the threshold of sensory receptors is lowered. Blood is shunted away from the brain and digestive system and directed to the muscles. Muscle tension is increased. We become hypervigilant, prepared for any change in the environment. In this heightened state of arousal, we may be unable to concentrate or focus on other ideas. Sleep is difficult or impossible.

**TABLE 8–1**    The Limbic System—The Emotional Brain (Responsible for Physical and Emotional Survival)

*Memory and Cognition*
- Stores memories with a social or emotional connection
- Monitors incoming information and "decides" what to remember
- Compares incoming information to previous information and "decides" how to respond
- Provides motivation for action

*Emotions, Mood, Social Skills*
- Regulates emotional state and mood
- Organizes social behaviors
- Facilitates self-concept and self-esteem
- Develops attitudes and opinions about the external world

*Autonomic System*
- Heart rate, blood pressure, breathing
- Hunger, thirst, digestion, elimination, fluid regulation
- Temperature regulation, sweating
- Attention, arousal, alertness, focus, concentration
- Muscle tone, posture, readiness to act
- Controls level of sensory stimulation allowed

This response is so powerful that people have been known to lift cars off victims in order to save lives. Without the assistance of the SNS, such feats of valor and strength would not be possible. Many of the stresses faced in daily life, however, are ongoing and continuous. It is generally not healthy to maintain the response over time. It activates the release of three hormones by the adrenal glands: epinephrine, norepinephrine, and cortisol. Epinephrine and norepinephrine produce the "adrenaline rush" that we feel when we are angry, afraid, or aroused. Cortisol initially produces anti-inflammatory effects, but when released over time, it acts to suppress the immune system. This can leave the body susceptible to infectious, autoimmune, and neoplastic disease (Koenig, 1999; Kremer, 1999).

While the SNS is responsible for mediating fight-or-flight reactions, the PNS supports the opposite responses. A calm, unchanging, nonthreatening environment allows the PNS to decrease the blood pressure, heart rate, and respiratory rate. Blood is shunted away from the muscles and directed to the brain and digestive system. Tension and muscle tone are reduced (Umphred, 1995). We no longer feel the need to escape from danger, so we can concentrate on learning and social activities. We are able to sleep. The contrasting functions of the SNS and PNS are outlined in Table 8–2.

It is important to realize that perceived stress, threat, or danger can trigger a SNS state. For example, for most adults, the sight of a young child rushing into the street in front of a car will trigger a SNS response and all of its uncomfortable sensations. The sight of a friendly

**TABLE 8–2**   The Autonomic Nervous System

| Sympathetic—Stimulating | Parasympathetic—Relaxing |
|---|---|
| Arousal, fight or flight response | Relaxation, focused attention |
| Stimulus: Fear, excitement, anger, pain | Stimulus: Safe, familiar, trust, lack of change |
| Sensory overload or bombardment overload | Lack of stimulation or sensory overload |
| Possible Responses: | Possible Responses: |
| • Increased respiratory rate | • Decreased respiratory rate |
| • Increased heart rate and blood pressure | • Decreased heart rate and blood pressure |
| • Blood gets shunted to muscles | • Blood gets shunted to brain and digestive system |
| • Increased glucose levels & energy | • Decreased glucose levels and energy |
| • Alert, aroused, focused on environment | • Calm, relaxed, content |
| • Cannot sleep | • Fatigue, enhanced sleep |
| • Quick responses, impulsiveness | • Maintained attention, concentration |
| • Enhanced sensory input | • Filtered-out sensory input |
| • Survival responses to change | • Slow, thoughtful responses |
| • Happy, angry, aroused, excited, afraid | • Focused, emotionally bonded |
| • Agitated, irritable, aggressive | • Bored, withdrawn, apathetic |
| • Hyperactive | • Lethargic, shut down, confused |
| • Disorganized responses | • Coma, catatonic |
| Sensory Input: | Sensory Input: |
| • Quick, fast, light, bright colors | • Slow, maintained, dull, pleasant |
| • Loud, fast-changing, movement | • Quiet, soft, smooth, warm, firm, rhythmic |
| • Hot, cold, forceful, unexpected, rough | • Moderate, unchanging, predictable |

dog could trigger the same SNS response if the person has a fearful memory of dogs. Conversely, when there is a perception of safety, the PNS maintains the bodily functions at a level that supports a calm, yet alert, state.

Both the SNS and PNS are needed to maintain homeostasis and to support our ability to respond appropriately to changes in the environment. The optimal healthy state is achieved when there is a balance between the two systems. The person is able to focus attention on the matters of everyday life but has a healthy readiness to react to stress. In our stressful, stimuli-filled culture, the SNS seems to be chronically overactive. Over time, this can create a constant state of hypervigilance and chronic stress, leading to an increased susceptibility to illness (Kabat-Zinn, 1990).

As mentioned earlier, the ANS is housed in the limbic system. The limbic system is the part of our brain where emotional memories are stored and emotional responses are mediated (Whybrow, 1997). Two important emotional functions occur here. One function allows us to make emotional attachments and bond with other people. This includes our ability to respond to others in a nurturing way. The limbic system also monitors the sensory information received and interprets it for emotional content. All incoming information is compared to emotional history. Through this process, we decide what to think and feel about new information based on our prior experiences, which influence our perception of new information. Does the current situation appear to be pleasant and something we want to approach? Is there a potential threat or harm we need to avoid? Based on our appraisal of the situation, we decide how to emotionally respond. The final perception of any situation causes a corresponding output from the ANS.

It is truly fascinating that the part of our brain that supports the automatic physical functions of our cardiopulmonary, digestive, musculoskeletal, and central nervous systems is the same area that controls our emotions, moods, and responses to emotional stimulation. At the most basic level of the brain, the mind, body, and spirit are intimately related. What affects one will inevitably affect the other.

Joan Borysenko, a cell biologist, psychologist, and yoga and meditation instructor, cites three intriguing anecdotes (Borysenko, 1987). In the first, a person with multiple personality disorder has diabetes in one identity but not in others. Second, a woman under hypnosis develops a blister on her skin when the hypnotist touches her with a "hot iron," which is really a pencil. Third, in one clinical test, one-third of the subjects in the placebo group lost their hair in response to "chemotherapy." Given these profound examples, it is easy to see that, as health care providers, we can access the interrelatedness of the body, mind, and spirit to help achieve desired treatment outcomes.

# Psychoneuroimmunology

To help us understand the interrelatedness between the mind, the body, and the spirit, psychologists, immunologists, and neuroscientists have teamed together to form the field of psychoneuroimmunology (PNI) (Borysenko, 1987). This area of study is concerned with the complex interactions between the central nervous system (CNS) and the immune system. These interactions are bidirectional. That is, the CNS, in mediating both physical and psychological control mechanisms, affects the immune system, and the immune system affects the CNS (Solomon,

1987). For example, personality factors, stress, and negative emotions such as anxiety, depression, and loneliness have been linked to the onset and course of autoimmune diseases, such as rheumatoid arthritis, allergies, systemic lupus erythematosus (commonly known as lupus or SLE), cancer, and acquired immune deficiency syndrome (AIDS) (Bahnson, 1980; Solomon, 1981, 1987).

The mechanisms that control psychoneuroimmunologic functions are quite complex. As we have already discussed, the limbic system monitors all incoming stimuli, controls our emotional state and responses, and supports all autonomic functions. When events occur that are perceived as stressful, the limbic system triggers the hypothalamus to secrete neuropeptides that activate the SNS and the pituitary gland. The pituitary gland releases adrenocorticotropic hormone, which stimulates the adrenal cortex to secrete cortisol and other corticosteroids. These neurohormones decrease immune system function and leave the body susceptible to infectious diseases, autoimmune diseases, and neoplastic disease (Kremer, 1999). Activities that diminish the stress response, such as religious attendance, prayer, counseling, and meditation, have a powerful effect on lowering circulating levels of immunosuppressive substances (Koenig, 1999).

The presence of chronic stress has been shown to influence how individuals respond to acute stress. People who have high levels of chronic stress respond to acute stress with higher levels of perceived distress, increased levels of stress hormone production, and decreased levels of natural killer cell production. Furthermore, recovery time from acute stress is delayed (Pike et al., 1997).

Studies have also shown that surgery depresses immune function. The combined effects of surgical trauma, anxiety, and postoperative pain increase the blood levels of stress hormones (Kremer, 1999). It has been proposed that administering effective levels of pain medication postoperatively, along with the practice of anxiety-reducing relaxation techniques, may decrease the stress response of the body and, in turn, decrease the postoperative susceptibility to infection.

When clients receive psychotherapy or psychotropic medications to reverse depressive symptoms, they experience a decrease in the immunosuppressive substances circulating in the blood (Stein, Keller, & Schleifer, 1985). Other stress-reducing strategies can also enhance the function and health of the immune system. Regular participation in a spiritual community and routine practice of meditation or prayer have been shown to effectively diminish the stress response (Koenig, 1999). In one particular study, an increased rate of healing was observed when standard psoriasis treatment was coupled with mindfulness meditation (Kabat-Zinn et al., 1998).

# Pulling It All Together

Today, I had the weirdest experience. I was doing an intake evaluation on this client, Dick. He recently experienced a right cerebrovascular accident and now has a significant left hemiplegia. He told me that twelve years ago he had been diagnosed with terminal pancreatic cancer. His only symptom was that he had become jaundiced. When he went to the doctor, he was given a full workup, which resulted in his being rushed into surgery for a Whipple procedure. The surgeon had to close him right back up because the cancer had completely consumed his pancreas and had spread to the surrounding organs. He was given six to eight weeks to live.

Now here's the strange part. He mentioned that he just prayed and prayed—he knew that he could beat the cancer. He opted to have chemotherapy and radiation to "extend his life." There was no promise for a cure. After nearly dying from the treatment, he has done reasonably well. His last MRI, done three years ago, showed that he is cancer-free! I don't know too much about cure rates in cancer, but it was my understanding that pancreatic cancer is usually terminal.

Now, he's had a fairly massive stroke. What makes it difficult for me is that he thinks his prayers will cure him once more. I've seen a few other clients who have had strokes. Although they did get some return of function, none were actually "cured," especially when they also had arteriosclerosis as bad as this client's. While I don't want to discourage him from his beliefs, I don't want to mislead him either. I wonder if it would be wrong for me to pray with him. I have a fair amount of faith myself, but I'm unsure how much I should incorporate this into our time together.

*—From the journal of Tom Chisholm, social work student*

It is inevitable that we will experience pain and suffering at some point in our lives. This universal experience provides us with a common language by which to communicate with our clients (Nouwen, 1979). It is important to be emotionally honest with our clients and let them know that we recognize and validate their pain whether it is physical, emotional, or spiritual. It is critical, however, to respect professional boundaries. To say, "I know what you're going through" or "I know what you feel" is dishonest and may even be perceived as condescending and patronizing. The fact is that we really do not know.

Each health care discipline has its own set of ethical guidelines. It is our duty to carefully consider these and any other applicable codes of conduct to ensure that the client–professional relationship is not breached. Our clients are dependent on us in many ways. They must never feel that the care to which they are entitled is dependent on meeting some unstated, but perhaps implied, expectation of the health care provider.

Clients' spiritual strength can help them overcome the limitations and disappointments inherent in situations of illness and injury. In spite of significant advances in medicine, there are still many diseases and conditions that cannot be cured, and many treatment options are accompanied by serious side effects. Diabetes, arthritis, mental illness, spinal cord injury, and AIDS, for example, cannot yet be cured, but the process of healing can be facilitated. Healing restores the person to a sense of wholeness, even if the disease or condition remains present. Clients who are able to draw effectively upon their spirituality can greatly benefit from this in their healing process. Anything that buffers stress or provides emotional support is important (Benson, 1996; Koenig, 1999; McColl et al., 2000).

It is appropriate for us to use all available therapeutic agents to help our clients recover. We commonly encourage good nutrition, exercise, stress-reduction techniques, and adequate sleep. Knowing that spirituality can positively influence healing, we must also address this. Determine how each client nourishes his or her spirit. Some may rely on the serenity of an afternoon walk on the beach, others may find peace in prayer or meditation, and still others may need to reconnect with a certain community for support or encouragement.

Many primary care providers have begun to incorporate spiritual assessment tools in the examination of their clients (Hatch, Burg, Naberhaus, & Hellmich, 1998; McBride, Pilkington, & Arthur, 1998; McKee & Chappel, 1992; Puchalski, 1999). The tools vary in specific design but seek to determine the client's spiritual beliefs, the significance of these beliefs to the client, and how the medical provider can best integrate these beliefs into the care of the client. Perhaps assessment of spirituality will be standard practice in the future. There is already evidence that including the healing powers of spirituality and faith into care plans can help improve quality of life and the outcomes of our interventions for some clients.

If you share common spiritual practices with your clients, and they initiate the request for your spiritual support, there is no legal or ethical reason to refuse. However, some health care providers are more comfortable with their own spirituality than others. If you believe that it is beyond the scope of your professional practice to address the clients' spiritual needs yourself, then you can politely decline. Either way, a referral to spiritual counsel would be appropriate. Regardless of how the task is accomplished, helping clients address mental or physical barriers that are blocking their access to spiritual practices is important.

Consider the client who has sustained a cervical level spinal cord injury whose spiritual practice involves weekly attendance at a local church. Physical accommodations, such as ramps or physical assistance to overcome stairs, would be relatively easy to arrange. However, if the client is experiencing anger as part of the grieving process or fear of facing the community with a new, fragile, and altered sense of self, the issues are more complex. As in every aspect of clinical practice, we must examine the needs of our clients as individuals, establishing an effective plan for each problem. At times, we can accomplish the problem-solving alone. Sometimes, referral to others who are better trained to deal with the problems is appropriate.

## SUMMARY

This chapter discussed the importance of viewing our clients as whole beings rather than focusing on illness or disability. The interrelatedness of the mind, body, and spirit is well documented and has been summarized here. The benefits of addressing each of these health dimensions can lead to significantly improved outcomes.

## REFLECTIVE QUESTIONS

1. What practices do you use to help yourself feel calm in a crisis or to overcome feelings of sadness or loss?
2. Do you use any of the mind–body–spirit techniques discussed?
   a. If yes, how often do you use these practices?
   b. If yes, describe them and their effect on you.
   c. If not, why not?
   d. If not, would you consider using them in the future?
3. a. Which mind–body–spirit techniques might you use with clients?
   b. How do you think you could incorporate them into your plan of care?
   c. What would you do if a client asked you to pray with him or her?

**4. a.** How do you think you might respond to someone whose beliefs or spiritual practices are different from your own?
  **b.** What if you found the beliefs or practices to be offensive?
**5. a.** Do you think your clients' spiritual or religious beliefs should be part of your examination and assessment?
  **b.** Why or why not?

## CASE STUDY

Ruth Parker is a 54-year-old woman who faces many stressors in her life, both at work and at home. She presents with a host of physical problems, including headaches, hypertension, generalized anxiety, and insomnia.

Her physician has recommended medications, but she is reluctant to use any of them. Instead, she asks if other alternatives are available.

**1. a.** What is there about Mrs. Parker's life circumstances that might be contributing to her health problems?
  **b.** Provide a physiological rationale for your response.
**2.** What interventions could you recommend for Mrs. Parker that do not include medications?
**3.** Provide a rationale for each intervention you identified in question 2.
**4.** Mrs. Parker tells you that her neighbor uses copper bracelets and magnets to treat her arthritis and asks whether this might be helpful for her. How might you respond?

## REFERENCES

Bahnson, C. B. (1980). Stress and cancer, state of the art (Pt. 1). *Psychosomatics, 21,* 975–981.

Benson, H. (1996). *Timeless healing: The power and biology of belief.* New York: Scribner.

Benson, H., & Stuart, E. (1992). *The wellness book: The comprehensive guide to maintaining health and treating stress-related illness.* New York: Fireside.

Borysenko, J. (1987). *Minding the body, mending the mind.* New York: Bantam Books.

Cannon, W. B. (1929). *Bodily changes in pain, hunger, fear and rage.* New York: Appleton.

Chauhan, P. S. (1998). Ayurveda: The traditional Indian medical science. In *Ayurvedic* [Online]. Available: http://www.ayurvedic.org/. Date accessed: 1/2/02.

Chen, K. M., & Snyder, M. (1999). A research-based use of tai chi/movement therapy as a nursing intervention. *Journal of Holistic Nursing, 17*(3), 267–279.

Chopra, D. (1993). *The healing mind: Ancient wisdom, modern insights* [Videotape]. Lancaster, MA: The Maharishi Ayurveda Health Center.

Cohen, M. H. (1998). *Complementary and alternative medicine: Legal boundaries and regulatory perspectives.* Baltimore: Johns Hopkins University Press.

Craigie, F. C., Jr., & Hobbs, R. F., III. (1999). Spiritual perspectives and practices of family physicians with expressed interest in spirituality. *Family Medicine, 31*(8), 578–585.

Donahue, M. J., & Benson, P. (1995). Religion and the well-being of adolescents. *Journal of Social Issues, 51*(2), 145–160.

Engel, G. L. (1977). The need for a new medical model: A challenge for biomedicine. *Science, 196,* 129–136.

Gallup Poll. (1999). Gallup Poll topics: A-Z. Religion. In *The Gallup Organization* [Online]. Available: http://www.gallup.com/poll/indicators/indreligion4.asp

Halstead, L. S. (2001). The power of compassion and caring in rehabilitation healing. *Archives of Physical Medicine and Rehabilitation, 82,* 149–154.

Hatch, R. L., Burg, M. A., Naberhaus, D. S., & Hellmich, L. K. (1998). The Spiritual Involvement and Beliefs Scale: Development and testing of a new instrument. *Journal of Family Practice, 46*(6), 476–486.

International Center for the Integration of Health and Spirituality. (2002). About ICIHS. In *International Center for the Integration of Health and Spirituality* [Online]. Available: http://icihs.org/abouticihs/abouticihs.asp

Jonas, W. B., & Levin, J. S. (1999). *Essentials of complementary and alternative medicine.* New York: Lippincott, Williams & Wilkins.

Kabat-Zinn, J. (1990). *Full catastrophe living: Using the wisdom of your body and mind to face stress, pain, and illness.* New York: Delta.

Kabat-Zinn, J., Wheeler, E., Light, T., Skillings, A., Scharf, M. J., Cropley, T. G., Hosmer, D., & Bernhard, J. D. (1998). Influence of a mindfulness meditation-based stress reduction intervention on rates of skin clearing in patients with moderate to severe psoriasis undergoing phototherapy (UVB) and photochemotherapy (PUVA). *Psychosomatic Medicine, 60,* 625–632.

Koenig, H. G. (1999). *The healing power of faith: Science explores medicine's last great frontier.* New York: Simon & Schuster.

Kremer, M. (1999). Surgery, pain and immune function. *CRNA: The Clinical Forum for Nurse Anesthetists, 10*(3), 94–100.

Matthews, D. A. (1998). *The faith factor: Proof of the healing power of prayer.* New York: Penguin Books.

McBride, J. L. (1999). The family practice residency curriculum: Is there any place for spirituality and religion? *Family Medicine, 32*(10), 685–686.

McBride, J. L., Pilkington, L., & Arthur, G. (1998). Development of brief pictorial instruments for assessing spirituality in primary care. *Journal of Ambulatory Care Management, 21*(4), 53–61.

McColl, M. A., Bickenback, J., Johnston, J., Nishihama, S., Schumaker, M., Smith, K., Smith, M., & Yealland, B. (2000). Changes in spiritual beliefs after traumatic disability. *Archives of Physical Medicine and Rehabilitation, 81*(6), 817–823.

McCullough, M., & Larson, D. (1999). Religion and depression: A review of the literature. *Twin Research, 2,* 126–139.

McKee, D. D., & Chappel, J. N. (1992). Spirituality and medical practice. *Journal of Family Practice, 35*(2), 201, 205–208.

Meyers, D. G. (1999, December). The pursuit of personal and social healing: What role for spirituality? In H. Benson (Chair), *Spirituality and healing in medicine.* Symposium conducted at the meeting of Harvard Medical School, Department of Continuing Education and Mind/Body Medical Institute, and CareGroup, Beth Israel Deaconess Medical Center, Boston.

Newman, B. (1998). *Voice of the living light: Hildegard of Bingen and her world.* Berkeley: University of California Press.

Nouwen, H. J. M. (1979). *The wounded healer.* New York: Doubleday.

Novey, D. W. (2000). *Clinician's complete reference to complementary/alternative medicine.* St. Louis, MO: Mosby.

O'Mathuna, D., & Larimore, W. (2001). *Alternative medicine: The Christian handbook.* Grand Rapids, MI: Zondervan.

Ornish, D. (1990). *Dr. Dean Ornish's program for reversing heart disease.* New York: Random House.

Pelletier, K. R. (1977). *Mind as healer, mind as slayer: A holistic approach to preventing stress disorders.* New York: Delta/Seymour Lawrence.

Pike, J. L., Smith, T. L., Hauger, R. L., Nicassio, P. M., Patterson, T. L., McClintick, J., Costlow, C., & Irwin, M. R. (1997). Chronic life stress alters sympathetic, neuroendocrine, and immune responsivity to an acute psychological stressor in humans. *Psychosomatic Medicine, 59,* 447–457.

Puchalski, C. M. (1999). FICA: A spiritual assessment. In H. Benson (Chair), *Spirituality and healing in medicine.* Symposium conducted at the meeting of Harvard Medical School, Department of Continuing Education and Mind/Body Medical Institute, and CareGroup, Beth Israel Deaconess Medical Center, Boston.

Reisser, P. C., Mabe, D., & Velarde, R. (2001). *Examining alternative medicine: An inside look at the benefits and risks.* Downers Grove, IL: Intervarsity Press.

Ross, M. C., Bohannon, A. S., Davis, D. C., & Gurchiek, L. (1999). The effects of a short-term exercise program on movement, pain, and mood in the elderly. *Journal of Holistic Nursing, 17*(2), 139–147.

Selye, H. (1974). *Stress without distress.* New York: J. P. Lippincott.

Solomon, G. F. (1981). Emotional and personality factors in the onset and course of autoimmune disease, particularly rheumatoid arthritis. In R. Ader (Ed.), *Psychoneuroimmunology* (pp. 159–179). New York: Academic Press.

Solomon, G. F. (1987). Psychoneuroimmunology: Interactions between central nervous system and immune system. *Journal of Neuroscience Research, 18*(1), 1–9.

Spencer, J., & Jacobs, J. J. (Eds.). (1999). *Complementary and alternative medicine: An evidence-based approach.* St. Louis, MO: Mosby.

Stefano, G. B., Fricchione, G. L., Slingsby, B. T., & Benson, H. (2001). The placebo effect and relaxation response: Neural processes and their coupling to constitutive nitric oxide. *Brain Research Reviews, 35,* 1–19.

Stein, M., Keller, S. E., & Schleifer, S. J. (1985). Stress and immunomodulation: The role of depression and neuroendocrine function. *Journal of Immunology, 135,* 827–833.

Umphred, D. (1995). *Neurological rehabilitation* (3rd ed.). St. Louis, MO: Mosby.

Whybrow, P. C. (1997). *A mood apart: The thinker's guide to emotion and its disorders.* New York: HarperPerennial.

# ADDITIONAL READINGS FOR PART II

Albert, S., & Logsdon, R. (2000). *Assessing quality of life in Alzheimer's disease.* New York: Springer.

Annas, G. (1992). *The rights of patients: The basic guide to patient rights (an American Civil Liberties Union handbook)* (2nd ed.). Totowa, NJ: Humana Press.

Baker, G. (2001). *Quality of life in epilepsy: Beyond seizure counts in assessment and treatment.* Newark, NJ: Harwood Academic.

Belknap, M. (1997). *Mind–body magic: Creative activities for any audience.* Duluth, MN: Whole Person Associates.

Benson, H. (1993). *The wellness book: A comprehensive guide to maintaining health and treating stress-related injuries.* New York: Simon & Schuster.

Benson, H. (1997). *Timeless healing: The power and biology of belief.* New York: Simon & Schuster.

Benson, H. (2000). *The relaxation response* (2nd ed.). New York: First Wholecare Printing.

Bowling, A. (2001). *Measuring disease: A review of disease-specific quality of life measurement scales* (2nd ed.). Milton Keynes, UK: Open University Press.

Butler, R., Jasmin, C., & Jasmin, C. (2000). *Longevity and quality of life: Opportunities and challenges.* New York: Plenum Press.

Callanan, M., & Kelley, P. (1997). *Final gifts: Understanding the special awareness, needs, and communications of the dying* (rev. ed.). New York: Bantam Books.

Caudill, M. (1994). *Managing pain before it manages you.* New York: Guilford Press.

Cote, L., Sprinzeles, L., Elliot, R., & Cote, L. (2000). *Parkinson's disease and quality of life.* New York: Haworth Press.

Diener, E., & Eunkook, S. (2000). *Culture and subjective well-being (well-being and quality of life).* Cambridge, MA: MIT Press.

Dossey, L. (1999). *Reinventing medicine.* New York: HarperCollins.

Dossey, L. (2001). *Healing beyond the body: Medicine and the infinite reach of the mind.* Boston: Shambhala.

Hanh, T. N. (1975). *The miracle of mindfulness.* Boston: Beacon Press.

Joint Commission on Accreditation of Healthcare Organizations. (1998). *Ethical issues and patient rights across the continuum of care.* Oakbrook Terrace, IL: Author.

Kabat-Zinn, J. (1990). *Full catastrophe living: Using the wisdom of your body and mind to face stress, pain, and illness.* New York: Bantam Books.

Kabat-Zinn, J. (1994). *Wherever you go, there you are.* New York: Hyperion.

Kapp, M. (1999). *Geriatrics and the law: Understanding patient rights and professional responsibilities* (3rd ed.). New York: Springer.

Keating, T. (1999). *Open mind, open heart* (3rd ed.). New York: Continuum.

Kessler, D. (2000). *The needs of the dying: A guide for bringing hope, comfort, and love to life's final chapter* (rev. ed.). New York: HarperCollins.

King, D. (2000). *Faith, spirituality, and medicine* (2nd ed.). New York: Haworth Press.

Koot, H. (2001). *Quality of life in child and adolescent illness: Concepts, methods, and findings.* Newark, NJ: Harwood Academic.

Lassey, W., & Lassey, M. (2000). *Quality of life for older people: An international perspective.* Upper Saddle River, NJ: Prentice-Hall.

Matthews, D. (1998). *The faith factor: Proof of the healing power of prayer.* New York: Penguin.

Matzo, M., & Shermann, D. (2001). *Palliative care nursing—quality care to the end of life.* New York: Springer.

Noelker, L., & Harel, Z. (2000). *Linking quality of long-term care and quality of life.* New York: Springer.

Payne, R. (1995). *Relaxation techniques.* Edinburgh, UK: Churchill Livingstone.

Peck, M. (1998). *Further along the road less traveled: The unending journey toward spiritual growth* (3rd ed.). New York: Simon & Schuster.

Remen, R. (1996). *Kitchen table wisdom: Stories that heal.* New York: Riverhead Books.

Rubinstein, R., & Moss, M. (2000). *The many dimensions of aging.* New York: Springer.

Schwartz, C., & Sprangers, M. (2000). *Adaptation to changing health: Response shift in quality-of-life research.* Washington, DC: American Psychological Association.

Shapiro, M. (1999). *What you need to know about HMOs and the patient's bill of rights.* Santa Cruz, CA: Crossing Press.

Siegel, B. (1990). *Peace, love and healing.* New York: Harper & Row.

Siegel, B. (1998). *Love, medicine and miracles* (2nd ed.). New York: HarperCollins.

Spiro, H., Curnen, M., Wandel, L., & Wandel, L. (1998). *Facing death: Where culture, religion, and medicine meet.* New Haven, CT: Yale University Press.

Sulmasy, D. (1997). *The healer's calling: A spirituality for physicians and other health care professionals.* Mahwah, NJ: Paulist Press.

VandeCreek, L. (1998). *Scientific and pastoral perspectives on intercessory prayer.* New York: Harrington Park Press.

Weil, A. (1996). *Spontaneous healing: How to discover and enhance your body's natural ability to maintain and heal itself.* New York: Ballantine Books.

Wilson, P. (1999). *Calm at work.* New York: Penguin.

# Part III

# *Changing Perspectives*

Health professionals actively foster clients' adjustment and acceptance of changes that occur, secondary to illness or injury. Part III focuses on personal changes related to body image and self-concept, condition-specific characteristics, and sexuality.

Psychosocial aspects of body image, highlighted in Chapter 9, form a complex framework by which people understand themselves and perceive how others understand them. Body image is so inextricably associated with self-concept, identity, and ego that a variation in one variable may modify others. This relationship affects a person's response to changes in body image from disease or injury and is influenced by many factors, such as prior loss, prognosis for treatment and recovery, personal control, and a host of other elements. People perceive the meaning of physical effects differently. The nature of the current loss, including if it is a sudden-onset, chronic, or progressive course, can alter how a person manages the changes in body image. Strategies for health providers to facilitate clients' adaptation and acceptance include communication, education and support, and emphasizing capabilities for life's activities.

Although there are common themes for psychosocial issues for people who have disease and injury, disability-specific characteristics exist. Chapter 10 focuses on a representative group of disabilities that affect people across the lifespan. Developmental disabilities influence growth and maturation and have an impact on all aspects of life. Sudden-onset disabilities may result in a disruption of body image, as well as temporal disorientation, a range of emotions, and grieving. People facing acute or rapidly progressive diseases may share these responses. Many deal with existential well-being, particularly when the situation is life threatening. Older people may have multiple problems with which to cope, including the possibility of dementia and death.

Another significant facet of understanding oneself is sexuality. As a determinant in interpersonal relationships, sexuality involves gender identity, attractiveness, attitudes, and practices. It is explored in Chapter 11, using a developmental context to integrate biological, psychological, social, cultural, and behavioral dimensions into each stage of life. Because clients are sensitive to the perceived and actual attitudes of health providers, effective care encompasses accurate knowledge, positive attitudes, and understanding. Clinical interventions, including the taking of a sexual history, are described.

# 9

# *Body Image and Self-Concept*

That could be me, sitting in a wheelchair with right hemiplegia and aphasia, waiting for speech therapy to begin. I take the same birth control pills that caused Lisa's stroke. I also have two young kids at home. Most of my clients who have had strokes are in their 60s, 70s, and 80s, not 35! This one's too close for comfort. I'm not used to working with a client whose life parallels mine.

When I brought Lisa into the treatment room and placed her in front of a mirror, she began to cry. I wondered if she was emotionally labile or if she's justifiably upset about how much her life has changed. Can she be both? To think, only last week she was juggling a career as an executive in this hospital, and a home, husband, and two preschool-age kids! I don't think I can handle this.

—*From the journal of Alma Jackson, speech-language pathology student*

Psychosocial aspects of body image form a complex framework by which a person understands the self and perceives how other people understand him or her. Body image, self-concept, identity, and ego are so closely entwined that a change in one of these elements can affect the others. When a person becomes ill or has an injury, he or she experiences change and loss. There may be changes in physical or mental function, independence, self-image or identity, and body image. This chapter describes the relationship between body image and self-concept, explores responses to changes in body image from disease and injury, and offers strategies to support adjustment to these changes.

In the first half of the twentieth century, it was believed that self-image was represented neurologically in the brain. The concept of body image was defined by postural and bodily movements (Head, 1920). Later, psychological constructs (Schilder, 1950) were added to the mix. Today's perspective recognizes that body image includes how people *look* and how they *think* they look (Laufer, 1991). Social, cultural, and personal attitudes and beliefs, plus an individual's internal history relating to the body, help form part of the self-concept. Elements of this aspect of the self-concept include physical strength, endurance, abilities, and perceptions of masculinity, femininity, and physical attractiveness. Consider a woman whose mother said to her, "Mildred, I don't care what anyone says, I think you're beautiful." What a message to give to someone! In trying to be supportive and complimentary, her mother was simultaneously imbedding a negative message that was to stay with this woman—*always!* We have a lifetime of receiving these messages and putting them into our gunnysack, incorporating them into our own body image.

Society strongly influences our view of ourselves (Monteath & McCabe, 1997). Many people, including Lisa herself in the journal entry at the beginning of this chapter, tend to regard her as not being "normal." Because Lisa's body image is intermingled with her personality, self-image, identity, ego, and sense of worth (Norris, 1970), alterations in her body and its function have the potential to damage more than her physical being (Bronheim, Strain, & Biller, 1991). Bodily changes and her altered self-image disrupt her social and vocational roles, compounding her situation (Drench, 1995).

# Sudden Onset versus Chronic or Progressive Course

Lisa's problems had a sudden onset. Might there be any differences in her situation if it were slowly developing, congenital, or chronic? The Body-Cathexis Scale and the Self-Cathexis Scale, developed by Secord and Jourard, and Kurtzke's Status Disability Scale were used to study perceptions of body image in men with multiple sclerosis (Samonds & Cammermeyer, 1989). Those who had the disease longer, with more physical problems, and were older were more satisfied with themselves and their bodies than other people in the study. Perhaps, unlike Lisa, they were able to adapt to their changes over time because their alterations were gradual.

Might Lisa's altered physical situation have had a different effect on her if she were *born* with the right hemiplegia, perhaps from cerebral palsy? There may be differences in body image between acquired and congenital impairments, but this may not be universal. People with acquired problems—quadriplegia secondary to traumatic spinal cord injury—were compared to people with congenital problems—cerebral palsy (Stensman, 1989). All of the people used wheelchairs and needed assistance with daily activities. No significant differences in body image were identified between the groups.

The sudden onset of acquired problems, such as trauma, can have a "shock value," leaving the person unprepared for the abrupt disruption in body image, self-concept, and lifestyle. Consider a client who was changing a car tire on the shoulder of the road when another car sped by him, ripping his right leg off below the knee. Unlike many other clients with severe vascular disease who faced surgical amputation, this man had no time to psychologically prepare for the traumatic loss of his limb and subsequent changes in his life. This "shock" hampered both his adjustment to the loss and his progress in rehabilitation.

Whether the injury or illness is acute, chronic, or progressive, physical changes have an impact on a person. Similar to other psychosocial aspects of health care, there is not one generic assessment, intervention, or answer that applies to everyone. This is why effective communication, comprehensive evaluation, and a host of possible strategies is so crucial to the quality of client care.

# The Meaning of Physical Change

Physical and psychological characteristics are not separate entities. Lisa may perceive her physical condition contaminating other aspects of her being. We tend to infer things about a person from sometimes just one characteristic. A server in a restaurant asks the dining companion for the order of the other person at the table who may be seated in a wheelchair or have no sight, as though that person could not independently handle the decision and order the meal. This phenomenon, known as "spread" (Dembo, Leviton, & Wright, 1956), can contribute to how a person perceives his or her impairment or disability.

If perceived negative changes can diminish self-concept and cause depression, can the converse also be true? Clients with paraplegia who participated in a walking training program with electric stimulation and an ambulation system, known as Parastep 1, had significant increases in physical self-concept scores and decreases in depression scores (Guest, Klose, Needham-Shropshire, & Jacobs, 1997).

What do physical changes mean to a person? What may the consequences of these changes entail? Is it something to which a person can adjust or is it a catastrophic loss? The answers to these questions are as unique as the individuals who are affected by changes and loss. A small scar on the face of a top fashion model might have more impact than it would on other people. To world-class violinist Itzhak Perlman, a finger deformity might have dire consequences for his career. Yet, as a result of poliomyelitis, this same man uses crutches and leg braces to come on stage to sit and play. Early in his career, he made sure that he was already seated in place, no crutches in sight, when the audience saw him. Over time, he has gained confidence to reveal his impairment, and his audiences have supported him.

The subconscious body image has a loud voice. It can also send messages that no change has occurred. Some clients deny that parts of their bodies are paralyzed. As long as they perceive themselves as looking normal, they may hold on to their premorbid body image (Schilder, 1964). In holding on to familiar negative perceptions, a person may lose 70 pounds and still have a "heavy" body image. Someone who elects to have cosmetic surgery might not necessarily "feel" different. Even desired changes in the body may be difficult to incorporate into the self-concept until the person relinquishes the past image (Safilios-Rothschild, 1970).

Psychosocial adjustment and physical functioning are intimately linked. Dissatisfaction with body image seriously affects the quality of life after a severe burn injury (Fauerbach et al., 2000). The greater the body image dissatisfaction, the lower the psychosocial adjustment and level of physical functioning. Comparing the self-concepts of people with and without physical disabilities, Tam (1998) found significantly higher ratings of total self-concept, material self-concept, and physical self-concept in people without physical disabilities. Health care practitioners need to understand the meaning of physical changes and the relationship between physical and psychological characteristics. How a person responds to changes in body image depends on numerous factors.

# Factors That Influence How a Person Responds to Changes in Body Image

## Prior Loss

Responses to changes in the body are influenced by many variables, such as prior losses, the nature of the current loss, and the outlook for improvement and adjustment (Cohen, 1991). Are there previous losses? Is this one of many? One woman had two colostomies, congestive heart disease, angioplasties, a triple coronary artery bypass graft, chronic thrombophlebitis in her lower extremities, and a stroke with some residual deficits, to highlight just a few of her problems. For her, it became a matter of one more scar, one more problem. Each loss provided skills for dealing with subsequent losses. Although additional circumstances did cause further bodily deterioration, they did not appear to further alter her body image.

## Nature of Current Loss

The nature of the current loss also has an impact on changes in body image. What else is going on? Are there more urgent issues? Consider a woman facing the prospect of prophylactic bilateral mastectomies for lobular carcinoma in situ. No guarantees of preventing the spread of the condition come with the surgery, but she says that she "would rather live without breasts than die with them!" Her outlook influences the way she responds to anticipated changes in her body and puts body image, sexuality, and potential life-saving issues into a balanced perspective.

## Prognosis for Treatment and Recovery

Another factor that influences body image is the prognosis for treatment and recovery. Will the issue at hand hinder or enhance the person's quality of life and functional activities? Will this be a problem in the short run but be "livable with" for the next twenty years?

Someone in the terminal phase of an illness may reject changes offered by the medical community. Consider a client whose physician told him that he had "only nine months to a year to live." He emphatically responded, "Why should I live my last year disfigured?" In response to the option of having his lower extremity amputated to eliminate the primary site of his bone cancer, this man evaluated his outlook for treatment and recovery. Learning that the drastic treatment would not result in his recovery, he decided to remain intact.

## Patterns of Development

Patterns of development also influence reactions to changes in body image. Clients may ask, "What has my lifestyle been so far? Have I had other problems with which to deal?" A family history of coping strategies is part of a pattern of development. Consider two sisters in their 30s who have had hearing loss since birth. As they get older, their hearing acuity is decreasing. They wear bilateral hearing aids, and so does their brother. Their brother was recently diagnosed with retinitis pigmentosa and may lose his sight. As a result of this finding, his sisters were tested. The women have an 80 percent chance of also developing this visual problem. As devastating as this news is to them, they both know they will deal with this if it happens because this is consistent with their pattern of development.

## Family and Cultural Values, Beliefs, and Attitudes

Family and cultural values, beliefs, and personal and societal attitudes also influence how people respond to changes in body image (Kolb, 1959). For some people, a change in appearance is the beginning of a new identity as a "sick person" (Register, 1987). Adjustment to a changed identity is influenced by how important the body was to the person prior to the illness or injury (Schoenberg & Carr, 1970). Consider an 82-year-old woman who is getting shorter and has a pronounced kyphosis from the effects of osteoporosis. She badly fractured her left wrist and forearm, which remain significantly deformed. Yet, she's more concerned with her loss of function than the aesthetics of the situation. A lifetime of family and cultural values of hard work, "pulling one's share," and "not fussin' about how we look" influence the manner in which she faces these changes.

## Personal Control

The sense of self is also influenced by changes in appearance and by the strength of the belief that the person has control of his or her health and circumstances. Some people quickly abdicate control, responsibility, and decision making, turning it over to health care providers: "Fix me. You make the decisions for me. Give me the silver bullet or magic potion." Other individuals have a strong need to take responsibility for their well-being and exercise control over what is happening to them.

Consider a woman in her 60s who highly valued attractiveness and fitness. She walked four miles daily, played tennis several times a week, and ate a diet low in calories, fat, and cholesterol. Acting responsibly for her health and quality of life, she worked to look and feel good and defy her family history. She did not want to have "strokes" like each of her parents. She made sure that she had yearly physical examinations and all the recommended medical screenings.

This woman took control of her health *until* her misdiagnosed low back pain was determined to be bone cancer. The medical community and her body were "betraying" her. Although her mammograms were always negative, breast cancer cells were found during a bone biopsy—in her thigh! Thyroid cancer was found. A benign brain tumor was discovered and surgically removed. As a result of that surgery, she developed neurological problems. She later developed pain that increased in intensity, frequency, and duration, and ultimately limited her activities and self-esteem. Her body was sadly and ironically raging out of her control!

This woman had highly valued personal control and taking charge of her life. Her belief that she had control over her health was dashed, and her self-concept and body image suffered, complicated by the attention she had given to her premorbid body. She began to feel hopeless and that further medical intervention was futile. The body weight that she had diligently controlled increased secondary to medications. Her hair that she always perfectly coiffed washed down the drain, replaced by a wig. As her personal control declined, her body image continued to deteriorate.

## Sin and Stigma

Additional factors that influence body image are people's concepts of sin and stigma, which are often viewed in the context of blame and fault, guilt and shame. Some people feel that their loss is a punishment for something real or imagined, perhaps some "sin" they may have committed. That can create a rift between what is real and what one hopes for or fantasizes about (Cohen, Krahn, Wise, Epstein, & Ross, 1991). A client who believed that his hands "did bad things" used a machine to cut them off. They were able to be reattached with adequate circulation, but they remained stiff and functionless. Although he was in an inpatient psychiatric unit, he managed to repeatedly attempt suicide.

In addition to an association between illness and sin, there is a relationship between the stigma of physical illness and social rejection (Crandall & Moriarty, 1995). Severity of a disease and illness perceived to be behaviorally caused, that is to say, under the person's control, are strong indicators leading to social, and perhaps personal, rejection or blame. Consider a client in his early 20s. By his own admission, he had used his handsome appearance to his advantage throughout his life, doing quite well for himself. At the time of health care intervention, he was facing painful and limiting arthritic changes. He blamed himself for causing the arthritis, since his Reiter's syndrome was associated with gonorrhea, a sexually transmitted disease.

Perceived stigma and the presence of illness contribute to negative psychosocial well-being and add to emotional distress. A laryngectomy may prolong life, but it leaves the person with a loss of speech and with physical disfigurement. Negative psychosocial impact is most catastrophic in clients with laryngectomies who have a highly stigmatized self-perception (Devins, Stam, & Koopmans, 1994).

Physical disfigurement need not be present for there to be a perceived stigma. Hearing impairment, a functional disability, can be perceived to be a threat to one's social identity. As such, people with hearing impairments may be reluctant to acknowledge their problem and refuse to seek treatment rather than face possible negative consequences from sharing their circumstances (Hetu, 1996).

There are also stigmas of visible (i.e., paraplegia), nonvisible (i.e., diabetes), and both visible and nonvisible (i.e., multiple sclerosis) chronic conditions (Joachim & Acorn, 2000). Having a condition that not only sets one apart from others but is also sustained over time can result in being stigmatized by others.

The decision to hide or disclose one's status can be very difficult—remain silent to possibly protect yourself from stigma and try to "pass for normal" or reveal information and face the possibilities of negative consequences. There are, however, potential positive aspects to disclosure. First, individuals may find support from others who share their difficulties, and second, disclosure can help foster positive attitudes toward people with illness and injury.

In responding to changes in body image from illness and injury, people may also face the relationship between disability, stigma, and perceptions of negative differences. These perceptions of negative differences often elicit adverse reactions, stigmas in both people with and without disabilities (Susman, 1994). Although people's perceptions are changing as society's attitudes toward impairments, functional limitations, and disabilities are becoming more en-lightened, people with functional limitations still face negative attitudes and perceptions.

## Social Support

Finally, the value of social support cannot be underestimated as a factor that influences how a person responds to changes in body image. When a person's abilities dramatically change due to an illness or injury, he or she often becomes unable to participate in usual life endeavors. As a result, the individual loses both the social support and satisfaction inherent in these ac-tivities. In the most extreme situation, the person may be abandoned.

Let's look at two similar, yet contrasting, examples of support. Laura was a prima balle-rina who fractured her cervical spine while performing in *The Nutcracker*. Because most of her friends were dancers who continued to perform, she gradually lost her social circle and its support and became lonely and depressed. In addition to her obvious physical losses, the in-jury led to social isolation. She lacked the emotional and practical support that might have bolstered her sense of purpose and worth, encouraged her recovery efforts, and helped with pragmatic needs, like groceries and meals. Her boyfriend, however, steadfastly stood by her, becoming her sole support system, a role that was very wearing on him. After many years, there is a positive footnote to this support. Reclaiming her life, Laura *was* able to perform again—this time as a country singer.

In contrast, many clients with acquired immune deficiency syndrome (AIDS) find them-selves completely abandoned. Craig had just graduated from college when his HIV infection developed into full-blown AIDS. Suddenly, his friends dropped him, and his parents refused to have any contact with him. His despair grew to such a degree that he attempted suicide. Social support might have made a difference in the way Craig faced his situation. He believed that he no longer had value as a person and that it did not matter whether he lived or died. Feeling like a social outcast, he saw no options open to him and no future. The messages he received from those around him validated those perceptions and fueled his convictions.

# Responding to Changes in Body Image from Disease and Injury

How do you think you would respond to a change in body image? What would a hand disease mean to *you*? A facial disfigurement? Radical neck surgery? A laryngectomy with an artificial voice box, especially if you have to communicate verbally with very distressed clients? What would be your straw that would break the proverbial camel's back? Using a wheelchair? Losing your sight? How would it affect you professionally? In functional daily living? Socially? Would you be angry at something being taken away from you? Would you wonder, "Why me?"

## Concern about Value and Normalcy

Adolescents and young adults with spinal cord injuries have concerns about being valued and feeling normal regarding their appearance and capabilities, relationships with others, and phys-ical and emotional independence (Dewis, 1989). Our contemporary society highly values physical beauty and ability (Porter & Beuf, 1991). If we forget that for one minute, the bill-boards, magazines, television, and movies quickly remind us. So consider what a visible physical impairment, with its psychosocial issues, may mean to a person.

As we know, there are no pat answers. Not everyone with a devastating injury has a negative outcome. Consider Michael, who sustained a T-6 spinal cord injury in a skiing accident when he was 16 years old. He felt that it was the "best thing that ever happened to him." Prior to the accident, Michael tended to fade into the background in social situations. Following the injury, he gained notoriety, being in the spotlight wherever he went. He flourished, becoming the life of the party. It is doubtful that he would have chosen the injury as a means for improving social acceptance, but he was able to adjust, accept, and thrive in the midst of his circumstances. Beware of making assumptions. It is wiser to maintain an open mind and initiate a dialogue with the client.

## Physical Appearance and Self-Esteem

Physical appearance is not always intricately related to self-esteem. One woman who has worn breast prostheses since she had bilateral mastectomies appears "normal" to others. On hot summer days, though, she's more comfortable going without the prostheses, but not everyone around her is ready for that. For her, appearance is not *who* she is.

In contrast, an illness or injury that alters the body may be the worst-case scenario to a person whose physical appearance is tightly linked with self-esteem. Accepting the impairment might injure the sense of self. What if that person premorbidly believed that disease or injury meant uselessness or ugliness? How do you think this belief system would affect the person's ability to realistically evaluate the situation and find solutions?

Our physical appearance is an expression of ourselves to others. Even early research on body image showed that appearance can bias impressions and serve to identify a person based on his or her loss (White, Wright, & Dembo, 1948). How many people think of Beethoven as a "deaf" composer, identifying him based on this one deficit? Sarah Bernhardt, the illustrious actress of a bygone era, continued to perform for theater audiences long after she had a lower extremity amputation. Yet, some people regard these individuals as people with impairments who achieved instead of as accomplished, talented people who happened to have impairments.

## Denial, Repression, Loss, and Grief

In trying to understand how people respond to changes in body image, remember that things are not always as they appear. Some clients seem to deny that there is a change, but it may be that they are repressing the emotions associated with those changes (Rochlin, 1965). Denial and repression can be barriers to motivation and, ultimately, to successful outcomes in rehabilitation. If a client does not recognize that there is a problem, he or she will not see that there is a need for intervention. But what happens when the person can no longer deny or ignore the reality of the situation? Feelings of loss and grief, discussed in Chapters 12 and 13, intertwined with depression, which is explored in Chapter 16, may develop.

## Dark Humor

Another response to changes in body image from illness and injury is the use of dark humor, also known as "gallows humor." Humor can bring people together by having them laugh with, not at, the person who is trying to cope with an altered image. Consider the client who used to say that he and Gertrude, the name he gave his leg prosthesis, were going to therapy. Students and staff members alike laughed and thought that he was in control of his situation, accepting the addition of the artificial limb into his life. However, by naming his prosthesis, he might have remained further detached from it. Using a woman's name could have reinforced the idea that it was not *part* of *him*. Yet, there are others who regard a prosthesis as an addition to the body, not a part of the body itself, like a shoe is useful for walking but not part of the body. There are no simple interpretations. Once again, we need to avoid making assumptions.

## Fears Related to Surgical Changes

Surgical changes in the body also evoke fears and concerns. There may be the fear of being useless, unattractive, unloved, unacceptable, and unworthy. Even a surgical scar from a relatively minor procedure can have a deleterious effect on a person who prizes his or her body. Location, size, and appearance of that scar can influence the degree of acceptance. The value or meaning of the altered function or body part is not the same for every person.

A colostomy and ileostomy are hidden underneath clothing, but they can elicit feelings of being dirty and repulsive. Adjustment may be hampered in people who pride themselves on cleanliness and grooming. For verbally expressive people, a laryngectomy might cause them to retreat from others. With a distorted or lost mode of communication, they may be afraid of losing not just the *expression* of their inner core but *part* of their inner core.

Clients facing a mastectomy, hysterectomy (Drench & Losee, 1996), orchidectomy, or prostatectomy may be afraid of losing their sexual identity. The fear may heighten if the person strongly associates his or her sense of masculinity or femininity with the lost body part (Morgan, 1985). According to responses on the body image index, women with total mastectomies were more afraid of losing their sexual attractiveness than were women with partial mastectomies (Lasry et al., 1987). Women who had total mastectomies were more depressed and dissatisfied with their body image than women who had lumpectomies. Negative body image was directly proportional to the extent of the surgery.

## Facial Disfiguration

The psychological impact of facial disfiguration can be traumatic. Disfigurement and dysfunction from head and neck cancer surgery severely and adversely affect quality of life (Dropkin, 1999). Altered body image, especially secondary to facial disfigurement, can result in profound distress for clients, affecting their social functioning (Newell, 1999). Common wisdom says that the eyes are the windows of the soul, and the face is the expression and representation of the person. What effect do you think a facial disfiguration has on a person's sense of self?

An early study showed that people with facial disfiguration never fully integrated it into their body image if they were brought up to hide the deformity (Macgregor, Abel, Bryt, Lauer, & Weissmann, 1953). People who are raised to have a realistic picture of their faces describe themselves more accurately. Adults who were born with craniofacial disfigurements report greater dissatisfaction with their appearance and lower self-esteem and quality of life than adults without facial disfigurations (Sarwer et al., 1999).

Facial deformities may be more difficult to cope with than deformities in other parts of the body because the face symbolically represents the self-concept (Wright, 1983). Consider a woman with a prior history of breast carcinoma who developed squamous cell cancer of the gum and osteoradionecrosis of the jaw. Surgeons removed her teeth and progressively more of her jaw. She has undergone major reconstruction for functional purposes, such as speaking and eating, as well as cosmesis. At 49 years of age, she is the object of staring wherever she goes. This bright, engaging woman recently took a job that entails going into "rough" neighborhoods in housing projects. She says, "I'll be safe—who would want to bother with *me?*"

## Shame, Embarrassment, Anger, Withdrawal, and Depression

In Chapters 12 and 13, we will see how depression, grief, anxiety, and fear are common reactions to loss. However, they do not exist in a vacuum. These feelings are often accompanied by shame, embarrassment, anger, and withdrawal. When the "what once was" and "now is" are assessed, the downside is usually more striking than the existing competencies (Vamos, 1990). The losses can color everything the person thinks about and does. At the extreme, he or she may perceive that values and roles once associated with the physical loss are also gone.

Gadow (1980) suggests that the ill or injured body speaks an "unfamiliar language" (p. 181). Learning that new language and integrating it into one's self can become easier if the person understands the changes and his or her role in coping with them. It also helps if the course is stable and the extent of the problems is predictable.

Depression may be another response to changes in body image. Men with chronic low back pain scored higher in depression than men with hypertension (Lisanti, 1989). In the same study, men with continuous chronic low back pain had higher scores in depression and lower scores in self-esteem than men with intermittent chronic low back pain. Possible contributing variables may be multifactorial. Is your client concerned with a visible versus nonvisible problem? Are diminished function and mobility key issues? Is pain an element? Is the temporal aspect important, as in a chronic versus an intermittent problem? Is there a combination of issues?

## Remaining Whole

The terror of loss can drive the need to remain physically and emotionally intact. A client who had gas gangrene of his lower extremities absolutely refused surgery to amputate his legs, even though the physicians explained that the spread of toxins from his legs to the rest of his body would kill him. Was he gambling with his life by keeping his body "whole"? He understood the situation and adamantly maintained control of his destiny, to the chagrin of his health care providers. Remaining "whole" was more important to him than remaining alive.

### Achieving "Success"

People, however, usually adapt to a greater or lesser extent to an altered identity, mastering their new roles. Overcoming obstacles, acquiring new skills, and achieving a level of success that they had not thought possible may enhance body image and self-concept. Many clients and their families have said that they consider the experience to be positive. Some have even considered it a gift.

We must not fall prey, however, to the common myth that adversity always makes you stronger. After two years of rehabilitation for a near-fatal war injury that resulted in the loss of both legs and parts of his hands, Lewis B. Puller, Jr., seemed to accept the changes in his life (Puller, 1993). He used a wheelchair to regain mobility and independence; reclaimed his family roles as husband, father, and breadwinner; and served as senior attorney in the Office of the General Counsel at the Department of Defense. Yet, less than one year after his inspiring keynote address to an audience of physical therapists at their annual conference, he ended his life. "Personal demons may be more complex and pervasive than we realize. Even 'success' stories carry scars" (Drench, 1994, p. 14).

# Strategies for Adapting and Accepting Changes in Body Image

Health care professionals assume important roles in helping clients adjust to and accept alterations in body image by supporting their feelings of loss, anxiety, and depression. We can help clients regain lost skills and emphasize their abilities. In addition, we can facilitate the grieving process by validating their loss. Grieving is an essential process that cannot be hurried. Clients may adjust physically to the changes, but without mourning the losses, an emotional acceptance cannot be attained (Olson, Ustanko, & Warner, 1991). The person needs to be able to dissociate from the past body image in order to integrate changes into the current self-concept.

### Communication

What we as health professionals say and do speak volumes. Notice how you and other health providers behave with clients. Do you talk with clients, actively listen, spend time with them, and touch them? Debbie, a psychiatric nurse, tells of extending her hand to shake the hand of a new client diagnosed with AIDS (Drench, 1998). The man told her that his doctor puts masks over his face *and* stethoscope and wears a gown and gloves each time he has to touch him. There are significant messages we send in a simple touch.

It is important for health care providers to be aware of different levels of meaning of communication with the client. Counseling and support groups have been very beneficial, especially with clients with low self-esteem (Porter & Beuf, 1991). People often feel relief to be with others who understand their difficulties. Speaking with people with similar problems who have active lives can provide emotional as well as practical support. Such a person can serve as a positive role model, one who has successfully "made it" (Drench, 1996).

Early assessment and intervention can ease the client's journey and should be everyone's responsibility within the scope of their discipline. Can you appropriately evaluate which clients need reassurance and who may need psychiatric intervention? The assessment may be beyond your scope of practice, but you can identify red warning flags that will compel you to seek assistance. After discharge from care, clients who are not coping well with dysfunction and disfigurement are at greater risk for problems, such as infection, noncompliance with therapeutic recommendations, depression, social isolation, and obsession with or denial of changes in body image (Dropkin, 1989).

## Education and Support

Client education and support is critical to quality of life. Learning postoperative self-care reduces anxiety and promotes body image reintegration (Dropkin, 1999). As a result of fear, clients may avoid being seen by others and performing self-care activities (Newell, 1999). The client may be reluctant to do dressing or ostomy changes, to look at and touch altered areas, or to try new skills, such as using a speaking device post-laryngectomy. Helping clients confront their fears and deal with practical challenges can ease those difficulties. Patience and a step-by-step teaching approach, with positive reinforcement for achieved goals, and compassionate support is beneficial.

Support from health care providers, friends, and family is very meaningful. In a study of adolescents and young adults with burns, those who perceived greater support from friends and family had more positive body images, increased self-esteem, and less depression than those who did not recognize this support. In addition, support from friends was considered to be of higher value to the adolescents and young adults than support from family (Orr, Reznikoff, & Smith, 1989).

Consistent and congruent verbal and behavioral messages can help a client adapt to a new body image (Cohen, 1991; French & Phillips, 1991). This is a critical time to make sure your actions match your words. Emotional honesty is also important. If you want the client to trust you, you cannot say that everything is fine, that nothing has changed. Alterations in the body have occurred that necessitate the client's attention (Drench, 1996).

The client needs to integrate the changes that have occurred to his or her body image into a new self-concept. As health providers, we need to listen to the clients' concerns, acknowledge the difficulty of their situations, and help them to know they will be able to do this. Our role as change agents is to help the client understand and appreciate the value he or she continues to have as a person.

## Emphasizing Capabilities

Clients can benefit from our help in emphasizing their capabilities rather than their deficiencies. Understanding their own inherent strengths and values, what Wright (1983) calls "asset values," can be motivating and promote a greater appreciation for "what is." In contrast, comparing themselves to other people (Wright's "comparative values") who have no or different disabilities can place obstacles in the path of recovery. If health providers and clients are aiming for a return to the premorbid state, anything short of that gold standard will be perceived as failure and cause frustration. Through the phenomenon of spread, the person may see other areas, besides the physical, as being inferior and unacceptable. Success in recovery, improving function, and overcoming obstacles is dependent on the person's feeling effective and capable.

We can help clients use an asset rather than comparative value system to place greater weight on nonphysical attributes. Sixteen-year-old Jim Langevin had spent his summer vacation working as a police cadet, dreaming of becoming a police officer or an agent of the Federal Bureau of Investigation. As two members of the SWAT team were examining a handgun in the police department locker room, it inadvertently discharged, sending a bullet ricocheting off a metal locker and ripping through the teenager's neck. Langevin became a person with quadriplegia. He not only survived but ultimately thrived, later becoming Secretary of State of Rhode Island. Twenty years after the accident, he became the first person with quadriplegia elected to the U.S. House of Representatives. Instead of enforcing the law, he is part of creating it.

Although initially Langevin reacted with disbelief, anger, and frustration, he was able to see possibilities and work toward them. He also hopes that his actions will inspire others to follow their dreams and not yield to their limitations (personal communication, April 4, 2002). Emphasizing a client's assets and sharing stories with "successful" outcomes, parts of which a client might be able to achieve, can also be motivating.

### Life's Activities

Becoming involved in life's activities and developing a sense of mastery and pride in one's abilities may minimize, prevent, or replace grieving and self-pity. A valuable lesson to share with clients is that they are people with disabilities rather than physically disabled individuals.

People with acquired and congenital disabilities recommend the value of other strategies for adapting and accepting changes in body image. They suggest maintaining a healthy level of fitness, playing sports activities for people with disabilities, having a broad social network with people with and without disabilities, dressing stylishly, and fostering self-confidence (Stensman, 1989).

## Summary

This chapter discussed the relationship between body image and self-concept, how clients respond to changes in body image, and strategies that health professionals can employ to help clients adjust to these changes. Because body image is so closely associated with self-concept and personal identity, a change of one aspect can affect the whole person. Health care providers are instrumental in fostering clients' adjustment and acceptance by recognizing and helping them work through their loss and emphasizing their strengths.

## Reflective Questions

1. Alma Jackson, the speech-language pathology student who wrote the journal entry at the beginning of this chapter, had a very powerful response when working with Lisa, a client with a serious impairment whose life paralleled her own.
   a. How would *you* feel if Lisa were your client?

    b. What do you think Lisa might be thinking or feeling about her abilities?
    c. What might you say or do to find out more?
2. a. Do you think people with a sudden onset of illness or impairment respond differently than those with a progressive condition?
    b. In what ways might they be similar or different?
3. Consider what is important to your body image and self-concept.
    a. What attributes do you most value?
    b. What impairments or deficits would you find most difficult to accept?
    c. How do you think you would feel about yourself if you had a disability?
    d. How do you think your beliefs and values affect the way you feel about clients? Do you think clients can sense this?
    e. How do you think your values and beliefs affect your ability to set goals for clients?
    f. How do you think your values and beliefs affect your ability to support clients' goals?
4. a. What factors influence a client's body image?
    b. What factors influence a client's self-concept?
5. a. How do you think a person's body image and self-concept affect motivation?
    b. How you think body image and self-concept affect the person's ability to comply with the treatment program?

## CASE STUDY

Marguerite Finley is a 36-year-old executive of an investment firm. Diagnosed with rheumatoid arthritis when she was 28, she has been progressively hampered by pain, deformity, and loss of functional mobility in her hands. She is now seeking surgery to improve function, pain, and appearance.

Marguerite enjoys a happy marriage, a wide circle of friends, and a highly satisfying career. However, she has become increasingly troubled by the appearance of her hands, seeing them as unattractive compared to her memory of her hands as they once were. Although she grooms her nails and wears nail polish, she no longer is able to wear rings. She now tends to hide her hands when she is with friends, as well as strangers, and is very sensitive to "looks of pity" from others.

1. What factors may influence how Marguerite responds to changes in her body image?
2. What impact might Marguerite's physical changes have on her self-concept and on her self-esteem?
3. Discuss the relationship between stigma, perceptions of negative changes, and impairment for Marguerite.
4. As a health professional, what can you do to foster Marguerite's adjustment and acceptance of the changes in her body image?

## REFERENCES

Bronheim, H., Strain, J. J., & Biller, H. F. (1991). Psychiatric aspects of head and neck surgery. Part II: Body image and psychiatric intervention. *General Hospital Psychiatry, 13*(4), 225–232.

Cohen, A. (1991). Body image in the person with a stoma. *Journal of Enterostomal Therapy, 18*(2), 68–71.

Cohen, C. G., Krahn, L., Wise, T. N., Epstein, S., & Ross, R. (1991). Delusions of disfigurement in a woman with acne rosacea. *General Hospital Psychiatry, 13*(4), 273–277.

Crandall, C. S., & Moriarty, D. (1995). Physical illness stigma and social rejection. *British Journal of Social Psychology, 34*(Pt. 1), 67–83.

Dembo, T., Leviton, G. L., & Wright, B. A. (1956). Adjustment to misfortune: A problem of social-psychological rehabilitation. *Artificial Limbs, 3*(2), 4–62.

Devins, G. M., Stam, H. J., & Koopmans, J. P. (1994). Psychosocial impact of laryngectomy mediated by perceived stigma and illness intrusiveness. *Canadian Journal of Psychiatry, 39*(10), 608–616.

Dewis, M. E. (1989). Spinal cord-injured adolescents and young adults: The meaning of body changes. *Journal of Advanced Nursing, 14*(5), 389–396.

Drench, M. (1994). Lewis B. Puller, Jr. [Letter to the Editors]. *PT—Magazine of Physical Therapy, 2*(10), 14.

Drench, M. (1995). Coping with loss—Adjusting to change. *International Society for Behavioral Science in Physical Therapy, 7*(2), 1–3.

Drench, M. E. (1996). Changes in body image secondary to disease and injury. In *Nursing focus: Psychosocial adaptation to disability and chronic illness* (pp. 15–19). Glenview, IL: Association of Rehabilitation Nurses.

Drench, M. (1998). *Red ribbons are not enough*. Wilsonville, OR: BookPartners.

Drench, M. E., & Losee, R. H. (1996). Sexuality and sexual capacities of elderly people. *Rehabilitation Nursing, 21*(3), 118–123.

Dropkin, M. J. (1989). Coping with disfigurement and dysfunction after head and neck cancer surgery: A conceptual framework. *Seminars in Oncology Nursing, 5*(3), 213–219.

Dropkin, M. J. (1999). Body image and quality of life after head and neck cancer surgery. *Cancer Practice, 7*(6), 309–313.

Fauerbach, J. A., Heinberg, L. J., Lawrence, J. W., Munster, A. M., Palombo, D. A., Richter, D., Spence, R. J., Stevens, S. S., Ware, L., & Muehlberger, T. (2000). Effect of early body image dissatisfaction on subsequent psychological and physical adjustment after disfiguring injury. *Psychosomatic Medicine, 62*(4), 576–582.

French, J. K., & Phillips, J. A. (1991). Shattered images: Recovery for the SCI client. *Rehabilitation Nursing, 16*(3), 134–136.

Gadow, S. (1980). Body and self: A dialectic. *Journal of Medicine and Philosophy, 5*(3), 172–185.

Guest, R. S., Klose, K. J., Needham-Shropshire, B. M., & Jacobs, P. L. (1997). Evaluation of a training program for persons with spinal cord injury paraplegia using the Parastep 1 ambulation system. Part 4: Effect on physical self-concept and depression. *Archives of Physical Medicine and Rehabilitation, 78*(8), 804–807.

Head, H. (1920). *Studies of neurology* (Vol. 1). London: Hodder & Stoughton.

Hetu, R. (1996). The stigma attached to hearing impairment. *Scandinavian Audiology Supplement, 43,* 12–24.

Joachim, G., & Acorn, S. (2000). Stigma of visible and invisible chronic conditions. *Journal of Advanced Nursing, 32*(1), 243–248.

Kolb, L. C. (1959). Disturbances of the body image. In S. Arieti (Ed.), *American handbook of psychiatry* (Vol. 1, pp. 749–769). New York: Basic Books.

Lasry, J. C., Margolese, R. G., Poisson, R., Shibata, H., Fleischer, D., LaFleur, D., Legault, S., & Taillefer, S. (1987). Depression and body image following mastectomy and lumpectomy. *Journal of Chronic Diseases, 40*(6), 529–534.

Laufer, M. E. (1991). Body image, sexuality and the psychotic core. *International Journal of Psychoanalysis, 72*(Pt. 1), 63–71.

Lisanti, P. A. (1989). Perceived body space and self-esteem in adult males with and without chronic low back pain. *Orthopaedic Nursing, 8*(3), 49–56.

Macgregor, F. C., Abel, T. M., Bryt, A., Lauer, E., & Weissmann, S. (1953). *Facial deformities and plastic surgery*. Springfield, IL: Charles C. Thomas.

Model, G. (1990). A new image to accept: Psychological aspects of stoma care. *Professional Nurse, 5*(6), 310–316.

Monteath, S. A., & McCabe, M. P. (1997). The influence of societal factors on female body image. *Journal of Social Psychology, 137*(6), 708–727.

Morgan, S. (1985). *Coping with a hysterectomy* (rev. ed.). New York: Signet.

Newell, R. J. (1999). Altered body image: A fear-avoidance model of psychosocial difficulties following disfigurement. *Journal of Advanced Nursing, 30*(5), 1230–1238.

Norris, C. (1970). The professional nurse and body image. In C. E. Carlson (Ed.), *Behavioral concepts and nursing intervention* (p. 43). Philadelphia: J.B. Lippincott.

Olson B., Ustanko, L., & Warner, S. (1991). The patient in a halo brace: Striving for normalcy in body image and self-concept. *Orthopaedic Nursing, 10*(1), 44–50.

Orr, D. A., Reznikoff, M., & Smith, G. M. (1989). Body image, self-esteem, and depression in burn-injured adolescents and young adults. *Journal of Burn Care and Rehabilitation, 10*(5), 454–461.

Porter, J. R., & Beuf, A. H. (1991). Racial variation in reaction to physical stigma: A study of degree of disturbance by vitiligo among black and white patients. *Journal of Health and Social Behavior, 32*(2), 192–204.

Puller, L. B., Jr. (1993). *Fortunate son: The autobiography of Lewis B. Puller, Jr.* New York: Bantam Books.

Register, C. (1987). *Living with chronic illness: Days of patience and passion*. New York: Bantam Books.

Rochlin, G. (1965). *Griefs and discontents: The forces of change*. Boston: Little, Brown, and Company.

Safilios-Rothschild, C. (1970). *The sociology and social psychology of disability and rehabilitation*. New York: Random House.

Samonds, R. J., & Cammermeyer, M. (1989). Perceptions of body image in subjects with multiple sclerosis: A pilot study. *Journal of Neuroscience Nursing, 21*(3), 190–194.

Sarwer, D. B., Bartlett, S. P., Whitaker, L. A., Paige, K. T., Pertshuk, M. J., & Wadden, T. A. (1999). Adult psychological functioning of individuals born with craniofacial anomalies. *Plastic Reconstructive Surgery, 103*(2), 412–418.

Schilder, P. (1950). *The image and appearance of the human body: Studies in the constructive energies of the psyche*. New York: International Universities Press.

Schilder, P. (1964). *Image and appearance of the human body*. New York: Wiley.

Schoenberg, B., & Carr, A. C. (1970). Loss of external organs: Limb amputation, mastectomy, and disfiguration. In B. Schoenberg, A. C. Carr, D. Peretz, & A. H. Kutscher (Eds.), *Loss and grief: Psychological management in medical practice* (pp. 119–131). New York: Columbia University Press.

Stensman, R. (1989). Body image among twenty-two persons with acquired and congenital severe mobility impairment. *Paraplegia, 27*(1), 27–35.

Susman, J. (1994). Disability, stigma, and deviance. *Social Science and Medicine, 38*(1), 15–22.

Tam, S. F. (1998). Comparing the self-concepts of persons with and without physical disabilities. *Journal of Psychology, 132*(1), 78–86.

Vamos, M. (1990). Body image in rheumatoid arthritis: The relevance of hand appearance to desire for surgery. *British Journal of Medical Psychology, 63*, 267–277.

White, R. K., Wright, B. A., & Dembo, T. (1948). Studies in adjustment to visible injuries: Evaluation of curiosity by the injured. *Journal of Abnormal Social Psychology, 43*, 13–28.

Wright, B. A. (1983). *Physical disability: A psychosocial approach* (2nd ed.). New York: Harper & Row.

# 10

# *Condition-Specific Characteristics*

I know that clients vary a lot in how they cope with and adjust to their illnesses or disabilities, but now that I've been working in rehabilitation for a while, I'm seeing some trends that I think will help me understand what my clients are experiencing. For example, clients who have traumatic injuries seem to have similar adjustment challenges, like the shock of having a sudden, significant change in their lives. One moment they're going about their business as usual, and in the next, their life is completely different. Similarly, all of my older clients have to cope with the inevitable changes associated with aging, causing so many of them to have multiple diagnoses. With each client I treat, I feel I'm a bit more prepared for the next.
—*From the journal of Marcy Guttadauro, speech-language pathology student*

This chapter addresses psychosocial issues related to a select group of disabilities. While generalizations are made about each group, it is important to recognize that outcomes of individual clients will vary widely. Livneh and Antonak (1997) attribute these differences to four categories of variables:

1. Demographics, such as age, sex, and marital status
2. Personality and temperament
3. External factors, such as socioeconomic status and availability of support
4. Disability-specific characteristics

The first three concepts have been discussed elsewhere in this book. The fourth, disability-specific characteristics, is the topic of this chapter.

The most significant types of disabilities that affect people from childhood through middle age are congenital or perinatal conditions, trauma, and acute or rapidly progressive diseases that lead to disablement or death (Ferrucci et al., 1996; Verbrugge, 1995). For most of these conditions, the disablement process is rapid and related to the underlying cause. Among older people, disability can be caused by specific medical conditions, which are often complicated by the aging process, leading to multiple comorbidities (Ferrucci et al., 1996). We discuss each of these major sources of disability, exploring psychosocial issues common to each.

# Congenital and Perinatal Conditions

I can't stop thinking about Jimmy, the client I met while doing my home care rotation. He's 56 years old and lives with his mother. Their family doctor called in a referral to see if we could help set up some kind of a plan for Jimmy's future. He has always lived at home with his mother, and she literally taught him everything he knows. From what we could gather, Jimmy experienced complications at birth, which left him with athetoid quadriplegia. He communicates with a simple, homemade word board and a series of audible sounds that I didn't recognize as words. During the day, he's propped up with pillows in the living room. Remarkably, his 85-year-old mother carries him from his bedroom to and from the living room daily! She reported that recently this has become difficult, prompting her to wonder how much longer she would actually be able to care for Jimmy alone.

—*From the journal of Anna Zimmerman, social work student*

A developmental disability is defined as any mental or physical impairment that is manifested early in development, results in significant functional limitations, and usually requires special services throughout the lifetime (Robinson & Harris, 1997). Examples of the broad range of diagnoses that are included under this umbrella are:

- Cerebral palsy
- Autism
- Seizure disorders
- Mental retardation
- Learning disabilities
- Muscular dystrophy
- Down syndrome
- Myelodysplasia (spina bifida)
- Traumatic brain injury, occurring before age 5
- Sensory impairments (vision, hearing, tactile defensiveness)

Each diagnosis has its own set of complex symptoms, which can range from mild to severe, and it is not uncommon for clients to have multiple diagnoses, such as cerebral palsy with mental retardation and a seizure disorder. Although each person's experience varies, some commonalities exist with regard to the client's psychosocial experience.

It is often difficult for people with severe congenital disabilities to establish meaningful relationships and the sense of security and belonging that develops from them (Holzbauer & Bervin, 1996; Kishi & Meyer, 1994; O'Brien & O'Brien, 1992; Schnorr, 1997). Clients with a diagnosis of cerebral palsy were studied to determine their perceived sense of belonging (Schaller & De La Garza, 1999). Basing their work on the hierarchy of needs developed by Maslow (1968), in which a sense of belonging is a necessary prerequisite for developing self-esteem and achieving self-worth, the investigators found that some of their subjects had a perception of being different, unsupported, and unaccepted from a very young age. For example, one subject described his parents' reaction to his diagnosis. In an attempt to assure him of their love, they indicated that they intended to love him "in spite of his disability." In this very mixed message, these parents made it clear that he was different from everyone else, and it seemed that their love was anything but unconditional.

It can be overwhelming for parents to adjust to having a child with a disability (Wolf, Fisman, & Speechley, 1989). Mothers and fathers appear to adjust at different rates. Frey, Fewell, and Vadasy (1989) found fathers adjusting as much as three years earlier than mothers. This difference was attributed to the mothers' more traditional, active role in their children's care. In addition, there may be a great deal of ambivalence. Parents may experience feelings of frustration and entrapment as a result of the time and energy required to care for a child with a disability, yet it can also yield exceptional rewards of affection and devotion (Brinchmann, 1999; Ehrenkrantz, Miller, Vernberg, & Fox, 2001).

Siblings of children with disabilities may experience differential treatment from their parents (McHale & Pawletko, 1992; Wolf, Fisman, Ellison, & Freeman, 1998). Children who do not have a disability may receive less parental attention, particularly if one or both parents are frequently engaged in the care of the child who has a disability (McKeever, 1983). In addition, siblings without disabilities may have excessive responsibility for household chores or the care of the child with the disability (McHale & Gamble, 1989). Siblings may also be socially isolated. Because of family stresses, there may be severely limited opportunities to participate in activities outside of the home or for the social interaction needed to develop friendships (Cadman, Boyle, & Offord, 1988; Dyson, 1989; Siemon, 1984). In addition, they may feel embarrassed or be stigmatized for having a sibling who is "different." All of these factors can lead to resentment of the sibling who has a disability, exacerbating sibling rivalry.

Once the child with a disability reaches age 3, he or she is entitled to receive services through the public school system. Since the enactment of the Education for All Handicapped Children Act [Public Law 94-142] (1975), public schools have been required to provide educational services in the least restrictive environment possible. However, problems exist in trying to make this mandate a reality (Gerry & McWhorter, 1991; Gerry & Mirsky, 1992). Many children with disabling conditions are still underserved and understimulated in the educational environment (Willard-Holt, 1998).

Schaller and De La Garza (1999) confirmed these findings in their study of children with cerebral palsy. The children reported feeling resentful that their parents were in frequent conflict with school personnel over issues of placement and educational plans. They also reported a sense of separation, few friendships, and frequent taunting from classmates without disabilities. Their most significant positive relationships were those with teachers who made them feel important or recognized. One girl reported spending most of her school experience in a segregated classroom, located in a separate wing of the school. This precluded any interaction with peers without disabilities. When she was mainstreamed into high school, she experienced a very difficult transition, and reported feeling anxious, self-conscious, and fearful that her classmates who were able-bodied were constantly judging her.

A major portion of time and effort in school may be spent learning methods to compensate or accommodate for the effects of disability (Willard-Holt, 1998). Identification of the cognitive abilities of children who are severely physically disabled can be very difficult, complicated by speech or language impairment and the limitations of existing screening and intelligence tests. Most tools assume all children have similar physical abilities and social experiences. As a result of these factors, cognitive abilities often go unrecognized and underdeveloped (Willard-Holt, 1998).

Children who have developmental disabilities often have very different life experiences than those who do not. They may be routinely excluded from many social events, such as clubs, sports, and birthday parties, because of mobility impairments or the need for therapies, doctors' visits, and/or hospitalizations. Wheelchairs or other assistive technology are visible reminders of being different, are sources of stigmatization (Cahill & Eggleston, 1995; Voll, Krumm, & Fichtner, 1999), and can limit accessibility. For example, wheelchairs cannot traverse stairs, uneven terrain, and narrow spaces.

It can be especially difficult to meet the therapeutic needs of adults who have developmental disabilities. Until the 1970s, institutional placement was common for all people with significant disabilities. Consider Steven, a young man who was born in 1974 and diagnosed with Down syndrome just after birth. The pediatrician sternly advised his parents to place Steven in an institution because it was unlikely that he would ever walk or speak and would be a burden to the family. The doctor implied that it would be in the best interest of the child, leaving the parents feeling guilty and confused. Fortunately for this child, his parents did not follow the physician's recommendation. That does not mean that there were no challenges in keeping him at home, but it is likely that his developmental experience was more positive than it would have been had his parents followed the advice of their doctor.

## Adults with Developmental Disabilities

The medical literature has little to report about the needs and concerns of adults with developmental disabilities (Rapp & Torres, 2000; Robinson & Harris, 1997). Formal education of health care professionals also appears to be quite limited (Walsh, Hammerman, Josephson, & Krupka, 2000). Existing literature is based primarily on clinical experiences of the authors, rather than controlled studies or structured observations. Likewise, our review is also based primarily on our own experiences, with supporting references made when available. It is important to address adults with developmental disabilities separately from children. Because many of today's adults were raised in residential institutions, there are vast differences between their developmental experiences and those of children raised in their parents' homes. It is important for clinicians to be sensitive to the unique psychosocial needs of this population (Robinson & Harris, 1997).

Clients often present with many predictable and unfortunate problems related to living in an institutional setting. Specific problems requiring intervention vary from client to client, but the most common fall into three broad categories: physical, cognitive, and psychosocial. Consider the experience reported in this journal entry:

Rachael grew up in a state school, which was closed many years ago. All of the residents were discharged. Because she could be taught to manage her own care, she was one of the lucky ones who could be sent to a group home. Many of her friends were sent to nursing homes because they were "not smart enough" to make it in the community. She described her life at the state school as "okay but boring." Each day was pretty much the same. Whoever was assigned to her that day—man or woman—would come in and get her dressed and up into her wheelchair, where she'd spend the day. The process was reversed at night. Some of the attendants would actually talk to her, but most seemed pretty busy and just assumed that she was "deaf, dumb, and blind." Although she experienced "funny feelings" and embarrassment when she had male attendants, there was nothing she could do about it. She recalled one attendant, Mary, whom she especially preferred. When I asked why she was a favorite, Rachael replied, "Mary was the only one who would clean up the food that I spilled on myself as I ate."
—*From the journal of Katia Corbett, counseling psychology student*

## PHYSICAL PROBLEMS

Physical problems can be due to a specific diagnosis, for example, spastic paraparesis related to brain injury in cerebral palsy. However, because of the relative immobility and limited personal care provided in institutions, various secondary complications are frequently seen (Robinson & Harris, 1997). Relative immobility can lead to limited strength, motor control, and perceptual motor development. Severe contractures can result from difficulty managing spasticity and poor positioning. Cardiopulmonary problems are also common, due to inactivity and/or scoliosis. Overuse of functional body parts can lead to degenerative joint disease and subluxed or dislocated joints. Finally, skin integrity may be altered by chronic skin breakdown. Cognitive and psychosocial issues can complicate all of these physical problems.

## COGNITION/COMMUNICATION

Like physical concerns, cognitive problems may have a primary source, such as mental retardation associated with Down syndrome. However, a phenomenon known as institutional retardation may also be present. This is the result of understimulation during the developmental process. Although residents of institutions were once typically assumed to be retarded, many were not. This was particularly true for clients with communication problems. Difficulties in communication can stem from physical impairment, such as the lack of motor control or breath support needed for verbal communication. Visual or hearing impairments can further complicate communication. There might also be an auditory processing problem—that is, the client can hear what is being said but cannot process it effectively or quickly enough for functional communication.

The subtleties of communication make a big difference in how we perceive each other. As outlined in Chapter 2, body language and facial expressions influence how others interpret our messages. People who lack control of their motor skills, such as those with athetoid cerebral palsy, have difficulty with communication because of involuntary movements, grunts, and other distracting behaviors that can be overwhelming to most observers.

Many adults with developmental disabilities have poor communication skills. It can be difficult to extract and interpret information appropriately during the examination process

(Robinson & Harris, 1997). It may be tempting, and at times helpful, to augment the client's reported history by speaking with care providers, but this requires particular caution. Just because personal care attendants accompany clients to the clinic, it cannot be assumed that they can accurately report the clients' hopes and dreams. They may be primarily concerned with one aspect of a client's life, such as finding an easier method of transfer. This may not be representative of the client's own goals, but because of learned passivity, difficulty with communication, or fear of repercussions, the client may not feel comfortable contradicting the attendant's report.

### PSYCHOSOCIAL CONCERNS

Adults with significant developmental disability have complicated psychosocial concerns (Robinson & Harris, 1997). Those raised in an institutional environment face additional difficulties. As infants, children, and adolescents, they lacked the daily nurturing love of family that is required to develop a sense of trust and security. Early experiences may have taught them to develop passive relationship roles (Minde, 1973). This can result in poor adult life-management skills, such as finding employment, managing personal care attendants, and being effective advocates for themselves. They may have little concept of how to plan for the future, including setting and reaching goals. Social skills are often extremely limited, and confusion about sexuality, dating, and friendships is common, with limited understanding and management of emotions (Konstantareas & Lunsky, 1997; Sulpizi, 1996).

Wellness is a concept that has not typically been addressed with this group of clients. For the general population, health is defined as the absence of illness, injury, and disability. Using this definition, people who have developmental disabilities cannot be considered healthy. Rather, society tends to categorize people in this group, based on their cognitive, emotional, or physical limitations. When addressing the needs of people with developmental disabilities, Zajicek-Farber (1998) proposes that we change our concept of health and wellness to incorporate a broad range of social criteria. Proposed criteria include level of satisfaction with personal relationships, education, work, standard of living, community interactions, creative expression, and future prospects for growth and development. This approach focuses attention on clients' capacity for self-direction and helps target interventions appropriately.

# Sudden-Onset Disability

The circumstances surrounding some of my patients' lives are so overwhelming. I received a referral to examine Mr. Byers, a 48-year-old man who was admitted for renal bypass surgery last Friday. He expected to go home on Monday morning, but something went terribly wrong during the surgery. The ventilator malfunctioned, and Mr. Byers was without oxygen for an extended period of time. Now, he presents with spastic quadriplegia, and he may not even make it! His wife reminds me so much of my mother, and his daughter is exactly my age. Life can change so quickly. I can't begin to imagine how they will cope with this.

*—From the journal of Althea Gerakas, physician assistant student*

The sudden onset of disability disrupts virtually every aspect of a person's life—self-concept, relationships, vocational and avocational pursuits, independence, and future plans. Trauma, such as spinal cord injury, stroke, or amputation, can be devastating. Acceptance and adjustment depend on many factors, including the diagnosis and degree of disability, perception of reality, flexibility in thinking, cognitive adjustment of self-image, awareness of situational demands, and judgment (Florian, Katz, & Lahov, 1991), and the responses of family, friends, and clinicians. Clients are often acutely aware of an observer's shock, fear, disgust, curiosity, or pity. As discussed in Chapter 13, most researchers agree that there is a temporal sequence to the psychological adaptation to disability, and not all phases are evident in each client. Reactions may overlap, fluctuate, and appear in a different order.

Lilliston (1985) identified four independent responses that commonly occur when a person experiences a sudden onset of disability. These include (1) disruption of body image; (2) change in experience and orientation of time; (3) grief and depression; and (4) fear, anxiety, guilt, and rage. Sensitive understanding of the clients' experiences will help health care providers support the process of adjustment.

## Disruption of Body Image

As discussed in Chapter 9, body image is the mental representation of the physical body (Head, 1920; Schilder, 1950). It reflects familiar visual and sensory perceptions and incorporates personal, interpersonal, environmental, and temporal criteria (Lilliston, 1985; Livneh & Antonak, 1997). Body image affects how people relate to themselves, to other people, and to the external environment (Bramble, 1995). Although it can be modified by psychological defense mechanisms such as denial, body image is thought to remain fairly constant. When a client's body image is suddenly altered by severe injury or illness, the visual and sensory feedback may be unfamiliar (Falvo, 1999; Livneh, Antonak, & Gerhardt, 1999). This can be very frightening to the client and may result in feelings of shame, anxiety, and doubt (Lilliston, 1985). Successful psychosocial adaptation is characterized by an integration of disability-related characteristics into a new body image and self-concept (Livneh & Antonak, 1997).

## Orientation to Time

Most individuals integrate concepts of past, present, and future into their daily functioning. We all experience a subjective sense of time, in terms of it moving slowly or quickly. Following sudden, severe injury or illness, clients may experience temporal disorientation. This can be due to hospitalization, pain, medication, and/or frequent disruptions in the sleep–wake cycle. In addition, the ability to manage one's own time is essentially taken over by others in the hospital.

Temporal disorientation is significant because there is often an incompatibility of the client's orientation to time compared to that of the staff and/or family. While the client's day may seem interminable, the staff experiences a hectic one. Although clients generally become very present-oriented because of the overwhelming nature of changes to which they must adapt, their support system may not be. Family members may be focused on losses (past-oriented) or the challenges to be faced when the client comes home (future-oriented). This disparity can lead the client to experience a sense of being a prisoner in time (Lilliston, 1985).

## Grief and Depression

As discussed in Chapters 12 and 13, grief is a normal reaction to significant loss. The loss associated with the onset of a disability differs from other losses because it requires an extended and indeterminate period of mourning (Davis, 1987). Grief is renewed as each and every loss is realized (i.e., the ability to walk, the ability to have children, loss of dreams, loss of income) (Gill, 1999). This type of grief is also known as chronic sorrow (Burke, Hainsworth, Eakes, & Lindgren, 1992; Davis, 1987; Olshansky, 1962).

Depression is an expected by-product of grief or chronic sorrow. Although not all clients experience severe depression, most display at least transient evidence of it (Frank, Elliott, Corcoran, & Wonderlich, 1987; Rybarcyzk, Nyenhuis, Nicholas, Cash, & Kaiser, 1995; Wortman & Silver, 1989). Great variability is reported for the incidence of depression among people with sudden-onset disabilities. However, for our purposes, it suffices to say that, compared to the general population, depression is significantly more common among people with disabilities (Friedland & McColl, 1992; Livneh & Antonak, 1997; Turner & Beiser, 1990; Turner & McLean, 1989; Turner & Noh, 1988; Turner & Wood, 1985).

Burke and coworkers (1992) point out that we cannot expect chronic sorrow to resolve with final acceptance, which typically occurs in other forms of grief, because the chronicity of the disability serves as a constant reminder of the loss. However, they do make a distinction between chronic sorrow and pathological grief. While pathological grief is characterized by unrelenting feelings of sadness, guilt, and/or anger, the presence of chronic sorrow still allows for an adaptation, characterized by a highly functional lifestyle.

## Fear, Anxiety, Guilt, and Rage

Shock is generally the first reaction to the overwhelming experience of sudden-onset disability. It is characterized by psychic numbness, dissociation, and cognitive disorganization (Gill, 1999; Livneh & Antonak, 1997). Defense mechanisms begin to emerge, protecting the client from full and sudden realization of the consequences of the illness or injury. As the full magnitude becomes apparent, anxiety is common. Physiological and psychological reactions associated with anxiety include rapid respiratory and heart rates, confusion, and purposeless overactivity. Anxiety is often experienced recurrently, in response to fears related to treatments, test results, and uncertainties about the future (Livneh & Antonak, 1997).

Internalized anger is often allied with feelings of self-blame and guilt. This is particularly true if the client feels responsible for the disability (Gill, 1999). Consider John, who blames himself for the car accident that resulted in the death of his girlfriend and the amputation of his left lower extremity. His anger and rage also extends to others. He filed a lawsuit against the driver of the other car involved in the accident, claiming that a delay in changing from high to low beams was the primary cause of the accident. In addition, he frequently displays anger and aggression toward his health care providers, asserting that if only a competent surgeon had been available, his leg could have been saved. This type of hostility is a form of retaliation, which the client directs at anybody or anything perceived to be associated with the disability (Lilliston, 1985; Livneh & Antonak, 1997).

## Adjustment

Adjustment entails the intellectual and emotional acceptance of present and future implications of the disability. As discussed in Chapter 14, it begins with acknowledgment of the permanency of the disability, as evidenced by self-acceptance, integration of a new self-concept, and adjustment of life-long aspirations and plans (Yoshida, 1994). According to Livneh and Antonak (1997), acceptance is evident when the client

- develops an integrated and positive sense of self;
- discovers new potentials;
- establishes and pursues social and vocational goals; and
- overcomes obstacles encountered in the pursuit of goals.

The best predictors of greater life satisfaction include optimism, higher levels of perceived health and social support, an internal locus of control, and the use of problem-focused, versus emotion-focused, coping behaviors (Chan, Lee, & Lieh-Mak, 2000; Gill, 1999; Lou, Dai, & Catanzaro, 1997). Problem-focused strategies are action-oriented and aimed at making changes within the self or in the environment. An example of this might involve a client who arranges for architectural modifications to the home to ensure wheelchair accessibility. Emotion-focused strategies are best suited for short-term or acute episodes over which the client has little control. Avoidance is one example. While it may not be particularly damaging for a client to avoid looking at and touching a mastectomy scar, long-term use of this coping strategy would be harmful and detrimental to successful adaptation.

# Acute or Rapidly Progressive Diseases

Today, I met with Joseph. I felt so inadequate, knowing that all that we can offer him at this point is experimental therapy. He's only 42 and has a wife and two young children, ages 2 and 4. A diagnosis of liver cancer was just made after exploratory surgery was done to determine the cause of acute jaundice. Although he has not felt well for a few weeks, it never occurred to him that he might have something as serious as cancer. He described feeling numb and unable to make any decisions. I'll meet with him again on Friday, after he and his wife have a chance to consider the treatment options.

—*From the journal of Libby Marshall, oncology medical resident*

The diagnosis of a life-threatening disease can be viewed as a psychological trauma, evoking many of the same reactions common to those who have sustained sudden-onset disability. The initial shock experienced with the diagnosis will generally have a more narrow focus than that experienced with traumatic physical injury (Livneh & Antonak, 1997). Anxiety and depression are frequently observed psychological reactions (Glanz & Lerman, 1992).

Anxiety typically stems from the numerous fears that the diagnosis activates. Fears may be related to losses of control, independence, bodily functions, income, or privacy. Additional difficulties are associated with altered role in the family, sexual dysfunction, social isolation, and pain (Freidenbergs & Kaplan, 1993; Stam, Bultz, & Pittman, 1986). Feelings of helplessness, uncertainty, and hopelessness all contribute to and are exacerbated by the client's struggle to understand the implications of the diagnosis, negotiate the health care system, and deal with an unpredictable future (Whyte & Smith, 1997).

Chronic stress is common, as clients may require repeated hospitalizations, surgery, or other intensive courses of treatment. Frequent exposure to the experiences of other clients can also be stressful (Whyte & Smith, 1997). As discussed in Chapter 8, if left unmanaged, physical, social, and emotional problems will occur (Greenberg, Kazak, & Meadows, 1989; Van Dongen-Melman & Sanders-Woudstra, 1986; Worchel, Nolan, & Wilson, 1988).

The emotional distress involved in dealing with a terminal illness is not limited to the client (Steele, Forehand, & Armistead, 1997). Parental and marital relationships often suffer from the increased demands of dealing with the illness (LaMontagne, Wells, Hepworth, Johnson, & Manes, 1999). It may be important to the client's well-being to recommend counseling for family members to facilitate their coping. Those who are able to effectively cope with situational demands are better able to provide physical and emotional support for the client (LaMontagne et al., 1999).

## Coping Strategies

Coping involves cognitive and behavioral changes in order to manage situational demands (see Chapters 13 and 14). For clients with acute or rapidly progressive diseases, both problem-focused and emotion-focused strategies can help meet the external demands of the situation while managing internal conflicts (Dunkel-Schetter, Feinstein, Taylor, & Falke, 1992; LaMontagne et al., 1999). Problem-focused strategies, aimed at changing something in the self or the environment, can be used to alter situations that clients view as controllable or amenable to change. Consider Sheila, who was recently hospitalized for an opportunistic infection related to AIDS. She asked each of seven friends to be available to sit with her children one day a week, so that she would not have to worry about that detail if she required emergency care at any time.

Emotion-focused strategies, which regulate the emotional or cognitive components of stressful situations, are best suited for short-term or acute episodes over which the client has little control. These strategies may be helpful in dealing with the pain or discomfort associated with a particular form of treatment.

Attitude seems to predict the response of people with acute or rapidly progressing diseases. Denial and a "fighting spirit" seem most beneficial in terms of ultimate survival. Clients with cancer who display these characteristics are significantly more likely to be alive and cancer-free in ten-year follow-up studies when compared to clients who are helpless and hopeless or stoical (Pettingale, Mars, Greer, & Haybrittle, 1985).

Hopefulness is particularly important to positive outcomes (Hinds & Martin, 1988) and has been linked to alteration in the progression of cancerous tumors (Hinds, 1988). In their study of adolescents with cancer, Hinds and Martin (1988) identified four sequential phases in the development of hopefulness. The first phase is cognitive discomfort, when the client activates personal survival tactics in an effort to obtain a reason to hope. Health care practitioners can provide information that is honest and accurate while allowing the client opportunity to hope. Consider the case of Mr. Fox, who asked his physician if he would live the six months needed to see his son graduate from high school. By responding that it was possible, even though not likely, Mr. Fox could still hope that this would happen.

The second phase in the development of hopefulness entails distraction. This requires concentration on neutral or positive thoughts, including "it could always be worse" or "God will take care of me." Peer counseling, to provide an awareness of others who have survived similar circumstances, is helpful at this time. The third phase is cognitive comfort. During this period, the client experiences a more positive attitude and develops the ability to consider the future. Finally, the fourth phase is personal competence, during which hopefulness is achieved. The client perceives him- or herself as resilient and resourceful, believing that a successful outcome is possible.

Although the issues people identify as being important to their quality of life are highly individualized, existential concerns are particularly relevant to this population (Cohen, Mount, Tomas, & Mount, 1996). These include the meaning of life and death, how people fit into the universe as a whole, and how clients make sense of their illness (Belcher, Dettmore, & Holzemer, 1989; Fryback, 1993; O'Connor, Wicker, & Germino, 1990; Reed, 1987; Yalom, 1980). As discussed throughout this book, it is critical that we treat the whole person, not just the medical condition. We need to address the client's suffering while improving the medical situation. This may be accomplished by arranging for pastoral counseling or other spiritual resources needed to explore issues of existential concern.

Clients with terminal illnesses define health as a sense of personal integrity and wholeness, rather than the view espoused by traditional Western medicine that focuses on maintaining physical, social, and emotional health (Kagawa-Singer, 1993). A compassionate care plan requires attention to the client's experience of the illness, not just the disease (Feifel, 1995). Therefore, a thorough assessment must include the existential domain.

The McGill Quality of Life Questionnaire (Cohen et al., 1996) is a clinically useful tool that goes beyond the physical, social, and emotional spheres to include the existential domain. Open-ended questions allow clients to provide answers specific to their personal experiences. Selected items from the tool appear in Table 10–1. The information can be used to provide individualized psychosocial interventions, such as health education, counseling, and/or stress management (Lutgendorf et al., 1997; Schneiderman, Antoni, Saab, & Ironson, 2001).

**TABLE 10–1**  McGill Quality of Life Questionnaire—Sample Questions

| | |
|---|---|
| One troublesome symptom is . . . | To achieve life's goals, I have . . . |
| Physically, I felt . . . | To me, every day seems to be . . . |
| When I think of the future, I am . . . | My life to this point has been . . . |

*(Adapted from Cohen et al., 1996)*

# Age-Related Disability

I'm really concerned about one of my favorite clients. My instructor has been treating her on and off for many years. She has diabetes, visual impairment, polyneuropathies, and a fairly recent amputation of her left lower extremity. It seems that every time she's admitted, there's a little more wrong with her and a little less that we can do to help her remain independent. It's very frustrating for us, and it must be even more so for her. What troubled me the most today was her mental status. She seemed very confused and asked for clarification of the same information over and over. Perhaps she's just overwhelmed by this hospitalization, but I called her primary physician, just in case.

*—From the journal of Nicole Jackson, occupational therapy student*

Modern medicine has prolonged life expectancy, but comparable progress has not been made toward making elder care the priority in public policy or medical practice. While only 12.5 percent of the population is currently over age 65, this group accounts for as much as 40 percent of the annual health care expenditures in the United States (Aldeman & Daly, 2001; Perel, 1998). There are a myriad of reasons why older people seek health care so frequently. Many experience chronic conditions, such as arthritis, coronary artery disease, and diabetes, and these conditions may be further complicated by acute episodes of illness and/or the natural processes of aging.

Because complex patterns of disability are encountered in older clients, treating any condition in isolation is likely to be ineffective (Ferrucci et al., 1996). In younger clients, the effect of minor pathologic events on functional status is often counterbalanced by physiological, behavioral, or social compensatory strategies (Fried, Herdman, Kuhn, Rubin, & Turano, 1991). These strategies are significantly less common in older clients because resilience generally decreases with age. Therefore, clients who acquire severe disability at an older age are more likely to experience a significant decline in functional status, becoming progressively more disabled over a shorter period of time.

When working with clients who are elderly, it is particularly important to take a careful history in order to identify all of the factors that may be contributing to the medical presentation. In this way, problems can be identified and treated early, and accommodations can be developed to compensate for lost function. Powerful predictors of overall health include the availability of social support, the ability to cope, mental health, and a positive attitude. Above all, it is important to involve the client as a partner in health maintenance (Aldeman, 2001).

The plan for health promotion and disease prevention in older clients must be carefully individualized. Healthy older clients, particularly those in the 65 to 75 year range, are often enthusiastic about planning for a healthy life. To achieve this, clients need to be educated on the importance of primary and secondary prevention strategies. Vaccines can prevent illnesses, such as influenza and pneumonia. Behavior modification can be implemented to eliminate smoking, limit the use of alcohol, and encourage exercise. Injury prevention is also important because falls, car accidents, fires, and gunshot wounds together represent the fifth leading cause of death among older people. Identification of risk factors, such as difficulty with night driving, also need to be addressed. Secondary prevention, in the form of screening, and early detection of problems, such as cancer, heart disease, dementia, depression, diabetes, and visual and hearing losses, is also essential (Daly, 2001).

Dementia is a common and perplexing problem among older clients. For example, as many as 4 million Americans currently have Alzheimer's disease (Garwick, Detzner, & Boss, 1994). The dementia associated with Alzheimer's disease is typically gradual in its onset and may not be diagnosed until significant deficits appear. Early signs may be dismissed as simple forgetfulness. Even early changes in mental function and personality can cause clients to lose their jobs, cease driving, and surrender financial management to another family member. These losses, coupled with concerns about what is happening to them, can cause clients to become depressed (Logsdon & Teri, 1997). Successful treatment of depression results in an improvement in self-care, reduction in the fears related to progression of the disease, and increased hopefulness (Cotrell & Schulz, 1993; McEvoy & Patterson, 1986). Treating the depression can avoid or minimize mental suffering, early institutionalization, and premature death in the approximately 30 percent of clients with a dual diagnosis of Alzheimer's disease and depression (Lyketsos & Rabins, 1994).

## SUMMARY

In this chapter, we addressed psychosocial issues related to condition-specific characteristics of select disabilities. Although individual responses vary according to many psychological and social factors, common threads are related to the nature of the disability or illness. A person's growth and maturation throughout the lifespan is affected by the presence of a developmental disability. This impacts all aspects of life, including relationships and social, educational, vocational, and avocational experiences. The aftermath of sudden-onset disability is characterized by disruption of body image, an array of emotional responses, temporal disorientation, and a grief response that helps to bring about adjustment. While the response to acute or rapidly progressive disease is similar to the experience associated with sudden-onset disability, existential well-being is particularly relevant when the disease is life-threatening. Older clients pose the challenge of treating multiple comorbidities, which can be complicated by dementia.

## REFLECTIVE QUESTIONS

1. Consider one key experience or activity you have enjoyed since childhood.
   a. How has this influenced the person you have become?
   b. How might you be different if you had been unable to participate in this experience or activity as a result of a developmental disability?
   c. How might your relationships have been different if you had a developmental disability?
2. How might your role in the family have changed if you had a sibling with a significant congenital problem?
3. Consider having a sudden-onset condition versus a progressive disorder.
   a. Which do you think would present a more challenging adjustment for you? Explain why.
   b. What types of coping strategies might you employ?
4. In the stereotypical American culture, lives are future-oriented. Clients, however, may be in a present-oriented timeframe.

   a. How might this discrepancy in time perception affect your ability to motivate a client?
   b. What strategies might you use to address these challenges?
5. Following the McGill Quality of Life Questionnaire, please complete these sentences:
   a. When I think of the future, I am _____.
   b. To achieve life's goals, I have _____.
   c. To me, every day seems to be _____.
   d. My life to this point has been _____.

## CASE STUDY

Michael Carnes is a 16-year-old boy who sustained a spinal cord injury at thoracic level 6 during a skiing accident. He was recently discharged from outpatient rehabilitation services and thinks that he is ready to return to the high school he attended prior to his injury. The rehabilitation team worked with the special educators at Michael's school to help ensure that the transition back to school would go as smoothly as possible.

A number of accommodations were arranged to improve physical accessibility of the school. In addition, all of the sophomore teachers attended a workshop designed to help them understand the physical limitations associated with spinal cord injury. Mrs. McGlathery, Michael's history teacher, asked Michael if he might like to meet John, a student from another school. She explained that John had used a wheelchair for mobility from a very early age because he has cerebral palsy. Knowing that Michael was still in the process of adjusting to his disability, she thought that meeting another student who uses a wheelchair would be helpful.

1. Based upon the developmental experiences of Michael and John up to this point, would you expect such an encounter to be helpful to Michael? Why or why not?
2. What kinds of behaviors might Michael display at school that would suggest adjustment to his new life circumstances?
3. What kinds of behaviors might Michael display at school that would suggest a failure to adjust to his new life circumstances?
4. Contrast Michael's experience of adjustment to that of someone who is experiencing a long, slow decline in function associated with aging and multiple comorbidities.

## REFERENCES

Aldeman, A. M. (2001). Managing chronic illness. In A. M. Aldeman & M. P. Daly (Eds.), *Twenty common problems in geriatrics* (pp. 3–16), New York: McGraw-Hill.

Aldeman, A. M., & Daly, M. P. (2001). *Twenty common problems in geriatrics.* New York: McGraw-Hill.

Belcher, A. E., Dettmore, D., & Holzemer, S. P. (1989). Spirituality and a sense of well-being in persons with AIDS. *Holistic Nursing Practice, 3,* 16–25.

Bramble, K. (1995). Body image. In I. M. Lubkin (Ed.), *Chronic illness: Impact and interventions* (3rd ed., pp. 285–299). Boston: Jones and Bartlett.

Brinchmann, B. S. (1999). When the home becomes a prison: Living with a severely disabled child. *Nursing Ethics, 6,* 137–143.

Burke, M. L., Hainsworth, M. A., Eakes, G. G., & Lindgren, C. L. (1992). Current knowledge and research on chronic sorrow: A foundation for inquiry. *Death Studies, 16,* 231–245.

Cadman, D., Boyle, M., & Offord, D. R. (1988). The Ontario child health study of social adjustment and mental health of siblings of children with chronic health problems. *Journal of Developmental and Behavioral Pediatrics, 9,* 117–121.

Cahill, S. E., & Eggleston, R. (1995). Reconsidering the stigma of physical disability: Wheelchair use and public kindness. *Sociological Quarterly, 36*(4), 681–698.

Chan, R. C., Lee, P. W., & Lieh-Mak, F. (2000). The pattern of coping in persons with spinal cord injuries. *Disability and Rehabilitation, 22*(11), 501–507.

Cohen, S. R., Mount, B. M., Tomas, J. J., & Mount, L. F. (1996). Existential well-being is an important determinant of quality of life. *Cancer, 77*(3), 576–586.

Cotrell, V., & Schulz, R. (1993). The perspective of the patient with Alzheimer's disease: A neglected dimension of dementia research. *Gerontologist, 33,* 205–210.

Daly, M. P. (2001). Health promotion and disease prevention. In A. M. Aldeman & M. P. Daly (Eds.), *Twenty common problems in geriatrics* (pp. 39–52). New York: McGraw-Hill.

Davis, B. H. (1987). Disability and grief. *Social Casework, 68,* 352–357.

Dunkel-Schetter, C., Feinstein, L., Taylor, S., & Falke, R. (1992). Patterns of coping with cancer. *Health Psychology, 11*(2), 79–87.

Dyson, L. L. (1989). Adjustment of siblings of handicapped children: A comparison. *Journal of Pediatric Psychiatry, 14,* 215–229.

Education for All Handicapped Children Act of 1975, Pub. L. No. 94-142, 20 *U.S. Code* § 1401 (1975).

Ehrenkrantz, D., Miller, C., Vernberg, D. K., & Fox, M. H. (2001). Measuring prevalence of childhood disability: Addressing family needs while augmenting prevention. *Journal of Rehabilitation, 67*(2), 48–60.

Falvo, D. R. (1999). *Medical and psychosocial aspects of chronic illness and disability.* Gaithersburg, MD: Aspen.

Feifel, H. (1995). Psychology and death: Meaningful rediscovery. In L. DeSpelder & A. Strickland (Eds.), *Readings on death and dying: The path ahead* (pp. 19–28). Mountain View, CA: Mayfield.

Ferrucci, L., Guralnik, J. M., Simonsick, E., Salive, M. E., Corti, C., & Langlois, J. (1996). Progressive versus catastrophic disability: A longitudinal view of the disablement process. *Journal of Gerontology, 51A*(3), M123–M130.

Florian, V., Katz, S., & Lahov, V. (1991). Impact of traumatic brain damage on family dynamics and functioning: A review. *International Disability Studies, 13,* 150–157.

Frank, R. G., Elliott, T. R., Corcoran, J. R., & Wonderlich, S. A. (1987). Depression after spinal cord injury: Is it necessary? *Clinical Psychology Review, 7,* 611–622.

Freidenbergs, L., & Kaplan, E. (1993). Cancer. In M. G. Eisenberg, R. I. Glueckauf, & H. H. Zuretsky (Eds.), *Medical aspects of disability* (pp. 105–118). New York: Springer.

Frey, K. S., Fewell, R. R., & Vadasy, P. F. (1989). Parental adjustment and changes in child outcome among families of young handicapped children. *Topics in Early Childhood Education, 8,* 38–57.

Fried, L. P., Herdman, S. J., Kuhn, K. E., Rubin, G., & Turano, K. (1991). Pre-clinical disability: Hypothesis about the bottom of the iceberg. *Journal of Aging and Health, 1*(3), 285–300.

Friedland, J., & McColl, M. (1992). Disability and depression: Some etiological considerations. *Social Science and Medicine, 34,* 395–403.

Fryback, P. B. (1993). Health for people with a terminal diagnosis. *Nursing Science Quarterly, 6,* 147–159.

Garwick, A., Detzner, D., & Boss, P. (1994). Family perceptions of living with Alzheimer's disease. *Family Process, 33,* 327–340.

Gerry, M., & McWhorter, C. (1991). A comprehensive analysis of federal statutes and programs for persons with severe disabilities. In L. Meyer, C. Peck, & L. Brown (Eds.), *Critical issues in the lives of people with severe disabilities* (pp. 495–525). Baltimore: Brookes.

Gerry, M., & Mirsky, A. (1992). Guiding principles for public policy on natural supports. In J. Nisbet (Ed.), *Natural supports in school, at work, and in the community for people with severe disabilities* (pp. 341–346). Baltimore: Brookes.

Gill, M. (1999). Psychosocial implications of spinal cord injury. *Critical Care Nursing Quarterly, 22*(2), 1–7.

Glanz, K., & Lerman, C. (1992). Psychosocial impact of breast cancer: A critical review. *Annals of Behavioral Medicine, 14,* 203–212.

Greenberg, H., Kazak, A., & Meadows, A. (1989). Psychological function in 8- to 16-year-old cancer survivors and their parents. *Journal of Pediatrics, 114*(3), 488–493.

Head, H. (1920). *Studies in neurology* (Vol. 2). London: Oxford University Press.

Hinds, P. (1988). Adolescent hopefulness in illness and health. *Advanced Nursing Science, 10*(3), 79–88.

Hinds, P., & Martin, J. (1988). Hopefulness: The self-sustaining process in adolescents with cancer. *Nursing Research, 37*(6), 336–340.

Holzbauer, J., & Bervin, N. (1996). Disability harassment: A new term for a long-standing problem. *Journal of Counseling and Development, 74*(5), 478–483.

Kagawa-Singer, M. (1993). Redefining health: Living with cancer. *Social Science and Medicine, 37,* 295–304.

Kishi, G., & Meyer, L. (1994). What children report and remember: A six-year follow-up of the effects of social contact between peers with and without severe disabilities. *Journal of the Association for Persons with Severe Handicaps, 19*(4), 279–289.

Konstantareas, M. K., & Lunsky, Y. J. (1997). Sociosexual knowledge, experience, attitudes, and interests of individuals with autistic disorder and developmental delay. *Journal of Autism and Developmental Disorders, 27*(4), 397–413.

LaMontagne, L. L., Wells, N., Hepworth, J. T., Johnson, B. D., & Manes, R. (1999). Parent coping and child distress behaviors during invasive procedures for childhood cancer. *Journal of Pediatric Oncology, 16*(1), 3–12.

Lilliston, B. A. (1985). Psychosocial responses to traumatic physical disability. *Social Work in Health Care, 10*(4), 1–13.

Livneh, H., & Antonak, R. (1997). *Psychosocial adaptation to chronic illness and disability.* Gaithersburg: Aspen.

Livneh, H., Antonak, R., & Gerhardt, J. (1999). Psychosocial adaptation to amputation: The role of sociodemographic variables, disability related factors, and coping strategies. *International Journal of Rehabilitation Research, 22,* 21–31.

Logsdon, R. G., & Teri, L. (1997). The pleasant events schedule—Alzheimer's disease: Psychometric properties and relationship to depression and cognition in Alzheimer's disease patients. *Gerontologist, 37,* 40–45.

Lou, M. F., Dai, Y. T., & Catanzaro, M. (1997). A pilot study to assess the relationships among coping, self-efficacy, and functional improvement in men with paraplegia. *International Journal of Rehabilitation Research, 20,* 99–105.

Lutgendorf, S., Antoni, M., Ironson, G., Klimas, N., Kumar, M., & Starr, K. (1997). Cognitive behavioral stress management decreases dysphoric mood and herpes simplex virus type-2 antibody titers in symptomatic HIV seropositive gay men. *Journal of Consulting and Clinical Psychology, 65,* 31–43.

Lyketsos, C. G., & Rabins, P. V. (1994). Psychopathology in dementia. *Current Opinions in Psychiatry, 7,* 343–346.

Maslow, A. (1968). *Toward a psychology of being* (2nd ed.). Princeton, NJ: Van Nostrand.

McEvoy, C., & Patterson, R. (1986). Behavioral treatment of deficit skill in dementia patients. *Gerontologist, 26,* 475–478.

McHale, S. M., & Gamble W. D. (1989). Sibling relationships of children with disabled and nondisabled brothers and sisters. *Developmental Psychology, 25,* 421–429.

McHale, S. M., & Pawletko, T. M. (1992). Differential treatment of siblings in two family contexts. *Child Development, 63*(1), 68–81.

McKeever, P. (1983). Siblings of chronically ill children: A literature review with implications for research and practice. *American Journal of Orthopsychiatry, 53,* 209–218.

Minde, K. K. (1973). Coping styles of 34 adolescents with cerebral palsy. *American Journal of Psychiatry, 135*(11), 1344–1349.

O'Brien, J., & O'Brien, C. (1992). Members of each other: Perspectives on social support for people with severe disabilities. In J. Nisbet (Ed.), *Natural supports in school, at work, and in the community for people with severe disabilities* (pp. 17–63). Baltimore: Brookes.

O'Connor, A. P., Wicker, C. A., & Germino, B. B. (1990). Understanding the cancer patient's search for meaning. *Cancer Nursing, 13,* 167–175.

Olshansky, S. (1962). Chronic sorrow: A response to have a mentally defective child. *Social Casework, 43,* 191–193.

Perel, V. D. (1998). Psychosocial impact of Alzheimer's disease. *Journal of the American Medical Association, 279*(13), 1038–1040.

Pettingale, K., Mars, T., Greer, S., & Haybrittle, J. (1985). Mental attitudes toward cancer: An additional prognostic factor. *Lancet, 1,* 750.

Rapp, C. E., & Torres, M. M. (2000). The adult with cerebral palsy. *Archives of Family Medicine, 9*(5), 466–472.

Reed, P. G. (1987). Spirituality and well-being in terminally ill hospitalized adults. *Research in Nursing and Health, 10,* 335–344.

Robinson, D., & Harris, M. H. (1997). An overview of age-related problems in people with developmental disabilities. *Orthopaedic Physical Therapy Clinics of North America, 6*(3), 369–381.

Rybarcyzk, B., Nyenhuis, D. L., Nicholas, J. J., Cash, S. M., & Kaiser, J. (1995). Body image, perceived social stigma, and the prediction of psychosocial adjustment to leg amputation. *Rehabilitation Psychology, 40*(2), 95–105.

Schaller, J., & De La Garza, D. (1999). It's about relationships: Perspectives of people with cerebral palsy on belonging in their families, schools, and rehabilitation counseling. *Journal of Applied Rehabilitation Counseling, 30*(2), 7–18.

Schilder, P. (1950). *The image and appearance of the human body.* New York: Wiley.

Schneiderman, N., Antoni, M. H., Saab, P. G., & Ironson, G. (2001). Health psychology: Psychosocial and behavioral aspects of chronic disease management. *Annual Review of Psychology,* 555–586.

Schnorr, R. (1997). From enrollment to membership: "Belonging" in middle and high school classes. *Journal of the Association for Persons with Severe Handicaps, 22*(1), 1–15.

Siemon, M. (1984). Siblings of chronically ill or disabled children. Meeting their needs. *Nursing Clinics of North America, 19,* 295–307.

Stam, H. J., Bultz, B. D., & Pittman, C. A. (1986). Psychosocial problems and interventions in a referred sample of cancer patients. *Psychosomatic Medicine, 48,* 539–548.

Steele, R. G., Forehand, R., & Armistead, L. (1997). The role of family processes and coping strategies in the relationship between parental chronic illness and childhood internalizing problems. *Journal of Abnormal Child Psychology, 25*(2), 83–94.

Sulpizi, L. K. (1996). Issues in sexuality and gynecologic care of women with developmental disabilities. *Journal of Gynecologic and Neonatal Nursing, 25,* 609–614.

Turner, R. J., & Beiser, M. (1990). Major depression and depressive symptomatology among the physically disabled: Assessing the role of chronic stress. *Journal of Nervous and Mental Diseases, 178,* 343–350.

Turner, R. J., & McLean, P. D. (1989). Physical disability and psychological distress. *Rehabilitation Psychology, 34,* 225–243.

Turner, R. J., & Noh, S. (1988). Physical disability and depression: A longitudinal analysis. *Journal of Health and Social Behavior, 29,* 23–37.

Turner, R. J., & Wood, D. W. (1985). Depression and disability: The stress process in a chronically strained population. In J. R. Greenley (Ed.), *Research in community and mental health* (Vol. 5, pp. 77–109). Greenwich, CT: JAI Press.

Van Dongen-Melman, J., & Sanders-Woudstra, J. (1986). Psychological aspects of childhood cancer: A review of the literature. *Journal of Child Psychology and Psychiatry, 27,* 145–180.

Verbrugge, L. M. (1995). Gender and health: An update on hypothesis and evidence. *Journal of Health and Social Behavior, 26,* 156–182.

Voll, R., Krumm, B., & Fichtner, H. J. (1999). Demand for psychosocial counseling of young wheel-chair users. *International Journal of Rehabilitation Research, 22,* 119–122.

Walsh, K. K., Hammerman, S., Josephson, F., & Krupka, P. (2000). Caring for people with developmental disabilities: Survey of nurses about their education and experience. *Mental Retardation, 38*(1), 33–41.

Whyte, F., & Smith, L. (1997). A literature review of adolescence and cancer. *European Journal of Cancer Care, 6,* 137–146.

Willard-Holt, C. (1998). Academic and personality characteristics of gifted students with cerebral palsy: A multiple case study. *Exceptional Children, 65*(1), 37–50.

Wolf, L., Fisman, S., Ellison, D., & Freeman, T. (1998). Effect of sibling perception of differential parental treatment in sibling dyads with one disabled child. *Journal of the American Academy of Child and Adolescent Psychiatry, 37*(12), 1317–1326.

Wolf, L., Fisman, S., & Speechley, M. (1989). Psychological effects of parenting stress on parents of autistic children. *Journal of Autism and Developmental Disorders, 19,* 157–166.

Worchel, F., Nolan, B., & Wilson, V. (1988). Assessment of depression in children with cancer. *Journal of Paediatric Psychology, 13*(1), 101–112.

Wortman, C. B., & Silver, R. C. (1989). The myth of coping with loss. *Journal of Consulting Clinical Psychology, 57,* 349–355.

Yalom, I. D. (1980). *Existential psychotherapy.* New York: Basic Books.

Yoshida, K. K. (1994). Institutional impact on self-concept among persons with spinal cord injury. *International Journal of Rehabilitation Research, 17,* 95–107.

Zajicek-Farber, M. L. (1998). Promoting good health in adolescents with developmental disabilities. *Health and Social Work, 23*(3), 203–213.

# 11

# *Sexuality*

Poor Mr. Michaels was so distressed today. He can't imagine how he can possibly resume a sexual relationship with his wife now that he has lost sensation below his chest, cannot maintain an erection, cannot ejaculate, and must wear an external condom catheter to manage urinary incontinence. It's difficult for him to even bring up the topic with her. Although he expects that Mrs. Michaels will be as disgusted as he is about the whole thing, he fears that she'll deny it "out of pity and embarrassment." After a very emotional session, Mr. Michaels finally agreed to ask his wife to meet with us next time to begin to talk about their options for resuming a sexual relationship.

—*From the journal of Teresa Dumont, counseling psychology student*

Sexuality is an important aspect of life and is strongly linked to many biological, psychological, social, cultural, and religious factors. It is an important determinant in all interpersonal relationships and encompasses all of the following:

- Gender identity
- Attractiveness
- Sexual attitudes and beliefs
- Sexual behaviors and practices

Our perceptions about sexuality are strongly affected by those expressed by our parents and a society that places value on certain body functions, body parts, and behaviors (Drench, 1992). For example, our society conditions men to prize physical performance (Anderson & Kitchin, 2000). Because of this, loss of the ability to perform sexually by achieving penile erection and ejaculation can have a devastating, demasculating effect, as illustrated in

Mr. Michaels's case above. Sexuality is influenced by many factors, including hormone levels, age, and health, and is closely linked to self-concept (Drench, 1992; Drench & Losee, 1996; Finan, 1997a).

Self-concept is a psychological construct that represents the way people feel about themselves (Super & Block, 1991). As discussed in Chapter 9, body image is one aspect of self-concept. It reflects the combined expectations that people have about how their bodies look and function to them with their perception of how others react to their bodies (McHugh, 1998). Because of the strong relationship between self-concept, body image, and sexual identity, when one factor is impaired, the others are affected, too. The problem then becomes a more global one, affecting all aspects of the client's life (Drench, 1992).

Healthy sexuality depends on the presence of three conditions: (1) the ability to enjoy and control sexual and reproductive behavior in a manner consistent with personal and social ethics; (2) freedom from psychological problems, such as fear, shame, guilt, and false beliefs, that could negatively affect sexual responses or relationships; and (3) freedom from illnesses, diseases, and impairments that interfere with physical aspects of sexual and reproductive function (World Health Organization, 1975).

In this chapter, we explore the importance of integrating sexuality in a holistic approach to client care. Because the development of healthy sexuality is a lifelong process, the major developmental tasks associated with each stage of life will first be reviewed. We also address the biological, psychological, social, cultural, and behavioral dimensions of sexuality and describe clinical interventions.

# Sexual Development

### Prenatal

Sexual development begins *in utero*. During the prenatal period, biological influences determine whether the embryo develops as male or female. This differentiation involves the genitals, internal reproductive organs (gonads), and the central nervous system. Sexual reflexes are all present at birth, except the male's ability to ejaculate, which depends on heightened levels of sex hormones that emerge during puberty. Following birth, psychological, social, and cultural factors become more significant than biological factors as sexual development continues (Masters, Johnson, & Kolodny, 1992).

### Early Childhood

The major sexual task of early childhood is to develop gender identity. This is the perceived sense of being male or female and is primarily shaped by psychosocial factors. Kohlberg (1966) proposes that gender development parallels intellectual development. He identifies three tasks that are involved in the process of developing gender identity:

1. Accurate identification of self and others as male or female (labeling).
2. The realization that boys become men and girls become women (stability).
3. The realization that gender is permanent and not changed by cultural gender cues, such as hairstyle or clothing (constancy).

Very young children understand gender in simplistic terms that match their views of the world. For example, preschool-age girls may believe that they can grow up to be fathers. By the age of 5 or 6, children understand that gender is constant. Through observation and imitation, they learn which behaviors are socially and culturally appropriate for each gender. Cognitive theorists, such as Kohlberg, believe that children mimic the behaviors of same-sex parents because it helps them achieve self-identity. In contrast, learning theorists believe that children are motivated to imitate same-sex parents simply because parents reward this behavior (Masters et al., 1992).

Healthy sexual development depends on the availability of appropriate same-sex role models. Parental attitudes, behaviors, beliefs, and values first influence a child's sexual identity. Children receive verbal and nonverbal messages about how their parents view themselves and their own bodies. As a child matures, use of proper vocabulary to describe body parts and functions may help to ensure ongoing effective communication about sexual issues between parents and children (Finan, 1997b; Masters et al., 1992).

During early childhood, sexual exploration takes the form of genital play. Parents' negative reactions to self-exploration can lead to feelings of guilt and a negative self-image. Rather, the child can be instructed to seek privacy for such exploration. The concept of appropriate versus inappropriate touching by others also needs to be clarified. Parents' general level of comfort with physical affection, the way they wash their children's genitals, and their responses to their children's genital exploration all provide signals to children about how they should feel about their own sexuality (Finan, 1997b).

Sexual development of children who have congenital disabilities may differ significantly from those who do not (Nosek et al., 1996). It may be difficult or impossible for children with mobility problems to imitate the behaviors of the same-sex parent. Sensory impairment, bowel and bladder incontinence, and abnormal muscle tone may interfere with normal self-exploration, making it difficult for the child to gain an early understanding of the anatomical and physiological functions of his or her body. A cognitive disability may also alter interactions between the parents and child. Onset of disability during the early childhood years can have a significant impact on sexual development throughout the lifespan.

Many parents have concerns about their child's sexuality but might be unsure about how to ask for information. They may fear that their child will never have an intimate relationship or that he or she will get emotionally hurt if involved with someone (Berman et al., 1999). Pediatric health care providers can help facilitate discussion by asking parents leading questions and by modeling appropriate sex education. Consider the approach taken by the Smiths' pediatrician. During their baby's recent visit to the Spina Bifida Clinic at a local teaching hospital, he offered the following:

> Some parents who have a child with spina bifida wonder what it will be like when their child grows up. Do you ever wonder if he'll be able to have a sexual relationship or a family of his own? Would you like to spend some time talking about this? Perhaps I can help you identify some appropriate reference materials that you might find helpful.

Kelton (1999) suggests creating the opportunity for discussion of sexuality at key points in the child's development, including just after diagnosis, immediately prior to puberty, during adolescence, and sometime prior to transferring care from a pediatric to an adult practitioner.

## Later Childhood and Adolescence

Adolescence represents the most dramatic period in sexual development. The goal of this period is for the child to emerge with a positive self-image, a strong sense of identity, the capacity to form intimate relationships, and to gain independence from the family (Blum, 1988; Haraguchi, 1981; McAnarney, 1985; Meeropol, 1991; Zajicek-Farber, 1998). The onset of puberty is brought about by a significant increase in sex hormones. Exciting physical and psychological changes occur as children of both genders experience rapid physical growth, maturation of the gonads and genitals, and the development of secondary sexual characteristics. Girls develop breasts and grow pubic and axillary hair. Boys experience increased muscle mass, growth of facial, pubic, and axillary hair, as well as deepening of the voice. Girls begin menstruation, and boys develop the ability to ejaculate, marking the onset of fertility. Hormonal changes are responsible for new sexual sensations and erotic thoughts and dreams in both boys and girls (Masters et al., 1992).

Sexual self-exploration continues, but more intimate interactions with partners emerge, including hand-holding, kissing, and other forms of physical closeness. These are early expressions of personal sexual identity and independent decision-making. The extent to which adolescents experiment with sexual behavior varies according to the individual's personal readiness, moral reasoning, fear of consequences, level of romantic attachment to the partner, and peer pressure. Those who seek complete personal independence from parental influences are more likely to engage in early sexual intercourse. Interestingly, these teens are also more likely to experiment with drugs and alcohol (Masters et al., 1992). Adolescents who have learned about sex at an early age from well-informed parents are more likely to abstain (Finan, 1997c; Masters et al., 1992).

Socially, adolescents experience many challenges, including developing progressive independence from parents, struggling to fit in with peers, and forming their own sets of values. While doing so, they must also cope with rapid physical changes and enhanced sexual feelings previously described. Many adolescents have incomplete or inaccurate information about sex that may cause them to feel anxious about how normal they are. The changes associated with puberty are closely linked to the development of body image and self-concept. Adolescents are particularly concerned about physical attractiveness, and any perception of being different threatens their self-image (Finan, 1997c; Masters et al., 1992). The influence of the media can be damaging, especially television, movies, and popular magazines, which place a premium on the young and beautiful, the strong and conspicuously muscled.

Adolescents who have chronic health conditions may need additional support and encouragement to develop a positive sense of self as a sexual person (Kelton, 1999). They face the same developmental tasks as their peers, but often have fewer opportunities to learn, practice, and perfect social skills (Blum, 1988; Cromer et al., 1990; Meeropol, 1991; Stevens et al., 1996). As we discussed in Chapter 9, body image and self-concept are often impaired, particularly if the disability is visible or if a wheelchair or other conspicuous assistive technology is required (Anderson & Kitchin, 2000; Cromer et al., 1990; Voll, Krumm, & Fichtner, 1999). Finding peer groups where they can fit in is extremely important because it is through group interactions that adolescents acquire sexual language, discuss sexual ideals, and form important relationships (Kelton, 1999).

Consider Tom, a 14-year-old boy with a diagnosis of Duchenne's muscular dystrophy. Until last year, he was able to walk around school independently. Now that he is in middle school, he requires the use of a wheelchair and occasional physical assistance of a personal aide. Although his classmates have been asked to "treat Tom like any other kid," this is not always practical. He is the only student in the school who uses a wheelchair. He is unable to pass through the busy halls during class changes without the assistance of his aide. In a recent conversation with his occupational therapist, Tom asked for ideas about how he could use his wheelchair to dance with a girl during the next school social. Without a peer group to model appropriate behavior, he had no idea how to begin to take social risks now that he required a wheelchair.

In addition, adolescents who have disabilities tend to receive less formal sexual education than their peers (Cromer et al., 1990; Kelton, 1999; Stevens et al., 1996). When they do receive information, the presented materials may not include disability-specific content (Berman et al., 1999; Blum, Resnick, Nelson, & St. Germaine, 1991; Kelton, 1999). This is unfortunate because adolescents with chronic conditions are at least as sexually involved as their peers and significantly more likely to be sexually abused (Choquet, Du Pasquier Fediaevsky, & Manfredi, 1997; Suris, Resnick, Cassuto, & Blum, 1996). It is critical to provide information regarding medically safe and appropriate contraception, reproduction, and genetics, as well as strategies to establish appropriate personal boundaries (Kelton, 1999).

Discussions with adolescents should not assume heterosexuality. Sexual orientation of teens with chronic conditions is believed to be comparable to the general population. Any information made available needs to include reference to appropriate gay, lesbian, or bisexual support groups because the client may be reluctant to ask questions directly (Kelton, 1999; Kreiss & Patterson, 1997).

Adolescents who have disabilities would like to discuss sexuality with their health care providers, but practitioners fail to offer the opportunity because of underestimating clients' sexual concerns, lack of knowledge, their embarrassment, or fear that the client will feel embarrassed (Wall-Haas, 1991; Waterhouse, 1993; Zajicek-Farber, 1998). Missed opportunities to discuss and solve adolescents' sexual concerns increase the likelihood of impaired sexuality as development continues.

## Early Adulthood

Early adulthood marks the time when important lifestyle choices are made and increasing responsibilities are assumed with respect to relationships. During this time, many young adults choose lifelong partners. Developing effective interpersonal skills is paramount because the ability to share feelings is essential to developing healthy, intimate relationships. Couples must openly explore topics, including sex outside of marriage, pregnancy, the use of contraceptives, monogamy, sexually transmitted diseases, future plans, and parenthood. The primary task of this period is to move from relationships characterized by infatuation and passion toward those that are more enduring and include mature love (Finan, 1997a; Rossi, 1994).

Often significant pressure is applied by well-meaning parents and peers for young adults to get married and start a family. Those who choose to remain single may have to deal with frequent questions about why they made this choice. Individuals who do choose marriage can expect to experience changes in their sexual relationship, particularly when they decide to start a family (Finan, 1997a).

Some young adults prefer to live with their partners without getting married. This concept emerged out of the radical political, social, and sexual revolutions of the 1960s and continues today. Masters and coauthors (1992) described three basic forms of cohabitation: (1) casual and temporary, (2) preparatory for marriage, and (3) alternative to marriage. The degree to which couples view cohabitation as an option depends on personal and family values (Blumstein & Schwartz, 1983; Masters et al., 1992).

Marriage has traditionally been associated with a higher degree of commitment than cohabitation, but there appear to be more subtle differences as well. When compared to married persons, people who cohabit are more likely to have lower quality and unstable relationships (Brown, 2000; Brown & Booth, 1996), are more likely to become depressed (Brown, 2000), and have a higher incidence of alcohol abuse (Horwitz & White, 1998). For these reasons, the choice of cohabitation may be particularly dangerous for young adults who have disabilities. The confluence of all potential negative influences could be overwhelming.

Major developmental tasks of this period, including attainment of physical and psychological independence, a career, and finding a lifelong partner, can be particularly challenging for young adults who have disabilities. As indicated above, developmental disabilities can have a negative impact on sexual development, causing fears and inhibitions about forming intimate relationships (Voll et al., 1999). An individual who acquires a disability during this period may face fewer challenges, particularly if there is already an established relationship, and the partner remains involved and supportive (Kreuter, Dahllöf, Gudjonsson, Sullivan, & Siösteen, 1998). However, the onset of illness or disability can leave a person vulnerable to feelings of shame, anxiety, doubt, and anger, which may place a significant psychological burden on the client and his or her partner (Kreuter et al., 1998; Lilliston, 1985).

Adults with disabilities are often regarded as disinterested in sexual and reproductive matters (Anderson & Kitchin, 2000; Sawin, 1986; Sulpizi, 1996). The attitudinal and physical barriers to reproductive health care that many clients encounter support this finding. Individuals with disabilities report both emotional and physical discomfort when they need to access the health care system (Becker, Stuifbergen, & Tinkle, 1997; Sawin, 1986). Common problems include inaccessible equipment and facilities, limited contraceptive options, health care providers' insensitivity and lack of knowledge about sexuality and reproduction for people with disabilities, and limited information tailored to their needs (Becker et al., 1997; Gans, Mann, & Becker, 1993; Tepper, 1992).

## Middle Adulthood

The middle-aged adult generally enjoys a time of sexual freedom and comfort. Most adults have established careers and/or families and can now spend more time and energy focused on themselves and their partners. Previous sexual experiences allow for more open and realistic sexual relationships. However, this is also an age when many adults begin to question their sexual attractiveness because of age-related changes. Reflection on past accomplishments and setting future goals are common themes. Identity and role confusion can occur and may give rise to a midlife crisis (Finan, 1997a; Masters et al., 1992).

Men seem to be more vulnerable to midlife crises than women. When men begin to question their sexual abilities and attractiveness, they are likely to experience sexual performance difficulties, which only adds to the crisis. In contrast, women often experience midlife as a time of self-discovery, enjoying unprecedented sexual openness that they were too inhibited to enjoy when they were younger and less sexually experienced. However, women are not immune to physical changes associated with aging (Masters et al., 1992).

Perimenopause generally begins when women reach their 40s, with menopause usually completed by age 55. The timing and symptoms vary, but most women will experience at least minor symptoms related to declining levels of hormones. Vaginal changes have the most significant effect on the sexual relationship at this time. Lower estrogen levels cause a reduction in vaginal elasticity and lubrication, which can cause pain during sexual intercourse. These problems can generally be eliminated with artificial lubricants and/or estrogen replacement. If a couple enjoys a loving and supportive relationship, they tend to discover means to adjust to age-related changes. Those who are unwilling to commit time or emotional energy to their relationships are more likely to experience waning sexual interest, seek extramarital affairs, and/or divorce during this time (Masters et al., 1992).

The onset of an illness or disability during this period may complicate midlife challenges. Rather than enjoying each other's company, the couple must adjust to changes associated with the illness or disability. Sexual changes associated with this phase of development may be exacerbated along with the emergence of new problems associated with the specific illness or disability encountered, as illustrated by Mr. Michaels in the journal entry at the beginning of this chapter.

## Older Adulthood

I met with the Arnolds today to discuss their discharge plan. As a routine question, I asked if either of them had any concerns about resuming their sexual relationship. Mrs. Arnold became flustered and got red in the face. She sputtered something that sounded like "those days are over." Mr. Arnold simply looked away. Since Mrs. Arnold was clearly upset and embarrassed, I dropped the issue and finished the meeting. As I continued my rounds, Mrs. Arnold's reaction bothered me. I waited until her husband left the room, then returned to talk with her. This time, I started by acknowledging her obvious discomfort with the subject and asked her if she had any questions or concerns that I might be able to address. Although she was still noticeably uncomfortable, she confided that she couldn't imagine how sexual intercourse would be possible in light of all the precautions she has to follow to avoid dislocating her new hip. We spent some time discussing alternative positioning and precautions. As we talked, she appeared more relaxed and at ease. She assured me that Mr. Arnold would be forever in my debt!

*—From the journal of Mitzy Riley, nursing student*

Older adulthood is characterized by numerous physical and mental changes and can also be emotionally difficult. Many older adults retire from their professional positions, which can lead to identity confusion. They are also burdened with the decline of physical and mental functions and are confronted with the real possibility of their own death or the death of their partners (Wainrib, 1992).

Older adults also face many myths and biases about sexuality. Until the 1950s, it was widely believed that interest in sex ended at the age of 50. Kinsey, Pomeroy, and Martin (1948), in their ground-breaking work on sexuality, concluded that people continue sexual interest and activity well into old age. This finding has been supported by many others (Brecher, 1984; Bretschneider & McCoy, 1988; Kinsey, Pomeroy, Martin, & Gebhard,

1953; Masters, 1986; McKinlay & Brambilla, 1993; Persson, 1980; Starr & Weiner, 1981; Wiley & Bortz, 1996). Contrary to popular belief, age does not eliminate the desire or ability to engage in sexual relationships or activities. However, age-related changes call for adaptations to ensure continued enjoyment and satisfaction (Drench & Losee, 1996).

Women who are postmenopausal may continue to experience some of the physical changes that began earlier during menopause. These changes may interfere with sexual functioning, but psychosocial issues are generally more of a concern. The primary issues include problems with sexual communication, commitment, and lack of enjoyment (Dunn, Croft, & Hackett, 1999; Wiley & Bortz, 1996).

Although men also face psychosocial concerns, they tend to center their problems on physical functioning. They experience more overt physical changes, including the need for longer and more direct stimulation to achieve erection, a reduction in the amount of semen, less intense sensations with ejaculation, and a longer recovery period after ejaculation before repeat ejaculation can occur (Dunn et al., 1999; Finan, 1997a; Masters et al., 1992). Erectile dysfunction can initiate a pattern of negativity involving expectation of failure, avoidance, and withdrawal. This can lead to blaming and anger in the relationship. Couples who view erectile dysfunction as a "couple's problem" versus a male issue can avoid the pattern of negativity and identify solutions and alternatives (Wiley & Bortz, 1996).

Declining health is one of the main problems associated with reduced sexual activity among older people (Diokno, Brown, & Herzog, 1990; Mooradian, 1991). Older adults are more likely to take medications, have chronic diseases, and undergo surgery. Table 11–1 outlines the most common problems experienced by older adults. Readers interested in more detailed information about the sexual implications of each of the disorders listed are referred to the summary provided by Arshag Mooradian (1991).

Because death is more likely as age progresses, loss of a partner is another leading cause of declining sexual activity in older age. Numerous social and cultural barriers exist that make it difficult or impossible for older adults to meet new sexual partners. Unfortunately, some health care professionals propagate the myth that older adults have no sexual needs or desires.

**TABLE 11–1**   Conditions Affecting Sexual Activity in Older People

| *Psychosocial* | *Diabetic Changes* |
|---|---|
| • Depression | • Vascular problems |
| • Poor self-concept | • Erectile dysfunction |
| • Social isolation | • Orgasmic impairment |
| • Poverty | • Neuropathies |
| *Hormonal* | *Medication Effects* |
| • Reduced testosterone | • Fatigue |
| • Hyperthyroidism | • Erectile dysfunction |
| • Hypothyroidism | • Premature or retrograde ejaculation |
| *Cardiopulmonary* | *Mobility Impairments* |
| • Arteriosclerosis | • Arthritis |
| • Decreased cardiac output | • Postsurgical limitations |
| • Dyspnea on exertion | • Paralysis |

## Clinical Interventions

Today, I attended a group therapy session that involved clients and their partners. Of all things, the topic was sexuality. All of the clients had experienced strokes. Some were several years poststroke, while others had only been living with the consequences of their strokes for a short time. I was a little surprised when I learned what the meeting was going to be about because all of the clients were well over age 65. I didn't expect the kind of discussion that ensued. They were talking about everything from extending the use of foreplay to ensure adequate vaginal lubrication to modifying positions needed to accommodate unilateral extremity weakness. At the end of the session, couples were discussing plans for practicing some of the techniques discussed. I was so impressed with their openness with each other. I never realized that people in this age group had the same sexual needs and desires that I do. I certainly have a new appreciation for my older clients now.

*—From the journal of Stephanie Ducey, social work student*

Clients are extremely sensitive to the perceived and actual attitudes of health care practitioners. For this reason, it is particularly important to become aware of our own biases, beliefs, and need for additional education before attempting to help clients with their concerns about sexuality (Drench & Losee, 1996). Health care providers are not immune to prejudices and misconceptions. Remember that a particularly common myth is that older adults or people with disabilities either have no sexual needs or desires or have excessive or perverted needs and desires (Anderson & Kitchin, 2000). Even when educated to the contrary, many providers remain influenced by their own experiences and still have difficulty understanding and accepting the needs of their clients (Eliason & Raheim, 2000). In addition, many practitioners fail to discuss sexuality with their clients because of their own embarrassment or lack of knowledge and the fear that their clients will be embarrassed (Wall-Haas, 1991; Waterhouse, 1993; Zajicek-Farber, 1998).

As illustrated in the journal entry, accurate practitioner knowledge is associated with more positive attitudes about the sexuality of clients (Kelton, 1999). Practitioners who understand that their clients have sexual needs can help them accommodate to changes of age, illness, and/or disability. Education can also help providers become more comfortable with sexuality, making it easier to facilitate discussions with clients.

Recognizing that many health professionals are uncomfortable addressing sexual issues with their clients, Kelton (1999) suggests a four-step approach to sexuality education:

1. Initiate a program of self-learning about sexuality by reading books and accessing other resources specific to the needs of the client population being treated.

2. Raise the consciousness of other members of the team by asking questions related to the impact that medications or other proposed treatments may have on sexual function and fertility.

3. Become comfortable discussing issues of sexuality with clients. Begin with topics that are easier for the clients to discuss and move toward more personal, intimate topics as clients invite you into their more private realms. Use correct scientific terms rather

than jargon or street language to maintain professional boundaries, but be prepared to offer alternate terminology if confusion is evident.

4. Document the topics discussed and create a written plan for the future. It is not necessary to discuss sexuality during every interaction nor is it appropriate to cover every aspect of sexuality in a single visit.

Resources related to sexuality are included among the additional readings listed at the end of this chapter. Readers may find these resources helpful for their own education. Providers should review sources before recommending them to individual clients. By doing so, resources that respect individual beliefs, values, and preferences can be selected.

Education can help providers develop knowledge, but a true sensitivity and respect for the individual needs of each client is needed in order to avoid imposing our own values. By obtaining a thorough history that reflects the client's beliefs, morals, and personal preferences, recommendations can be "tailor-made" to fit each client.

## Taking a Sexual History

Mrs. O'Leary was referred to physical therapy for lymphedema management. As she was reporting her social history to me today, she began to weep. Although she and her husband have always enjoyed an open and satisfying sexual relationship, she has been avoiding any intimate contact with him. She said that Mr. O'Leary is very supportive and has approached her many times just to "cuddle and be close," but she just has no interest. Her left upper extremity is "ugly and swollen," and she still can't bear to look at the mastectomy site. I thought she seemed pretty open to suggestions, and I offered ideas that would help her progress to more intimate contact with her husband. She seemed so relieved when she left. As we talked, she remembered that one of the nurses made some of the same suggestions before the surgery, but at the time, she really didn't think they applied to her. Because of the close relationship she and her husband had always enjoyed, she never expected any of these problems.

*—From the journal of Maria Menendez, physical therapist student*

A sexual history can be taken in conjunction with the medical and social history. It is best to begin with nonthreatening information and move toward more intimate details. This progressive approach to history-taking provides an opportunity for clients to share verbal and nonverbal feedback that establishes boundaries based on their comfort level (Drench, 1992; Drench & Losee, 1996; Shell & Miller, 1999).

It is important to remain objective, nonjudgmental, and sensitive throughout the discussion. Clients need to believe that the information they are sharing will remain confidential. Embarrassment is a common barrier. It may be more comfortable for some clients to respond in writing. Many published questionnaires can be used to obtain information about sexual concerns, fears, and preferences (McCabe, Cummins, & Deeks, 1999; Schover & Jensen, 1988; Siösteen, Lundquist, Blomstrand, Sullivan, & Sullivan, 1990). Written responses can then be used as the basis for discussion.

Practitioners need to refrain from judging clients based on their own beliefs and values about what is normal or abnormal, right or wrong. Each client has his or her own value system, and caution must be taken to respect individual differences. Consider the client's and his or her partner's cultural, social, sexual, and religious orientations. What is perceived to be moral and right varies according to these factors. What one client will find to be an acceptable expression of sexuality, another may find abhorrent. For example, some cultures consider kissing to be vulgar and dirty (Drench & Losee, 1996; Kaye, 1993; Kripke & Vaias, 1994; Masters et al., 1992; Rose & Soares, 1993).

There may or may not be a need to focus attention on sexuality and sexual function during the examination or treatment session. The subject can be presented along with other functional issues in a matter-of-fact manner. Clients who trust their health care practitioners will be open to counseling and assistance. It is important that they know that this subject can remain open for future discussion. Some clients may be initially reluctant to discuss sexuality and sexual function. However, if given another opportunity, they may decide to accept the invitation to discuss their concerns.

## SUMMARY

Sexuality is an integral component of health. Until recently, health care practitioners have overlooked this component of wellness, particularly for their clients who are older than 60 and/or those who have chronic health conditions. In this chapter, we discussed the importance of addressing clients' sexuality, regardless of their age. The stages of sexual development were presented and the impact of disability or illness discussed. Evidence exists that not all health care providers have the knowledge needed to effectively address the sexual needs of their clients. Guidelines for professional development were outlined. A sensitive, progressive approach for obtaining a sexual history was described.

## REFLECTIVE QUESTIONS

1. Reflect on the cultural, religious, family, and social influences in your life.
   a. How have these shaped your attitudes, beliefs, and values about sexuality?
   b. How have these shaped your beliefs and comfort level when discussing sexuality with clients?
2. What do you believe are your responsibilities for discussing issues of sexuality with clients?
3. Consider gender identity, attractiveness, sexual attitudes and beliefs, and sexual behaviors and practices. How might each of the following conditions affect these aspects of a person's sexuality?
   a. a congenital disability, such as spina bifida
   b. a progressive disorder, such as multiple sclerosis
   c. an acute onset of lower extremity amputation
   d. end-stage renal disease
4. What strategies might you use to discuss sexuality with someone whose opinions, beliefs, and attitudes are different from your own?

**5.** a. How do *you* differentiate between sexuality and sexual function?
   b. Provide examples to support your beliefs.

# CASE STUDY

Lucy Bluecreek is a 13-year-old girl with a hearing impairment. She recently received a new hearing aid that markedly improves her ability to hear, but it is significantly larger than her previous one. Lucy feels embarrassed about wearing the new hearing aid, feeling certain that everyone notices it. Her parents made her promise that she would wear it at school, but she often removes it, especially when she's in the company of boys.

**1.** Discuss the developmental factors that are likely to be influencing Lucy's feelings and behaviors.
**2.** How and why might Lucy's perspective be changed if a boy that she liked asked her to go out with him?
**3.** In what ways might Lucy's response to this new device be different if she were a student about to graduate from college? A middle-aged woman who was married with children? Explain the reason(s) for the differences.
**4.** If you were Lucy's teacher and were aware of her apparent discomfort with this new device, what kind of interventions might you suggest?

# REFERENCES

Anderson, P., & Kitchin, R. (2000). Disability, space, and sexuality: Access to family planning services. *Social Science and Medicine, 51,* 1163–1173.

Becker, H., Stuifbergen, A., & Tinkle, M. (1997). Reproductive health care experiences of women with physical disabilities: A qualitative study. *Archives of Physical Medicine and Rehabilitation, 78*(Suppl. 5), S26–S33.

Berman, H., Harris, D., Enright, R., Gilpin, M., Cathers, T., & Bukovy, G. (1999). Sexuality and the adolescent with a physical disability: Understandings and misunderstandings. *Issues in Comprehensive Pediatric Nursing, 22,* 183–196.

Blum, R. (1988). The intricate challenge of disability and adolescence. *Connections: The Newsletter of the National Center for Youth with Disabilities, 1*(1), 3, 7.

Blum, R., Resnick, M., Nelson, R. & St. Germaine, A. (1991). Family and peer issues among adolescents with spina bifida and cerebral palsy. *Pediatrics, 88,* 280–285.

Blumstein, P. W., & Schwartz, P. (1983). *American couples.* New York: William Morrow.

Brecher, E. (1984). *Love, sex, and aging.* Boston: Little, Brown.

Bretschneider, J., & McCoy, N. (1988). Sexual interest and behavior in healthy 80–102 year olds. *Annals of Sex Behavior, 17,* 108–129.

Brown, S. L. (2000). The effect of union type on psychological well-being: Depression of cohabitants versus married. *Journal of Health and Social Behavior, 41,* 241–255.

Brown, S. L., & Booth, A. (1996). Cohabitation versus marriage: A comparison of relationship quality. *Journal of Marriage and the Family, 58,* 668–678.

Choquet, M., Du Pasquier Fediaevsky, L., & Manfredi, R. (1997). Sexual behavior among adolescents reporting chronic conditions: A French national survey. *Journal of Adolescent Health, 20,* 62–67.

Cromer, B. A., Enrile, B., McCoy, K., Gerhardstein, M. J., Fitzpatrick, M., & Judis, J. (1990). Knowledge, attitudes, and behavior related to sexuality in adolescents with chronic disability. *Developmental Medicine and Child Neurology, 32,* 602–610.

Diokno, A. C., Brown, M. B., & Herzog, A. R. (1990). Sexual function in the elderly. *Archives of Internal Medicine, 150,* 197–200.

Drench, M. E. (1992). Impact of altered sexuality and sexual function in spinal cord injury: A review. *Sexuality and Disability, 10*(1), 3–14.

Drench, M. E., & Losee, R. H. (1996). Sexuality and sexual capacities of elderly people. *Rehabilitation Nursing, 21*(3), 118–122.

Dunn, K. M., Croft, P. R., & Hackett, G. I. (1999). Association of sexual problems with social, psychological, and physical problems in men and women: A cross-sectional population survey. *Epidemiology and Community Health, 53,* 144–148.

Eliason, M. J., & Raheim, S. (2000). Experiences and comfort with culturally diverse groups in undergraduate pre-nursing students. *Journal of Nursing Education, 39*(4), 161–165.

Finan, S. L. (1997a). Promoting health sexuality: Guidelines for early through older adulthood. *The Nurse Practitioner, 22*(12), 54–60.

Finan, S. L. (1997b). Promoting health sexuality: Guidelines for infancy through preschool. *The Nurse Practitioner, 22*(10), 79–88.

Finan, S. L. (1997c). Promoting health sexuality: Guidelines for the school-aged child and adolescent. *The Nurse Practitioner, 22*(11), 62–68.

Gans, B. M., Mann, N. R., & Becker, B. E. (1993). Delivery of primary care to the physically challenged. *Archives of Physical Medicine and Rehabilitation, 74,* 15–19.

Haraguchi, R. S. (1981). Developing programs meeting the special needs of physically disabled adolescents. *Rehabilitation Literature, 42,* 75–78.

Horwitz, A. V., & White, H. R. (1998). The relationship of cohabitation and mental health: A longitudinal study of a young adult cohort. *Journal of Marriage and the Family, 60,* 505–514.

Kaye, R. A. (1993). Sexuality in later years. *Aging and Society, 13,* 415–426.

Kelton, S. (1999). Sexuality education for youth with chronic conditions. *Pediatric Nursing, 25*(5), 491.

Kinsey, A. C., Pomeroy, W. B., & Martin, C. E. (1948). Age and sexual outlet. In A. Kinsey, W. Pomeroy, & C. Martin, *Sexual behavior in the human male* (pp. 218–262). Philadelphia: W. B. Saunders.

Kinsey, A. C., Pomeroy, W. B., Martin, C. E., & Gebhard, P. H. (1953). *Sexual behavior in the human female*. Philadelphia: W. B. Saunders.

Kohlberg, L. (1966). A cognitive-developmental analysis of children's sex-role concepts and attitudes. In E. Maccoby (Ed.), *The development of sex differences* (pp. 82–172). Stanford, CA: Stanford University Press.

Kreiss, J. L., & Patterson, D. L. (1997). Psychosocial issues in primary care of lesbian, gay, bisexual, and transgender youth. *Journal of Pediatric Health Care, 11,* 266–274.

Kreuter, M., Dahllöf, A. G., Gudjonsson, G., Sullivan, M., & Siösteen, A. (1998). Sexual adjustment and its predictors after traumatic brain injury. *Brain Injury, 12*(5), 349–368.

Kripke, C. C., & Vaias, L. (1994). The importance of taking a sensitive sexual history. *Journal of the American Medical Association, 271,* 713.

Lilliston, B. A. (1985). Psychosocial responses to traumatic physical disability. *Social Work in Health Care, 10*(4), 1–13.

Masters, W. H. (1986). Sex and aging—expectations and reality. *Hospital Practice, 15,* 175–198.

Masters, W. H., Johnson, V. E., & Kolodny, R. C. (1992). *Human sexuality* (4th ed.) New York: HarperCollins.

McAnarney, E. R. (1985). Social maturation: A challenge for handicapped and chronically ill adolescents. *Journal of Adolescent Health Care, 6,* 90–101.

McCabe, M. P., Cummins, R. A., & Deeks, A. A. (1999). Construction and psychometric properties of sexuality scales: Sex knowledge, experience and needs scales for people with intellectual disabilities (SexKen-ID), people with physical disabilities (SexKen-PD), and the general population (SexKen-GP). *Research in Developmental Disabilities, 20*(4), 241–254.

McHugh, J. P. (1998, Fall). Sexuality and ostomy surgery. *Ostomy Quarterly,* 24–25.

McKinlay, J. B., & Brambilla, D. (1993). Where do we go from here? Disentangling aging processes from the processes of aging. In J. Schroots (Ed.). *Aging, health, and competence* (pp. 223–242). New York: Elsevier.

Meeropol, E. (1991). One of the gang: Sexual development of adolescents with physical disabilities. *Journal of Pediatric Nursing, 6*(4), 243–250.

Mooradian, A. D. (1991). Geriatric sexuality and chronic diseases. *Geriatric Sexuality, 7*(1), 113–131.

Nosek, M. A., Rintala, D. H., Young, M. E., Howland, C. A., Foley, C. C., Rossi, D., & Chanpong, G. (1996). Sexual functioning among women with physical disabilities. *Archives of Physical Medicine and Rehabilitation, 77,* 107–115.

Persson, G. (1980). Sexuality in a 70-year-old urban population. *Journal of Psychosomatic Research, 24,* 334–342.

Rose, M. K., & Soares, H. H. (1993). Sexual adaptations of the frail elderly: A realistic approach. *Journal of Gerontological Social Work, 19*(3), 167–178.

Rossi, A. S. (1994). Eros and caritas: A biopsychosocial approach to human sexuality and reproduction. In A. S. Rossi (Ed.), *Sexuality across the life course* (pp. 3–36). Chicago: University of Chicago Press.

Sawin, K. J. (1986). Physical disability. In J. Kenney-Griffith (Ed.), *Contemporary women's health* (pp. 237–254). Menlo Park, CA: Addison-Wesley.

Schover, L. R., & Jensen, S. B. (1988). *Sexuality and chronic illness: A chronic approach.* New York: Guilford Press.

Shell, J. A., & Miller, M. E. (1999). The cancer amputee and sexuality. *Orthopedic Nursing, 18*(5), 53.

Siösteen, A., Lundquist, C., Blomstrand, C., Sullivan, L., & Sullivan, M. (1990). Sexual ability, activity, attitudes and satisfaction as part of adjustment in spinal cord injury subjects. *Paraplegia, 28*(5), 285–295.

Starr, B., & Weiner, M. (1981). *The Starr–Weiner report on sex and sexuality.* New York: Stein & Day.

Stevens, S. E., Steele, C. A., Jutai, J. W., Kalnins, I. V., Bortolussi, J. A., & Biggar, W. D. (1996). Adolescents with physical disabilities: Some psychosocial aspects of health. *Journal of Adolescent Health, 19*(2), 157–164.

Sulpizi, L. K. (1996). Issues in sexuality and gynecologic care of women with developmental disabilities. *Journal of Obstetric, Gynecologic, and Neonatal Nursing, 25,* 609–614.

Super, J. T., & Block, J. R. (1991). Self-concept and need for achievement of men with physical disabilities. *Journal of General Psychology, 119*(1), 73–80.

Suris, J. C., Resnick, M. D., Cassuto, N., & Blum, R. W. (1996). Sexual behavior of adolescents with chronic disease and disability. *Journal of Adolescent Health, 19*(2), 124–131.

Tepper, M. S. (1992). Sexual education in spinal cord injury rehabilitation: Current trends and recommendations. *Sex and Disability, 10,* 15–31.

Voll, R., Krumm, B., & Fichtner, H. J. (1999). Demand for psychosocial counseling of young wheelchair users. *International Journal of Rehabilitation Research, 22,* 119–122.

Wainrib, B. R. (1992). Introduction: Gender issues in the aging population. In B. R. Wainrib (Ed.), *Gender issues across the life cycle* (pp. 159–162). New York: Springer.

Wall-Haas, C. (1991). Nurses' attitudes toward sexuality in adolescent patients. *Pediatric Nursing, 17,* 549–555.

Waterhouse, J. (1993). Discussing sexual concerns with health care professionals. *Journal of Holistic Nursing, 11,* 125–134.

Wiley, D., & Bortz, W. M., II. (1996). Sexuality and aging—usual and successful. *Journal of Gerontology, 51A*(3), M142–M146.

World Health Organization. (1975). *Education and treatment in human sexuality: The training of health professionals* (Technical Report Series No. 572). Geneva, Switzerland: Author.

Zajicek-Farber, M. (1998). Promoting good health in adolescents with disabilities. *Health and Social Work, 23*(3), 203–213.

# ADDITIONAL READINGS FOR PART III

Albom, M. (1997). *Tuesdays with Morrie.* New York: Doubleday.

Baier, S. (1986). *Bed number ten.* New York: Holt, Rinehart, and Winston.

Bauby, J. D. (1997). *The diving bell and the butterfly.* New York: Random House.

Bouris, K. (1993). *The first time: Women speak out about "losing their virginity."* Berkeley, CA: Conari Press.

Buzzco Associates, Inc. (Producer), Kugel, C. & Cafarelli, V. (Directors). (1996). *Talking about sex: A guide for families* [Videotape]. (Available from Planned Parenthood Federation of America, Inc.)

Harris, R. (1994). *It's perfectly normal: Changing bodies, growing up.* Cambridge, MA: Candlewick Press.

Hickling, M. (1996). *Speaking of sex: Are you ready to answer the questions your kids will ask?* Vancouver, BC, Canada: Northstone.

Hingsburger, D. (1993). *I openers: Parents ask questions about sexuality and children with developmental disabilities.* Vancouver, BC, Canada: Family Support Institute Press.

Jeffes, S. (1998). *Appearance is everything: The hidden truth regarding your appearance discrimination.* Pittsburgh, PA: Sterling House.

Kaufman, M. (1995). *Easy for you to say.* Toronto: Key Porter Books.

Kroll, K., & Klein, E. L. (1992). *Enabling romance: A guide to love, sex, and relationships for the disabled.* New York: Harmony Books.

LeShan, L. (1989). *Cancer as a turning point: A handbook for people with cancer, their families, and health professionals.* New York: E.P. Dutton.

Levin, R. F. (1987). *Heartmates: A survival guide for the cardiac spouse.* New York: Pocket Books.

Maksym, D. (1990). *Shared feelings: A parent guide to sexuality education for children, adolescents and adults who have a mental handicap.* North York, Ontario, Canada: G. Allan Roeher Institute Press.

McDermott, J. (2000). *Babyface.* Bethesda, MD: Woodbine House.

Michael, R. T., Gagnon, J. H., Laumann, E. O., & Kolata, G. (1994). *Sex in America: A definitive survey.* Boston: Little, Brown.

Moffatt, B. C. (1986). *When someone you love has AIDS: A book of hope for family and friends.* New York: Plume.

Moglia, R. F., & Knowles, J. (Eds.). (1997). *All about sex: A family resource on sex and sexuality.* New York: Three Rivers.

Monette, P. (1988). *Borrowed time: An AIDS memoir.* New York: Harcourt Brace Jovanovich.

Nessim, S., & Ellis, J. (1991). *Cancervive: The challenge of life after cancer.* Boston: Houghton Mifflin.

Newell, R. (2000). *Body image and disfigurement care.* Leeds, UK: Routledge.

Peabody, B. (1986). *The screaming room: A mother's journal of her son's struggle with AIDS—A true story of love, dedication, and courage.* New York: Avon Books.

Rekers, G. (Ed.). (1995). *Handbook of child and adolescent sexual problems.* New York: Lexington.

Sipski, M. L., & Alexander, G. J. (Eds.). (1997). *Sexual function in people with disability and chronic illness.* Gaithersburg, MD: Aspen.

Strong, B., & DeVault, C. (1994). *Human sexuality.* Mountain View, CA: Mayfield.

Williams, M. (1922). *The velveteen rabbit or how toys become real.* Garden City, NY: Doubleday.

# Part IV

# *The Continuum of Loss, Grief, and Adjustment*

When people think of loss and grieving, they often relate these phenomena to dying and death. Loss also encompasses meaningful separations, dashed dreams, revised expectations, and shattered conceptualizations of independence, strength, and security. In addition, illness, impairments, and disability involve loss, even without death being part of the equation. Reactions to loss are affected by how individuals perceive it and the meaning they attach to what is lost. Although responses to loss are as individualized as those who experience it, grieving is both natural and universal. It is a psychological and physiological response to loss that befalls every age group and culture.

Part IV discusses loss, grief, and adjustment on a continuum, acknowledging that this is a process rather than finite stages in time. Chapter 12 discusses primary and secondary types of losses that can cause psychological distress and pose issues for clients and their personal and professional caregivers. Many factors influence the outcome of a loss experience, including the distress and deprivation of the loss, diminished cognition, and the chronicity of the loss and grief.

To provide sensitive care that addresses the whole person, health professionals need to understand the types of grief, including anticipatory, acute, chronic, and delayed or suppressed grief, presented in Chapter 13. They must also be aware of grieving behavior, recognizing that a grieving person's outward behavior can be deceiving. The three summarized models of bereavement, including the stage theory, the integrative theory, and the tasks of mourning, reinforce the nonlinear nature of the process.

Health providers can support and facilitate clients' progress along this continuum, helping them understand the meaning of their loss and accept its finality. Their adjustment includes awareness, knowledge, growth, and an adaptation to a new set of circumstances. Some individuals need to adjust to altered relationships, employment, financial resources, and insurance. Others face chronic symptoms or a loss of function. Still others must adjust to uncertainty, anticipating a progression or recurrence of an illness. Chapter 14 describes this coping behavior, psychosocial adaptation strategies, and implications for health care providers.

This exploration of the loss–grief–adjustment continuum can assist health professionals in identifying and integrating the client's sources of support into a plan of care. It can also facilitate the development of a therapeutic response to loss and grief.

# 12

# *Loss*

My client Anita had a miscarriage, and it was an early miscarriage at that. I don't want to seem insensitive, but it's not like she lost an actual baby. You should have seen her. She was hysterical! On her follow-up appointment today, she was in the throes of grief. If anyone has a reason to grieve like that, it would be my other client Priscilla. I can't even imagine carrying a baby to term and then discovering that the umbilical cord had become wrapped around a foot. I still don't understand why the doctor kept her in the hospital for 12 hours, with a dead baby inside of her, before finally delivering it.

*—From the journal of Linda Whitehead, nursing student*

Who can say which loss is more valid? A response to a loss is influenced by how people perceive the loss and the meaning they attach to what is lost. Although reactions to loss are as unique as the people who experience it, the process of grieving is a universal and natural phenomenon. Linda Whitehead, the nursing student who wrote this journal entry, is only partially right. Stillbirth *and* miscarriage both initiate feelings of despair and confusion, just at the vulnerable moment when families are expecting happiness. Far more is lost than the loss of the awaited child. Perinatal loss results in the loss of dreams, self-esteem, the parental role, and the confidence in the ability to create and deliver a healthy baby (Weiss, Frischer, & Richman, 1989).

This chapter begins the discussion of the continuum of loss, grieving, and adjustment, which will be continued in the following chapters. It explores loss from the perspective of the "three Ds"—disease, disability, and death—and recognizes loss, grieving, and adjustment as a process rather than finite stages.

# Loss Is a "Four-Letter Word"

By the time we assume our professional roles, we have experienced many changes, which we often perceive as losses. To the adage that "the only constants in life are death and taxes," we can add loss. People experience "separations and departures from those we love, our conscious and unconscious losses of romantic dreams, impossible expectations, illusions of freedom and power, illusions of safety—and the loss of our own younger self, the self that thought it always would be unwrinkled and invulnerable and immortal" (Viorst, 1986, p. 2).

## Cure, Goal, and Fail Are Also "Four-Letter Words"

As health care professionals, we do not always understand the meaning and value that loss of health or function holds for both the client and those who provide personal support. We may not value the need for a client to have a support system. Do we focus on a "cure," thereby giving credence to what Siegal (1986) calls a "failure orientation"? He believes that many physicians focus on physiology and overlook the impact that the client's attitude has on the outcome of treatment and the quality of life. "Physicians (are) praised for expertise in technical ability to save lives" (Munley, 1983, p. 16). If we believe in the primacy of the medical model, do we overlook clients' needs and desires in our goal setting and treatment intervention?

Hospice clients in the terminal phase of their illnesses, for example, benefit from palliative care, not a "cure" mentality. They will not have the same therapeutic goals that may be applicable for clients with short-term, reversible problems. Comfort measures, rather than aggressive medical therapies, form the plan of care. Health professionals need to adjust their sights and goals accordingly to deal with individuals' losses.

Many insights in health care are afoot, but people's attitudes are still slow to change. In the 1960s, sociologist Coser (1963) reported that nurses were strongly influenced by the medical model's orientation toward cure. Nurses in a rehabilitative setting were challenged by the therapeutic goals of helping clients achieve positive outcomes and return home. Their work afforded them a measure of self-esteem and satisfaction. In contrast, nurses working with clients who were terminally ill and/or had custodial needs did not derive professional gratification or self-esteem. Rather than being challenged by the different goals and needs, these nurses perceived their work as mechanical and routine. They did not experience the same degree of involvement with the clients. In *today's* health care arena, *some* things have changed.

Contemporary studies recognize that the prospect of progressive debilitation and dependency on a caregiver add to the anguish of clients with advanced diseases who are facing death (Cheville, 2000). The health care team can work to mitigate these issues. Many of these same concerns also apply to losses other than death.

## Types of Loss

While some losses are expected, predictable, and integral parts of life and growth, others are not. Losses may be *sudden,* like a child flying over the bicycle's handlebars, hitting the pavement, and sustaining a traumatic brain injury. Others are *gradual,* like the progressive loss of function, speech, and breathing of amyotrophic lateral sclerosis, commonly known as Lou Gehrig's disease, or ALS.

Some losses are *anticipated* because the disease process is more predictable, such as in cystic fibrosis. Others are associated with *uncertainty,* as in the form of multiple sclerosis characterized by remissions and exacerbations.

Loss may be *total,* like the death of a loved one or the anticipated death of oneself. It may be *partial,* like a severely damaged rotator cuff in a pitcher's shoulder.

Loss may also be *permanent,* like the paralysis resulting from a complete spinal cord injury, or *temporary,* like the paralysis often seen in the neurological syndrome Guillain-Barré.

Age-related changes in function represent another type of loss. Even a healthy older person experiences alterations in hearing, vision, and the musculoskeletal system. Osteoarthritis, for example, is a significant source of disability and functional limitation in older people (Burke & Flaherty, 1993). In older people with declining physical health, there can also be a loss of vitality and increased risk of disease.

A person can lose external objects, such as one's home. A move to an assisted environment, when a person is no longer able to independently function in his or her home, is a loss. In addition to the physical loss of the home and all of the memories associated with it, this may also be a symbolic loss, representing loss of some aspect of oneself. Perhaps it is loss of personal freedom and control, self-worth, or life role, such as that of breadwinner or head of the household.

Primary internal losses can result in secondary external losses. For example, a person who is diagnosed with acquired immune deficiency syndrome (AIDS) may experience physical and/or mental deterioration (primary loss), which necessitates assistance from others. Even with legislation to protect people's rights, the person with AIDS may face many secondary losses, such as employment, residence, and insurance, as a result of the primary physical and/or mental deterioration. Although new and effective treatments have helped some people return to the workforce, employment may no longer be possible for others. Loss of friends and family may occur. Social isolation may become a factor due to the stigma and discrimination that still surround this medical disease (Drench, 1998).

Illness takes its toll on the body. Loss of health, even in small degrees, can result in changes, such as those in the musculoskeletal, neurological, and pulmonary systems. Muscle strength, coordination, endurance, and balance may be partially or completely lost. Loss of bowel and bladder function diminish personal control and may affect one's social activities. One loss often produces other losses.

Memory, cognitive, and intellectual losses and functional limitations may have a negative impact on social roles, self-esteem, and independence. Consider people who have cerebrovascular accidents (strokes) and experience a loss of freedom. As a result of their strokes, they may have difficulty going outside their homes, walking and communicating as they once did, and participating in the leisure activities that they enjoyed prior to the neurological insult. They may experience confusion and deteriorating memory. Activities of daily living, such as washing, bathing, and dressing, may pose other problems. All of these changes can result in the loss of social contact and the once-valued roles that they previously held (Pound, Gompertz, & Ebrahim, 1998).

The loss of these social roles is also a reflection of a loss of autonomy, which negatively influences personal decision making and control of one's life. For example, cancer can result in a loss of occupational identity, control, and "normalcy," which can lead to anxiety and depression (Peteet, 2000). There may also be concerns about the side effects and efficacy of treatment. Many clients are distressed by the possibility of uncontrolled pain. This is actually two blended issues, pain and loss of control. Fears are related to the loss of autonomy, as well as impending isolation (Breitbart, Chochinov, & Passik, 1998). Sometimes it feels like there is little "choice" to be made between certain death and the acceptance of painful, debilitating cancer treatments. In addition, clients consider the "loss of the ability to do what one wants" a significant issue (Axelsson & Sjoden, 1998). These losses can be sufficiently distressing for the person to consider suicide or assisted suicide (Breitbart, 1990; Breitbart & Rosenfeld, 1999; Fairclough, 1998).

We see physical, psychological, symbolic, or a combination of these losses in clients with whom we work, secondary to their pathology and injuries. As a result of their losses, they may encounter additional losses in independence, body parts and/or function, and a sense of wholeness (Drench, 1995). These losses disrupt a person's present timeframe and can have far-reaching effects. The losses also change the future that the person had envisioned.

## Loss Associated with Chronic Conditions

Chronic medical conditions are long-term issues to manage. They tend to affect mental health, although the level of psychological distress varies with the type of condition and the individual person. Hearing and vision impairments and neurological, pulmonary, and cardiac diseases have strong correlations with psychological distress, perceptions of disability, and, to a lesser extent, with a sense of capability and competency (Ormel et al., 1997).

The sustained or relapsing aspects of chronic conditions can be wearing on an individual and may directly lead to depression. In addition, this depression can also be *indirectly* exacerbated by the effect that a chronic condition has on relationships, occupational changes, and emotional and economic status. Diminished self-esteem, personal control, and mastery can also indirectly fuel depression (Vilhjalmsson, 1998).

Any type of psychological distress is influenced by the loss of resources associated with the chronic medical condition. In addition, the severity of the disability can also be a factor, with more severe conditions creating greater psychological distress. Finally, the psychological attributes of the client play a role in the degree of distress that is experienced. As discussed in Chapter 9, those who are able to adopt effective coping strategies generally experience less psychological distress. The idea of a condition or disease being chronic means that the people involved have to make long-term adjustments.

A nurse told a client that his AIDS was now considered a chronic, rather than terminal, disease. She indicated that he could live with this for a long time instead of dying "within a month or two, like it had been in the early days of the disease. You can live with the idea of a chronic disease because it means you can live" (Drench, 1998, p. 137). Helping the client to understand the diagnosis and prognosis facilitates adaptation and coping.

Some chronic conditions can have positive manifestations. For example, following a stroke, a person faces unfamiliar restrictions and losses and may experience sorrow. Yet, hope for the strength to endure the situation can entwine with dreams of what may come. Perspective can change, and the person may appreciate life in a different light. Suddenly, the ordinary in life is not so "ordinary." In addition, nurturing relationships can be supportive and give the person a much-needed boost (Pilkington, 1999).

We will be discussing grieving and the therapeutic response to grief and loss in the following two chapters. At this point, though, suffice it to say that to grieve effectively, people need to integrate the losses into their lives. The individuals first need to come to terms with both the reality of the situation and the symbolic meaning of the loss. They must reframe their goals, priorities, and values to incorporate the person(s) they have become. Only then can they work to accommodate the loss into their existence.

Consider, for example, people with an acquired hearing loss, a common long-term condition. They may perceive a loss of control caused by insecurity in social encounters (Eriksson-Mangold & Carlsson, 1991). Yet, some people integrate the hearing loss into their lives, making the necessary lifestyle changes (Herth, 1998). This calls for modifying one's perspective on life and making some practical accommodations, such as minimizing distracting sounds and positioning oneself to read lips or hear to one's best advantage. However, not everyone is willing or able to make accommodations. Some people react with strong feelings of fear and sadness, which can produce a stress response.

> **M**rs. Williams is 60 years old. She's absolutely beside herself! I saw her today in the clinic, and she continued to complain about dizziness and ringing in her right ear. She says that she doesn't sleep well, has increasing headaches, and can't concentrate on her bridge game. She feels like she's not fun to be with any more, not even for herself. Her quality of life is going down the tubes, and I feel so helpless.
> —*From the journal of Robert Evans, audiology student*

Perceptions about loss of control, fear of serious illness, and anticipation of a severe episode of vertigo (dizziness) may be associated with an intensifying cycle of vertigo, anxiety, and restriction of activity (Yardley, 1994). The frequency of headaches is significantly related to the severity of the tinnitus (ringing in the ears), which strongly correlates with perceived attitudes (Erlandsson, Hallberg, & Axelsson, 1992). If Mrs. Williams can change her perceptions, perhaps the relationship between the audiological, psychological, dizziness, headaches, and tinnitus may be altered. A person's perceptions and feelings can often influence how he or she copes, grieves, and adjusts to a loss.

In some conditions, the precipitating loss is not chronic but the resulting feelings may become long-lasting. In an *acute loss,* low self-esteem and loss of personal control can become *chronic feelings.* These perceptions of inadequacy, which can include feeling anxious and depressed, are directly proportional to the intensity of stress, bereavement, and psychological suffering. If not addressed, they can last for years or even a lifetime. For example, four years after perinatal loss of a baby due to congenital abnormalities, parents can continue to experience these feelings (Hunfeld, Wladimiroff, & Passchier, 1997) and become "stuck" in their lives. This phenomenon, known as chronic sorrow, will be discussed in Chapter 13.

There are no hard and fast rules for negative feelings resulting from loss. Sometimes having more information about the condition can reduce the psychological distress. For instance, women who experience miscarriage may have feelings of anxiety, depression, grief, worry, and/or self-blame, which seem to diminish over time (Nikcevic, Tunkel, Kuczmierczyk, & Nicolaides, 1999). When they learn the cause of their miscarriage, commonly a fetal chromosomal abnormality, they experience less self-blame. Healing may begin. While there are no guaranteed outcomes, client education can reduce the devastating feelings accompanying loss.

## Loss for the Personal Caregiver

It is important to note that the individual personally facing the illness or injury is not the only one experiencing loss. Often, it is the significant others who we expect to administer medications, perform home care procedures, and enforce exercise regimens who are also grieving. Sadly, the needs of this group are often neglected. For example, caregivers of their life partners with Alzheimer's disease experience a loss of intimacy and shared mutuality. Communication, decision making, relationships, and the typical frustrations and joys of daily life are all altered (Garner, 1997). This seems to be true even if the caregivers are not life partners of those in their care.

Regardless if the caregiver is a sibling, son or daughter, niece or nephew, friend, or other relation, they, too, may endure this kind of personal loss and grief. They also tend to lose part of themselves in their role as caregiver, as they become enmeshed in attending to the needs of the other person (Loos & Bowd, 1997). White and Grenyer (1999) report that while clients with end-stage renal disease experience feelings of anger, depression, and hopelessness, their partners feel sadness, resentment, guilt, and loss.

Personal caregivers can face significant losses. For example, in a study by Sirki, Saarinen-Pihkala, and Hovi (2000), similar findings were noted between family members who lost children after terminal care and during active anticancer therapy. Parents report physical and/or mental problems with similar frequency, similar self-reported recovery times, and similar times for returning to work. Mothers, however, need longer recovery times and greater intervals of time before returning to work than do fathers. Siblings of children who die during active anticancer therapy have more difficulties than brothers and sisters of children who die after terminal care. Their issues include fear, behavioral and social problems, and problems associated with school. The good news is in knowing that mothers, fathers, brothers, and sisters of children who die (from cancer) have the ability to move through the grieving process and recover. They are, however, forever changed.

---

**B**obby threw his sister's stuffed bears against the walls and on the floor. He was yelling, "She wasn't supposed to die! All those months of throwing up. Going bald. Missing school. It seems like Mom and Dad spent years at the hospital with her, while the rest of us tried not to feel ignored. They said we should understand. It was temporary. She'd get better, and everything would be back to normal. The leukemia would be history. Well, it's not. Things will never be normal again." I let Bobby rant until he collapsed in my arms. We sat on the floor and wept together.

*—From the journal of Sanjay Patel, nursing student*

---

Caregivers and other family members and friends are in a position of good news–bad news. The intensity, duration, and meaning associated with their loss can result in negative outcomes of grieving, which may put them at a higher risk for their own illness and even death. In contrast, loss and grief can also have positive outcomes for those whose family members and friends die, by giving them the "gifts" of a clearer appreciation for their own lives and the lesson to enjoy themselves (Lev & McCorkle, 1998). A psychiatric nurse said, "I see people every day who wish that they could go back in time and have moments to live over again or wish they could have done things differently" (Drench, 1998, p. 172). A developing sense of gratitude and a healthy perspective of life are often part of the legacy left behind.

Grief holds possibilities for empowering people to grow and mature, but again, it can be a double-edged sword. Psychiatrist Viktor Frankl (1984), who survived the concentration camps of Auschwitz and Dachau during World War II, asserts that despair can occur when people suffer and perceive no meaning in the experience. However, a painful and lingering experience *can* facilitate self-discovery of one's deepest beliefs and overturn negative experiences.

# Loss for the Health Care Professional

**M**rs. Moriarty was a pale, shrinking form, lying in a sea of white sheets. We were working so hard to wean her off the ventilator, at first for only moments at a time. Finally, success! I felt strong and empowered. When she died, I was crushed. After work, I cried on the bus the whole way home.
*—From the journal of Dinah Rogers, respiratory therapy student*

Dinah's reflections illustrate that health care providers also experience loss. Oncology nurses, for example, who frequently confront different kinds of losses, have high levels of despair, social isolation, and somatization (Feldstein & Gemma, 1995). A nurse who works with patients in a long-term care setting speaks about the small losses often being more difficult than death itself.

When they die, it's hard, but it's not that hard. It's not as hard as having them lose control of their bladder and bowels. This is real sad. It's hard for us because we're talking to an otherwise competent client about Depends® saying, "Are you going out? Do you have enough diapers with you?" Or they'll be talking to you and say, "God, I had an accident," and sometimes you have to clean them up. It's the day-to-day stuff that's the hard part. By the time they get around to dying, it's almost easy. It's not easy, and it's sad, but the things you have to do to them while they're living are much harder than watching them die (Drench, 1998, p. 97).

Confronting these many small losses along the continuum of loss, grief, and adjustment can take its toll. Health professionals sometimes feel anxious or guilty that they are unable to respond to all of the clients' needs (Drench, 1992), especially in a health system where there is a premium placed on cost-effectiveness, budgeted time, and volume of clients, translated into reimbursement costs.

Care providers who work with clients over a long period of time, such as in a rehabilitation setting or skilled nursing facility, often develop relationships with the clients and deeply feel the losses. When clients with whom strong bonds are shared die, the losses can be acutely felt. Says one health provider:

> I knew when I left work he wasn't going to make it through the night. Fortunately, I don't get that involved with very many people. I've cried with some patients. I cry when patients with whom I'm close die, but I usually cry with other people. I don't generally go home and cry alone (Drench, 1998, p. 166).

Yet, an ambivalence may exist. As sad as it feels to lose a client, health care providers occasionally feel a sense of relief when a struggle is over: "Sometimes you feel sad, and sometimes you feel relief because you feel like, 'My God, they're fighting too hard, why don't they give up?' " (Drench, 1992, p. 156).

Health care providers encounter loss daily, from A to Z—from anterior cruciate ligament tears in athletes' knees to the "zoning out" of a client with mental deterioration. They need to handle the loss and reactions of clients and significant others, as well as of themselves. Part of their occupational core identity is that of a "helping" person. An effective helping relationship includes a certain level of sharing the clients' feelings of loss. Although their work may yield professional and personal satisfaction, health care providers may also perceive defeat and ineffectiveness as clients' losses amass (Drench, 1992).

Health care providers may also experience depression in response to dealing with clients' losses, treating a client who is terminally ill, and losing a client. We are educated and socialized to maintain a professional distance in order to minimize personal involvement. This is designed to help us make objective decisions regarding client care and prevent an unhealthy level of involvement. While emotional detachment can be a protective insulator against loss and separation, it can also compromise compassion and sensitivity. A certain degree of therapeutic bonding makes the relationship more effective. The other side of this "therapeutic coin" is that a sense of loss is a by-product of that emotional bonding between professional and client.

In addition, new loss can spark old losses. Unresolved loss in the health care provider's personal history may also be triggered by a client's loss if the professional overidentifies with the client. A social worker recalls,

> An older client reminded me of the way my father looked not long before he died. It stirred up a lot of feelings over a great and painful loss, including aspects that I buried or tried to shield myself from. It caused me to let a little more of that pain into my life. I also connected to this client in a different way and felt a little sadder about him (Drench, 1992, p. 115).

These unresolved loss and mourning experiences can come back and jar us awake when we least expect it. We grieve for the client. We grieve for others we may have personally lost. We grieve for ourselves.

These losses, with or without death, are very real to the health care providers. They experience personal and professional stresses, which can motivate or cause "singe-out," "rust-out," or in the extreme, burnout. When the demands and stress in the workplace become too great, the healer may become overwhelmed (Hall, 1997).

Hainsworth (1998) studied eight nurses, asking them to reflect on their experiences working with clients in acute care who had sustained catastrophic loss through severe brain injury. The nurses perceived their overall work experiences as negative, as they struggled to connect with clients and get support from colleagues and physicians. They experienced empathy but also felt vulnerable and futile, and abused by clients' families, who were struggling with their own dynamics. Although these acute care nurses sometimes felt ineffective and unsupported, they continued to seek professional satisfaction through their work. Overall, they wrestled with poor workplace experiences with patients who were neurologically devastated.

One loss is hard. Two is more difficult. Never-ending losses, especially with people with whom you work closely, can be devastating. Too many negative grieving outcomes or not grieving at all can lead to burnout. There must be an opportunity to grieve and to reach a balance in work and life. Health professionals working with people with AIDS report feelings of frustration, pervasive sadness, and anger, as well as gratification, challenges, and joy (Drench, 1998).

As health care professionals we need to confront and understand our own responses to loss and openly acknowledge them. In doing so, we become more aware and sensitive to the needs of others, develop empathy for their losses from illness or injury, and clarify the impact of our clinical interventions.

## SUMMARY

This chapter introduced the continuum of loss, grief, and adjustment as a process rather than finite stages. Everyone experiences loss in their lives, and clients are challenged by additional losses from injury, disease, disability, and death. Primary and secondary types of losses were discussed, both of which can cause psychological distress. These losses pose issues for the client as well as for the personal and professional caregivers. In the following chapter, we will move along the continuum and further investigate grief as a universal and natural response to loss.

## REFLECTIVE QUESTIONS

1. a. What activities, functions, or people are most important to you?
   b. Which are you most afraid of losing? Why?
   c. What would this loss mean to you?
   d. How do you think you might react to this loss?
2. a. Describe a significant internal loss you have experienced.
   b. Why was it significant?
   c. How did you react?
3. a. Describe a significant external loss you have experienced.
   b. Why was it significant?
   c. How did you react?
4. How might the losses you described in Question #2 and/or #3 affect your ability to support certain client situations?
5. Consider the multiple combined problems facing people as they age.
   a. What do you think it would be like to wonder what you might "lose" next?
   b. What could you do to maintain meaning in your life?
   c. What would motivate you to get out of bed in the morning?

# CASE STUDY

*Note:* Because loss, grief, and adjustment are presented on a continuum as a process rather than finite stages in time, there is only one Case Study in Part IV to reflect this. It is, however, told in parts, each with its own set of questions that pertain to the information in the particular chapter.

Cynthia Osbourne is a survivor. In a fiery blaze at a nightclub that killed 100 people and injured hundreds more, she lost her fiancé and was burned over more than 30 percent of her body. First rushed to a nearby hospital, then moved to an out-of-state burn center and then another hospital, she was kept unconscious so that she would not have to endure the unbearable pain from the burned areas. During this time, surgeons performed ten skin grafts on her body, including her hands.

Three months after the fire, she was transferred to a rehabilitation hospital, still in a neighboring state. Her 10-year-old and 7-year-old sons have been in the care of their grandparents. Now that she is out of the induced coma, Cynthia has flashbacks to the flames, the screaming in the inferno, and seeing piles of bodies being trampled as people tried to exit the building.

Lying in bed for three months resulted in heterotrophic ossification in both knees and an elbow, caused by a build-up of calcium that accumulated due to inactivity. Unable to bend her knees, she had generalized limited function, mobility, range of motion, and strength. She doubted that she would ever walk again. In addition, scar tissue on her hands limited her ability to feed herself and perform other self-care activities. Therapy included very painful stretching, attempts at standing, and eventually walking a few steps. Because she could not flex her knees, she had to descend stairs backwards and had difficulty getting into and out of a car from/to a wheelchair.

1. a. Describe Cynthia's losses.
   b. Identify which losses are internal losses and which are external losses. Provide a rationale for your decisions.
   c. Identify which losses are primary and which are secondary types of losses. Provide a rationale for your decisions.
2. Discuss the impact of Cynthia's losses and limitations on her self-esteem, independence, and social roles, including those of parenting and vocation.
3. What effect might pain have on Cynthia's circumstances?
4. What effect might Cynthia's losses have on her sons?

# REFERENCES

Axelsson, B., & Sjoden, P. O. (1998). Quality of life of cancer patients and their spouses in palliative home care. *Palliative Medicine, 12*(1), 29–39.

Breitbart, W. (1990). Cancer pain and suicide. In K. Foley, J. J. Bonica, & V. Ventafridda (Eds.), *Advances in pain research and therapy* (Vol. 16, pp. 399–472). New York: Raven Press.

Breitbart, W., Chochinov, H., & Passik, S. (1998). Psychiatric aspects of palliative care. In D. Doyle, G. Hanks, & N. MacDonald (Eds.), *Oxford textbook of palliative medicine* (pp. 933–954). New York: Oxford University Press.

Breitbart, W., & Rosenfeld, B. (1999). Physician-assisted suicide: The influence of psychosocial issues. *Cancer Control, 6*(2), 146–161.

Burke, M., & Flaherty, M. J. (1993). Coping strategies and health status of elderly arthritic women. *Journal of Advanced Nursing, 18*(1), 7–13.

Cheville, A. L. (2000). Cancer rehabilitation and palliative care. *Rehabilitation Oncology, 18*(1), 19–20.

Coser, R. L. (1963). Alienation and the social structure. In E. Friedson (Ed.), *The hospital in modern society* (pp. 231–265). Glencoe, IL: Free Press.

Drench, M. E. (1992). A phenomenological study of the lived experience of health care professionals working with people with acquired immune deficiency syndrome. *Dissertation Abstracts International* 53(5), 25.82B. (University Microfilms No. 9226096)

Drench, M. E. (1995). Coping with loss—Adjusting to change. *International Society for Behavioral Science in Physical Therapy, 7*(2), 1–4.

Drench, M. E. (1998). *Red ribbons are not enough: Health caregivers' stories about AIDS.* Wilsonville, OR: BookPartners.

Eriksson-Mangold, M., & Carlsson, S. G. (1991). Psychological and somatic distress in relation to perceived hearing disability, hearing handicap, and hearing measurements. *Journal of Psychosomatic Research, 35*(6), 729–740.

Erlandsson, S. I., Hallberg, L. R., & Axelsson, A. (1992). Psychological and audiological correlates of perceived tinnitus severity. *Audiology, 31*(3), 168–179.

Fairclough, D. L. (1998). Quality of life, cancer investigation, and clinical practice. *Cancer Investigative, 76,* 478–484.

Feldstein, M. A., & Gemma, P. B. (1995). Oncology nurses and chronic compounded grief. *Cancer Nursing, 18*(3), 228–236.

Frankl, V. E. (1984). *Man's search for meaning: An introduction to logotherapy* (3rd ed.). New York: Simon & Schuster.

Garner, J. (1997). Dementia: An intimate death. *British Journal of Medical Psychology, 70*(Pt. 2), 177–184.

Hainsworth, D. S. (1998). Reflections on loss without death: The lived experience of acute care nurses caring for neurologically devastated patients. *Holistic Nursing Practice, 13*(1), 41–50.

Hall, J. (1997). Nursing stress: Applying the wisdom of the wounded healer. *Lamp, 54*(8), 24–25.

Herth, K. (1998). Integrating hearing loss into one's life. *Quality Health, 8*(2), 207–223.

Hunfeld, J. A., Wladimiroff, J. W., & Passchier, J. (1997). Prediction and course of grief four years after perinatal loss due to congenital anomalies: A follow-up study. *British Journal of Medical Psychology, 70*(Pt. 1), 85–91.

Lev, E. L., & McCorkle, R. (1998). Loss, grief, and bereavement in family members of cancer patients. *Seminars in Oncology Nursing, 14*(2), 145–151.

Loos, C., & Bowd, A. (1997). Caregivers of persons with Alzheimer's disease: Some neglected implications of the experience of personal loss and grief. *Death Studies, 21*(5), 501–514.

Munley, A. (1983). *The hospice alternative: A new context for death and dying.* New York: Basic Books.

Nikcevic, A. V., Tunkel, S. A., Kuczmierczyk, A. R., & Nicolaides, K. H. (1999). Investigation of the cause of miscarriage and its influence on women's psychological distress. *British Journal of Obstetrics and Gynaecology, 106*(8), 808–813.

Ormel, J., Kempen, G. I., Penninx, B. W., Brilman, E. I., Beekman, A. T., & van Sonderen, E. (1997). Chronic medical conditions and mental health in older people: Disability and psychosocial resources mediate specific mental health effects. *Psychological Medicine, 27*(5), 1065–1077.

Peteet, J. R. (2000). Cancer and the meaning of work. *General Hospital Psychiatry, 22*(3), 200–205.

Pilkington, F. B. (1999). A qualitative study of life after stroke. *Journal of Neuroscience Nursing,* *31*(6), 336–347.

Pound, P., Gompertz, P., & Ebrahim, S. (1998). A patient-centered study of the consequences of stroke. *Clinical Rehabilitation, 12*(4), 338–347.

Siegal, B. S. (1986). *Love, medicine and miracles: Lessons learned about self-healing from a surgeon's experience with exceptional patients.* New York: Harper & Row.

Sirki, K., Saarinen-Pihkala, U. M., & Hovi, L. (2000). Coping of parents and siblings with the death of a child with cancer: Death after terminal care compared with death during active anticancer therapy. *Acta Paediatrics, 89*(6), 717–721.

Vilhjalmsson, R. (1998). Direct and indirect effects of chronic physical conditions on depression: A preliminary investigation. *Social Science and Medicine, 47*(5), 603–611.

Viorst, J. (1986). *Necessary losses: The loves, illusions, dependencies and impossible expectations that all of us have to give up in order to grow.* New York: Fawcett Gold Medal.

Weiss, L., Frischer, L., & Richman, J. (1989). Parental adjustment to intrapartum and delivery room loss: The role of a hospital-based support program. *Clinical Perinatology, 16*(4), 1009–1019.

White, Y., & Grenyer, B. F. (1999). The biopsychosocial impact of end-stage renal disease: The experience of dialysis patients and their partners. *Journal of Advanced Nursing, 30*(6), 1312–1320.

Yardley, L. (1994). Contribution of symptoms and beliefs to handicap in people with vertigo: A longitudinal study. *British Journal of Clinical Psychology, 33*(Pt. 1), 101–113.

# 13

# *Grief*

It's difficult for me to take care of dying patients. Frankly, I've never made peace with death. My grandmother lived with us, and we were inseparable. Gram taught me how to braid my hair, make strudel, and sew. I guess she was my best friend. When I was in my seventh-grade history class, the school secretary came to our room and took me out into the hall to privately talk to me. She told me that my grandmother had collapsed and died about an hour before. I was told that I could stay in her office until my father came to pick me up. Sitting with my bookbag on my lap, I quietly sobbed. I remember feeling so numb inside, like part of me had been swallowed up. When my father arrived, I barely had enough energy to get up and walk outside to the car.

—*From the journal of Anna Sorensen, respiratory therapy student*

As we discussed in the previous chapter, living with chronic illness or disability brings loss. Medical technology provides the means to make early diagnoses of many diseases, prolong life, and enhance the quality of life for people with chronic conditions. As part of life's journey, though, people still experience losses of many kinds, including those from death. Where there is loss, there is the universal human phenomenon of grief, a psychological and physiological process that occurs in response to loss in every age group and culture. It is a painful process during which those who have a loss experience powerful and confusing emotions. Hopefully, they come to understand the meaning of their loss and accept its finality. This chapter addresses grief, another part of the loss-to-adjustment continuum. It discusses types of grief, grieving behavior, stages of grieving and models of bereavement, grieving outcomes, and chronic sorrow.

# Types of Grief

In his seminal work on attachment and loss, British psychologist John Bowlby (1980) described the goal of mourning as accepting the reality of loss. The purpose of cultural traditions and rituals associated with death, such as wakes and funerals, is to help mourners face their losses. They create an acceptable opportunity for individuals to express feelings and receive comfort. They also "bring home the fact that a loss has in fact occurred" (p. 234). Yet, the process of grieving is also one of healing and recovery, helping people feel better. In today's fast-paced society of immediate gratification, people tend to underestimate the intensity of their distress, the problems that they face, and the length of time that the distress and problems will endure. In addition, Western culture can be death-denying, with people minimizing the time, duration, and potency of the experience.

In response to loss, grief is a natural phenomenon and is part of the period of adjustment. Although the need to grieve is universal across cultures, the grieving process is influenced by religious and social mores. However, regardless of the manner in which someone grieves, there are typical psychological and physical reactions. Psychological signs include an initial shock and disbelief, followed by sorrow and often regret. Grief-related emotions, such as anger, guilt, despair, sadness, depression, denial, and fear, tend to be powerful, confusing, and overwhelming. Physical signs associated with a grief reaction include fatigue, sighing, hyperventilation, feelings of physical emptiness in the abdomen and chest, and a sense of a lump in the throat. Anorexia, insomnia, and disorientation may also be present.

> I am new to this thing called widowhood.
>
> No one can tell you about grief, about its limitless boundaries, its unfathomable depths. No one can tell you about the crater that is created in the center of your body, the one that nothing can fill. No matter how many times you hear the word *final*, it means nothing until final is actually final.
>
> It has been just over four months since the day Bill died, and still I am paralyzed. I am a woman without a country, an alien who has dropped to earth from some other planet. I am in a capsule on the moon, bouncing from side to side, floating in space, but I cannot imagine emerging from the capsule to offer one small step for mankind. I keep thinking I will see a 224-point headline that reads DERANGED WIDOW FOUND SUSPENDED IN OUTER SPACE, and then realize that the headline refers to me (Coughlin, 1993, p. 3).

Just as there are different types and reactions to loss, there are different types and responses to grief: anticipatory, acute, chronic, and delayed or suppressed grief. Grief has typically been considered to have two temporal phases. Anticipatory grief is experienced prior to the actual loss, and "conventional" grief occurs after the fact, following a loss. There are similarities and differences between them. For example, although anticipatory and conventional grief are similar in expression and duration among husbands and wives whose spouses die, anticipatory grief is associated with greater intensities of anger, loss of emotional control, and atypical grief responses (Gilliland & Fleming, 1998).

Both anticipatory and conventional grief affect the survivors prior to and following a death. It is important to remember, though, that the client undergoing loss also grieves. Anticipatory grief includes preparing for losses that will occur as a result of surgery and disease progression as well as death. It may have similar signs to acute grief, but the timing is different.

Anticipatory grief is derived from the biomedical model that includes a predictable course of the behavior, feelings, and symptoms of the grieving process. Although widely accepted as a phenomenon in the literature, anticipatory grief can be a confusing concept. It is not always clearly distinguished from a "forewarning of loss" (Fulton, Madden, & Minichiello, 1996). In addition, it is not experienced in the same way by everyone. For example, in palliative home care, family members vary in their anticipatory grief patterns in several key areas. Interestingly, it is the adult children, those with more education, those not living with the person who is sick, nonprimary caregivers, and women who express more anger and hostility than other family members (Chapman & Pepler, 1998).

Conventional grief, which develops following a loss, can be acute, chronic, and delayed or suppressed. In contrast to anticipatory grief, acute grief begins following a recent or sudden loss. The loss could be the death of a loved one. It could be the loss of an important function, such as vision or the loss of perfect health due to a chronic illness. It could be a devastating diagnosis that disrupts one's life. The severity of the grief tends to be directly proportional to the perceived void resulting from the loss. The person who is acutely grieving may experience profound sadness, anxiety, denial, anger, and depression. He or she may feel overwhelmed, confused, numb, helpless, and hopeless.

Grief can also become chronic. The person enters a state of perpetual mourning. In some cultures, widows dress completely in black for the rest of their lives. Although the attire does not necessarily indicate that their grief continues at the same intensity over time, it does serve as an outward symbol of their position in the community.

Not everyone, though, allows themselves to grieve in the moment. Grief may be delayed or absent. Some people suppress their grief; however, it can be triggered at a later date. This may occur when the individual perceives the time and environment are safer or when the grief can no longer be inhibited. Consider the woman who suppressed her grief at the time of each of her three miscarriages. Years later, when her daughter had a miscarriage, she was overcome with grief, not only for her awaited first grandchild, but also for her three previous losses. She said, "I honestly thought I was over it. I can now see that I never even dealt with what happened. I buried my babies inside, just as if I buried them in the ground."

# Grieving Behavior

Although many people may grieve the same information or event, not everyone grieves as intensely as others. There are typically primary and secondary mourners. Primary mourners are people who perceive that they have lost the most, that is the client, the family, close friends. Secondary mourners also despair, but there is less of a void in their lives. They are likely to be coworkers and less close friends.

Grief or sorrow (emotional suffering) caused by bereavement (having something taken away) have come to be used interchangeably. Like other lifespan issues, bereavement behaviors as a response to loss are influenced by religious beliefs, age, cultural and community aspects, the personality of the grieving person, and the relationship between who is grieving and what is lost. Cultural healing rituals help mourners face their loss. These include practices such as photographic collages or collections at memorial services, candlelighting, charitable funds, condolence visits, specific prayers, and the AIDS quilt of memorial panels (coordinated by the Names Project).

However, in our fast-paced society, mourners are "allowed" only a few days of grief and are quickly encouraged to "get on with life." In contemporary, industrialized societies, the mourner is perhaps allotted two or three days away from the workplace. Mourning is considered morbid, and some people grow impatient with the time others need. Many people do not view grief as normal. Prolonged grief (timing is in the minds of the beholder), therefore, becomes pathological. The message is firm—if you need all this time and have all this pain, you are not adjusting well; you are somehow deficient.

In some societies, people minimize the loss they feel from a death. To reinforce these concepts, people euphemistically refer to the death experience in indirect terms, such as "returning to one's Maker," "entering the Kingdom," and "passing away (on or over)." In our efforts to protect children, such as excluding them from the bedside of a dying person or a funeral, we rob them of the opportunity to say goodbye, gain closure, and understand the process of living and dying. We want to quickly replace the loss—a hamster, a mother—as though someone or something else could be substituted. This behavior is not reserved only for children. Sometimes during the grieving period, we hear, "You're young. You'll marry again." This mentality provides little comfort.

Some cultures have even abdicated many of the rituals that comforted and helped move people through the mourning process. It is no longer common to see people wearing black armbands or dressing all in black for an extended period of time. Black wreaths and banners may be hung on public buildings for some losses but not typically on homes. Bodies are generally not laid out in the house; vigils are no longer the rule.

In a highly mobile society, people often live a distance from their extended family and friends. The built-in support that was once common in one's own neighborhood or town is rare today. Because so many of us do not live in insular communities, we do not grow up exposed to loss and death experiences. We often grieve alone, no longer blanketed by those around us. In addition, we usually relinquish the duties of washing and preparing the body of a loved one to strangers who are "professionals." We foresake the opportunity to be personally responsible, to lovingly touch and care for the person one last time, and to work toward closure. The physical connection also provides us with the unquestionable awareness and acceptance of the finality of the situation.

The society in which one lives also influences outward behavior of a grieving person. Clear messages in mainstream U.S. culture are: "You have to be brave for the children"; "Big boys don't cry"; and "You're young; you can have another baby" (Cable, 1998, p. 63). Therefore, it is no surprise that the outward behavior of a grieving person can be deceiving. Some people keen and wail, while others remain in control. "Quiet" mourners may cry in private or not at all. Some people stoically harbor their grief, but it can be prompted later by a memory, an association, or a subsequent loss. Sometimes the loss is met with ambivalence, with both grief and relief—grief over the loss and relief, especially after a particularly prolonged, painful, or deteriorating death.

Behaviors associated with acute grief frequently include crying, wailing, and agitation. There may be wringing of the hands, deep sighing, and general tension. This grief response usually happens immediately after the loss has occurred. The grieving person may become withdrawn, not eat, have difficulty sleeping or sleep more than usual, pace frenetically or sit lethargically, and lose interest in pleasurable things. He or she may express feeling numb, hopeless, helpless, and exhausted. It may seem that life no longer has any meaning. The world feels like an empty place. There is a loss of connection between the person in mourning and the rest of the world. They often wonder how others can go about "business as usual" while they are "dying inside." Mourners feel as though they are on the outside looking in.

If the mourning is in response to the loss of a person, there is often a tendency to place the person on a pedestal, idealizing the individual who has died. In contrast, some deaths, illnesses, or circumstances carry a stigma that compounds the complexities faced by the grieving people and often yields less compassion and support. People are sometimes blamed for their own happenstances, if their losses or deaths are perceived as resulting from poor lifestyle choices, such as substance abuse, AIDS, suicide, or foolish accidents (Cable, 1998).

I'm working with two high school students now in the burn unit. At a party, their boyfriends decided to pour grain alcohol into a dish to see if it would continue to burn on its own once they lit it. They lit the bottle from which it was poured, and suddenly, the bottle exploded, engulfing the girls in flames. One girl's parents are at the hospital every day, supporting and loving her. The other girl's parents yelled at her, "How could you do this?" She's lying there so badly burned, and her own parents are blaming the victim!

—*From the journal of Melanie Haber, nursing student*

Because individual perceptions vary greatly, no discussion of grieving behavior can really be exhaustive. However, themes emerge across the spectrum of problems. For example, a person may experience different reactions upon learning of the possibility of a diagnosis of cancer and throughout the course of the disease, such as those listed in Table 13–1.

These feelings and losses are not unique to cancer. They are universal and apply to other life-threatening illnesses or disabilities. When facing a loss, an individual's sense of personal control and well-being may be replaced by feelings of fear, helplessness, and anger. The latter is often directed at God, health care providers, family, and friends. A person may also encounter anxiety and depression (Maguire, Walsh, Jeacock, & Kingston, 1999).

**TABLE 13–1**    Reactions to a Diagnosis of Cancer

| Upon learning of the possibility of a diagnosis of cancer: | After the diagnosis is made and throughout the course of the illness: |
| --- | --- |
| • fear of death | • loss of control |
| • fear of disfigurement | • anger |
| • fear of disability | • guilt |
| • fear of abandonment | • fear of abandonment |
| • fear of disruption in relationships and role functioning | • fear of pain |
| • fear of loss of finances | • psychiatric disorders |
| • loss of independence | • other psychosocial factors |
| • denial | |
| • anxiety | |
| • anger | |

*(Sussman, 1995)*                    *(Blanchard & Ruckdeschel, 1986).*

Furthermore, some people may deny the reality of their situation, as well as the fears and thoughts associated with it. Other people *appear* to be in denial, but they are actually repressing these thoughts and fears, submerging them in their unconscious mind for the present time. Let us take a closer look at grieving behavior.

## Denial

Denial of the situation, fears, and thoughts may be another behavioral response to a disabling loss and is the first stage of the grieving process, as conceptualized by Kübler-Ross in her formative work on the subject (1969). It can be present even when the circumstances are visible and difficult for *others* to deny. Consider Richard, a 35-year-old man who was unsuccessfully treated for a glioblastoma. His brain tumor resulted in seizures, weakness, and functional limitations. Despite being told that he would not live much longer, he persisted in making long-range plans for when he "got better."

Upon receiving "bad" news—a diagnosis, prognosis, statement of complications—it is not unusual for a client or someone in the personal support system to react with surprise and *denial.* "It can't be true!" "I just had a mammogram (or electrocardiogram or some other test), and it was fine. You must have someone else's test results." "I will walk again. Can't you see that my toe just moved?"

Denying that there is a change or loss is not a conscious decision; rather, it is a form of self-preservation. Denial is not necessarily counterproductive to accepting one's reality. Like so much else in life, it is a matter of degree of intensity and duration. Initially, denial is a protective reaction, cushioning someone against shocking or discouraging news. It affords time to compose oneself, and in time, employ other defense mechanisms, hopefully on the road forward. It permits time to adjust to the reality of the loss. When denial goes beyond the initial phase, though, it can be detrimental. For example, seeking a second medical opinion is wise. "Shopping around for doctors," looking for "good" news, is part of an active denial system, which may ultimately hamper adjustment and acceptance.

Initially, I thought Julia accepted the fact that her child had been born deaf and blind when she said that she would grow up like Helen Keller. I now believe she was in denial. Just because she can't hear or see doesn't mean that she can or will achieve the unusual accomplishments of Ms. Keller, who also couldn't speak. That's a huge leap of faith!

—*From the journal of Matthew Mulcahey, medical student*

Denial is not necessarily a one-time response. It can reappear whenever there are new challenges to face. Consider Leslie, a client with multiple sclerosis. When he first attended rehabilitation, he worked on improving independent ambulation. As his disease progressed, he required a cane, and later a walker. Over time, he was referred for wheelchair mobility and transfer training. Each time he faced additional functional limitations, his denial resurfaced.

Although all team members may share the responsibility of dealing with denial, it is generally the purview of the mental health professional (i.e., psychotherapist, psychologist, psychiatric nurse, social worker) to decide how best to manage denial to meet the client's needs.

For example, the mental health professional may decide to confront the denial to mitigate its effect or maintain it as a productive defense mechanism, beneficial in adapting to life (Langer, 1994). Both schools of thought have their supporters and detractors, a discussion that is beyond the scope of this book.

It is the job of other health care providers to deal with denial within the boundaries of their practice. They can support the person and provide hope. When clients sense that the environment and conditions are safe, denial sometimes begins to dissipate.

## Anger

When dealing with loss and grief, anxiety and depression often pale in comparison to anger. Clients may feel anger toward their own bodies for betraying them. They may feel angry at being cheated out of a "normal" life, one without illness, injury, or premature death. At times, anger may also be based on fear. Clients often say, "It can't be me!" or "Why me?" Once the news is absorbed and is beginning to be processed, the client typically feels anger and sometimes even rage, during what Kübler-Ross (1969) recognizes as the second phase of her model of grieving. There can also be resentment—"What did I do to deserve this? Why couldn't it have been him (or her)?" "Life isn't fair!"

Martha Beck (1999) shares her personal story of being pregnant with a child who has Down syndrome. In a bookstore, she selected a book on the subject with a cover that horrified her: "two children, lumpish and awkward-looking, stared dully at the camera through small, misshapen eyes. I cannot tell you how much it hurt me to look at that picture. It was like getting my heart caught in a mill saw. Beneath a thin façade of polite pity, I found in myself a roiling sea of fear and loathing" (p. 196). After she purchased the book, she hurried into a small elevator where her feelings exploded.

> I . . . hit the stop button with a closed fist . . . Then, I leaned back against the wall and covered my face with my hands, trying to control myself. I felt as though some evil ogre had killed my "real" baby—the baby I'd been expecting—and replaced him with an ugly, broken replica. My grief at losing that "real" baby was as intense as if he had been 2 years old, or 5, or 10. The whole thing seemed wildly unfair to me: My baby was dead, and I was still pregnant. I was suddenly seized by a rage so strong I wanted to bash in the elevator walls (p. 196).

Anger can appear when a person no longer fits society's picture of "normal." It may fester when a client can no longer do the same activities in the previous way. The rage and resentment may be displaced onto family, friends, and health care providers. Anger may seem inappropriate and take the client, significant others, and health professionals by surprise.

I couldn't believe what I was hearing! Every day, in his aphasic way, Mr. Farmer would yell, scream, and shake his left fist at his wife. I asked her why he was so angry and why he was taking everything out on her. She hung her head and quietly told me that the stroke happened while they were having sex, and he was blaming her for it.
—*From the journal of Kia Lupen, social work student*

Clients may lash out at health professionals or be excessively demanding. It can become disabling when clients scream at you, "Get out of here!" (Drench, 1998). Care providers find it difficult to accept a client's rejection. Ruth Purtilo, a medical ethicist and physical therapist, espouses five plausible reasons for this rejection (1984). First, the client "rejects" the health care provider because of the displaced anger that the client, friends, or family put on the professional. Second, the client may consider that there is no longer a need for the care provider, thinking that he or she has come to terms with the anticipated death or other loss. Third, the client may have little energy and selectively chooses to use it on family and friends. Fourth, the client may have difficulty separating from or showing affection to the health care professional. Finally, the client may be separating from anything or anybody related to the health care setting.

Any one or a combination of these possibilities may explain the apparent rejection. It is natural for the health care provider to feel hurt, rejected, and confused and to suspect that he or she has somehow failed the client. However, it is important for the care provider to understand the behavior rather than judge it or take it personally.

As uncomfortable as it may be for health professionals to witness and deal with anger, deal with it we must. Anger that is not recognized and confronted tends to impede the grieving process. If ignored, it can be camouflaged and appear in other ways, such as in disabling illness, maladaptive behavior, and chronic unhappiness (Cerney & Buskirk, 1991). In Chapter 14, we will be discussing therapeutic responses to loss and grief. We can help clients acknowledge their anger and make referrals to appropriate team members, if the situation is outside the scope of our practice.

## Guilt

Anger and guilt are natural parts of the grieving process. Irrational anger may even be directed toward the deceased. "He left me with all these bills to pay and no insurance policy." "She said she'd take me to buy my prom dress. How could she just leave me like that?" Unresolved feelings of guilt may follow the anger.

Guilt also comes into play upon someone's death, if the grieving people feel as though they have wronged, disappointed, neglected, or been angry with the deceased. "I should have taken her to chemotherapy." "I could have brought meals over to the house." "I never did give him the money I owed him." "I never told my son that I loved him." If the bereaved person perceives the loss as punishment, guilt may also be a factor. "I should have insisted that she go to the hospital." "If I had used a condom, I wouldn't have AIDS, and I wouldn't be blind."

Guilt and shame often are intertwined. Following acute myocardial infarctions, women may feel guilty and ashamed about being tired and weak (Svedlund & Axelsson, 2000). They often feel "distressed," "vulnerable," and useless as they grapple with the fear of what their cardiac condition means to them. While adjusting to their heart attacks, they may develop insights of how to adapt and live "normally." It is interesting to note that these women do not always share their thoughts and feelings with their partners, suggesting a lack of communication, perhaps another loss.

## Bargaining

We learn to negotiate early in life. "If I get ready for bed now, can I have a story?" "If I clean my room, can I sleep over at Robin's house?" In clients with illness or injury, following Kübler-Ross's (1969) phases of denial ("It can't be me!") and anger ("Why me?"), the third stage of bargaining sounds like, "If I can just live long enough to walk my daughter down the aisle on her wedding day." This is often a short-term strategy (it is one thing if the wedding is imminent, it is another if the daughter is currently only 7 years old). Bargaining with God, health care providers, family members, or themselves is done to postpone an anticipated loss. Impairments and disabilities often steal some of a person's control over their lives and environment. Bargaining is one way to reassert some control.

For example, over the course of chemotherapy, a client with a diagnosis of lymphoma had lost both his appetite and significant weight.

> Over the weeks that we worked together, he got his appetite back and was starving all the time. I had never seen such a skinny man eat so much. He would hoard food all the time. I swear he was stealing it from other people's trays. One day, he was complaining about being hungry, and I made the big mistake of giving him something to eat. We'd had a party in the morning, and there were some bagels left over. The next day, when he came for exercise, he looked at me and said, "What, no bagels? No bagels, no exercise. If I'm going to do all this work, I want to be fed." It was the funniest thing—here was this "Mr. No Bagels, No Exercise". . .
>
> I, of course, bought into this entitlement and would bring him food. This tall, totally wild-looking man would be lounging on the mat table, licking his fingertips and wiping the cream cheese off the corner of his mouth. He reached a point of ambulating a few hundred feet and was really making some gains. When he left to go to another facility, we gave him food as a going-away present (Drench, 1998, p. 73).

This man's bargaining helped him gain some control and dignity while he accomplished short-term gains. Unfortunately, shortly after being transferred to another facility, he developed more problems with gait and balance. There had been a recurrence of his lymphoma, and he entered a hospice. Less than two weeks later, he died.

## Sadness and Depression

Grieving behavior also includes sadness and sometimes depression (see Chapter 16 for a detailed discussion of depression). After the stages of denial, anger, and bargaining, Kübler-Ross (1969) identifies a period of depression, the fourth stage of grieving and dying. Perhaps much of what Kübler-Ross describes as depression may really be profound sadness rather than clinical depression. Everyone feels sadness to a certain degree, but not everyone experiences depression as part of grieving behavior in response to loss. Sometimes there is also a sense of "why bother?"

A few years after struggling with and surviving breast cancer, 49-year-old Julie Maloney developed squamous cell cancer of the gum and osteoradionecrosis. Because of her necrotic jaw, she had teeth and much of her jaw removed. Periodically depressed over the course of many surgical interventions, Julie valiantly fought to overcome her trials and regain her life, despite difficulty eating, speaking clearly, and having a visibly deformed face. Her "straw that broke the camel's back" was that she couldn't find employment or a social life. She struggles with depression.

Depression may coexist with other reactions to loss and hinder adjustment to illness. For example, clients with end-stage renal disease and their families are overwhelmed by the intrusion, lifestyle adjustments, and significance that kidney dialysis has on their lives (White &

Grenyer, 1999). In addition to depression, these clients often experience anger and hopelessness. Although dialysis technology can be life-sustaining, it can have a negative impact on lifestyle. Framing the experience differently can help clients cope in positive ways, as described in Chapter 14. It is also interesting to note that depression can be mitigated by physiological changes. Consider the woman with end-stage renal disease who is no longer depressed since her electrolytes have been stabilized.

Depression can be an offshoot of loss. It may be clinical depression or depressed bereavement patterns, the ways in which people grieve for their losses (Langer, 1994). Either way, it justifies diagnostic and therapeutic intervention. For example, between 25 percent and 79 percent of people who have strokes are depressed (Gordon & Hibbard, 1997). If health professionals fail to identify the depression and provide appropriate intervention, the depression may impede functional and emotional recovery (Hermann, Black, Lawrence, Szekely, & Szalai, 1998). Our role as health care providers is to be able to recognize the signs and make referrals to appropriate team members, such as a psychotherapist, psychologist, psychiatric nurse, or social worker, as indicated.

## Anxiety

Psychological distress complicates one's ability to cope with the physiological changes associated with illness or injury. Although depression is not widely experienced, anxiety may be. Remember that depression and sadness are not synonymous. However, both anxiety and depression can be intermittent or constant, such as that seen over the course of breast cancer and its treatment (Longman, Braden, & Mishel, 1999). They may also persist through the final phase of a terminal illness.

Anxiety, as well as depression, may be long-lasting. For example, men who perceive loss secondary to their myocardial infarctions have greater levels of anxiety and depression, even three to four years after their heart attacks (Waltz, Badura, Pfaff, & Schott, 1988).

## Diminished Problem Solving

Any type of loss can result in a period of distress. A person can feel confused and defeated. The feelings of grief that accompany the loss tend to be affiliated with diminished cognitive effectiveness and problem-solving abilities, which vary in intensity and length of time (Caplan, 1990). As such, grieving persons often have difficulty acquiring, storing, and processing information. This can add to the distress. Consider the 36-year-old mother of two young children whose husband had recently died. Although she needed to return to work to support her family, she worried that she would not be able to adequately perform her job because she felt "dull."

During the grieving process, people tend to lose some level of ability to clearly define their sense of purpose and meaning in life, as well as the ability to continue in the face of adversity—"I just can't go on," "I can't live without," "I can't handle this." These thoughts and feelings can be associated with diminished energy. Such attitudes and perceptions weaken a person's sense of capability and resolve to "fight the good fight."

The grieving behaviors we have discussed are the more typical responses to loss. However, some clients have maladaptive reactions, that diminish their ability to function and can lead to other problems. Other types of grief behavior include medical symptomatology and illness, stemming from a decreased immune system response and resistance to infection; psychophysiologic reactions, such as essential hypertension, ulcerative colitis, and neurodermatitis; maladaptive behavior, such as sexual promiscuity and drug use; and neurotic and psychotic manifestations, such as schizophrenic and phobic reactions, which may begin or are exacerbated by severe loss (Peretz, 1980).

Therapeutic intervention that acknowledges the importance of psychosocial factors and incorporates them into the plan of care can help minimize a sense of helplessness for the clients and their families. We will be discussing these issues in Chapter 14.

# Conceptual Models of Grieving

## Stages of Grieving and Dying

In the second half of the 1960s, Swiss psychiatrist Elisabeth Kübler-Ross began to work with clients who were dying and, before the end of the decade, produced what was to become the formative work on the subject. *On Death and Dying* (1969) details the emotional process of dying, described in five stages: *denial, anger, bargaining, depression,* and *acceptance.* This widely, though not universally, accepted framework has also become a model for facing a loss in which no death is involved, such as those of functional limitations and disabilities. For example, the diagnosis of lifelong conditions in children, such as Type 1 (childhood) diabetes, may represent multiple losses for parents. Upon learning of the newly diagnosed diabetes, parents' grief reactions are similar to those of bereavement due to death (Lowes & Lyne, 2000).

It is critical to realize that not every person moves through all five stages and that the progression is not linear. The stages actually occur as more of a process. There is also no time sequence that accompanies the passages. These stages, however, are typical, in varying degrees. There is a great deal of back-and-forth movement. People often find themselves in one stage, only to slip back into a previous stage. Not everyone reaches acceptance. Some people remain depressed. Others never stop denying the reality of their situation. Anger becomes a constant and counterproductive companion for other people, while some never cease to bargain and negotiate.

Consider again Martha Beck (1999), pregnant with a child with Down syndrome:

> I remembered . . . the final stage was acceptance. But . . . that was when the tragedy was a death . . . What if the tragedy was born alive? I tried to force myself to reach acceptance immediately, right there in the elevator. . . . I wondered why the psychological stages of loss didn't include fear. Maybe it was because fear pervades and overwhelms everything else. I mashed my hands against my eyes and shook so hard that the elevator compartment trembled on its cable (p. 197).

The acceptance that was eluding this expectant mother was a premature expectation. It is when a client no longer denies the reality, has come to terms with anger, is not trying to bargain with good behavior to "buy" more time or easier circumstances, and is not depressed, that the person enters what Kübler-Ross (1969) calls the fifth stage: acceptance. Acceptance, however, is more than the absence of the other stages. It represents an advanced degree of the continuum of personal healing. For people with disabilities, it may be learning how to cope and adjust with situations. If impending death is the issue, acceptance is not synonymous with joy or satisfaction. It is sometimes a sense of resignation, devoid of feelings. Sometimes, it is a sense of peace.

Mr. Carlson was a 50-year-old man with lung cancer who was ventilator-dependent. Several times each day, he received treatment to clear his pulmonary secretions. One afternoon, he refused treatment. The health professional explained that lack of treatment would hasten his death, and visions of "drowning in your own secretions" were described. She educated, cajoled, and begged the client to allow treatment. The client adamantly refused. Mr. Carlson understood the facts, but he had had enough. He wrote the words on his notepad, "Let me go." They wept together, knowing that this was their goodbye. He died that evening.

## Integrative Theory of Bereavement

In addition to Kübler-Ross's five stages of grieving and dying, another way to understand bereavement is to examine an integrative theory of bereavement (Sanders, 1989). Refer to Table 13–2 for a comparison of the theoretical concepts of grieving. This model also has five phases, which are correlated with emotional, biological, and social factors. In the beginning, the person experiences *shock*. He or she responds to the loss with disbelief: "It can't be happening; "It's not true." The person numbly moves through this initial phase, often unable to complete the simplest tasks or make any decisions.

During the second phase, the person develops an *awareness of the loss*. Reality is beginning to "set in," and the person is starting to understand the meaning of the loss and the extent of the void caused by it.

In the third phase of *conservation and withdrawal*, the individual may feel fatigued, even listless: "I feel like a rag doll"; "I can barely get through the day. I don't have energy to spare." This is a period of conserving personal resources and avoiding tasks perceived as "extra" or unnecessary. The person may even isolate him- or herself from others and the everyday routine.

As time passes, the fourth phase of *healing* begins. It is a time of adjusting to a new reality. Activities are resumed, and the individual may be surprised to hear his or her own laughter. Sometimes, however, this realization of self-enjoyment can trigger feelings of guilt, and the person may retreat.

Finally, there can be *renewal*. During this fifth phase, the person is reaching resolution of his or her grief and emerging at the other end, engaged in life, often enthusiastically.

The integrative theory of the bereavement model recognizes that there are variables from both the individual and the environment that influence the grieving process. Both sets of me-

**TABLE 13–2** Comparative Models of Grieving

| Phases | Stages of Grieving and Dying (Kübler-Ross, 1969) | Integrative Theory of Bereavement (Sanders, 1989) | Tasks of Mourning (Worden, 2002) |
|---|---|---|---|
| 1 | Denial | Shock | Accept the reality of loss |
| 2 | Anger | Awareness of loss | Experience the pain associated with grief |
| 3 | Bargaining | Conservation and withdrawal | Adjust to circumstances created by loss |
| 4 | Depression | Healing | Emotionally relocate the person who has died and progress with life |
| 5 | Acceptance | Renewal | |

diating variables operate from the outset of grief. For example, external mediators include social support, sudden versus chronic illness, socioeconomic status, religion, concurrent crises, culture, and stigmatic death, such as AIDS. In addition, internal mediators are also at work, such as age, gender, personality, health, ambivalence toward the deceased person, and dependency behavior.

Outcomes of bereavement in this model are similar to those already discussed above. There may be personal growth (positive), a downward shift in general health or life's activities (negative), or no change in behavior or thinking (neutral).

## Tasks of Mourning

In addition to Kübler-Ross's five stages of grieving and dying and Sanders's five phases in the integrative theory of bereavement, there is another model to consider. Worden (2002) believes that grief is a process that involves learning to master four tasks of mourning. First, the person needs to *accept the reality of the loss.* The disbelief that accompanies a loss or a death is compounded if the incident is sudden, such as the unexpected death of a teenager on a basketball court. To accomplish this task, the person comes out of denial (Kübler-Ross's first stage of grieving) and shock (Sanders's first phase).

Once the person accepts the loss as real, the grieving person needs to *experience the pain associated with grief,* the second task of mourning. If the individual is part of a society that does not encourage people to express their feelings and emotions around the loss, there may be a temptation to lightly touch upon or even skip this mourning task. Although initial brief denial can comfort and shield the person from the loss, it limits the individual from moving on and completing the process. Avoiding the pain can also lead to depression or other psychiatric problems, as discussed in Chapter 16.

Worden's (2002) third task of mourning is *adjusting to circumstances created by the loss.* This could mean adjusting to life without a right arm or assuming different roles in life that were once fulfilled by the person who has died. For example, a young widow may need to learn to manage a household budget and be "both a mother and a father" to her children. A new sense of self, including one's perceived worth and esteem, may be a healthy by-product. There are both physical and emotional tasks to be mastered.

Finally, the fourth task of mourning in this model is *"emotionally relocating the deceased" and progressing with life.* Relocating does not connote erasing the person and the corresponding memories from one's life. Rather, it means giving those memories a different emotional role so that the individual may resume life's activities, that is, to "go on" despite the loss. It also means assigning meaning to the loss and integrating it into his or her belief system.

Common themes emerge across the conceptual models of grieving. There is an initial period of shock, disbelief, or denial. In order to progress through the grieving process, a person needs to become aware of the situation and accept the reality of the loss. The grieving individual needs to experience the pain of the reality, which may involve profound distress, including sadness or depression. There is little energy, and personal resources are used sparingly, even to the point of social isolation.

In order to emerge at the other end of the grieving tunnel with psychological and physical health intact, the person needs to find ways to adjust to circumstances, in light of the loss, to find other means of accomplishing things and discover alternate ways "to be." The goal is to heal, accept, and progress with life, in a word, to be renewed.

# Grief Outcomes

The perception of how severe a functional loss is will be influenced by both psychodynamic and pragmatic issues. The nature and severity of physical obstacles and the dependency caused by the loss affect one's perception (Hirst, 1989). There may be isolation, loneliness, and loss of social support. Consider the college student with paraplegia, secondary to a motor vehicle accident. His primary goal was to ambulate. The reality was that, although he could ambulate very short distances using crutches, the enormous energy expenditure compromised his health status. He was not able to walk functionally. Rather than being able to accept using the wheelchair as a means of mobility, he viewed it as a failure of his rehabilitation team. He also could not accept that there were fewer, and different, available options in life.

Negative reactions of other people also have an impact on a functional loss and how the person copes with it, as we described in our discussion on stigma in Chapter 9. These factors, acting singly or in combination, can become a social disability, impeding the quality of one's social life (Hirst, 1989).

There are other contributing aspects that may color how a person responds to a loss, including the premorbid personality and personal coping styles. Prior life history and cultural issues both play a role in one's perception of loss, as well as strategies to adjust to it. The roles that people have, such as head of the household, athlete, or beauty queen, and the attributes assigned to or assumed by them are part of a person's core identity. Being able to integrate the loss into their current lives is challenging. Sometimes a person will say, "I don't even recognize myself any more. Who is this person I've become?"

Sufficient resources, such as social and economic support, are also key elements that can influence the degree and type of other life stressors (Langer, 1994). Consider the family who cannot afford to make their home wheelchair accessible or to purchase a van. In addition, they were socially introverted before the illness that was to change their lives and do not have a network of friends to emotionally or practically help them. Everything is a struggle for them, which adds to their isolation and stress.

Following a loss, three interdependent elements influence outcome: (1) the pain of the loss of attachment and anguish of dealing with the situation, (2) the "handicapping" deprivation of not having what you once had before the loss, and (3) the deterioration of cognitive capabilities, including problem solving, and the will to struggle or live (Caplan, 1990).

These three elements, working alone or together in varying degrees, may affect grieving outcomes, which may be positive or negative. Some individuals may develop an acute adjustment disorder or chronic psychopathology, that is to say, psychiatric illnesses where they manifest maladaptive behavior to avoid reality or isolate oneself. Another poor outcome of grieving would be the development of a physical illness. Grief is considered pathological when it becomes excessive, protracted, or blocked. This is more likely to occur when social support is lacking. In contrast, these three elements may also produce a healthy grieving outcome, wherein the person enlists effective coping strategies and develops personal fortitude and self-mastery of the situation.

People may develop and affirm negative (perpetually mourning) or positive attitudes (engaging in life to the best of the person's ability) (Frankl, 1984). However, attitudes are dynamic and, therefore, changeable. People may vacillate between poles or have elements of both positive and negative attitudes concurrently. Consider Lucy Grealy (1994), who was diagnosed with Ewing's sarcoma at the age of 9. As a result of this primary malignant bone tumor, she underwent surgery to remove a significant section of her jaw, endured years of radiation and chemotherapy, and had thirty corrective operations that were not cosmetically successful. Although she ultimately accepted this as part of the person she was, during active cancer treatment, she established a protective barrier by wearing a large hat.

> My hat was my barrier between me, and what I was vaguely becoming aware of as ugly about the world, and me. It hid me, it hid my secret, though badly, and when people made fun of me or stared at me, I assumed it was only because they could guess what was beneath my hat (p. 107).

Frears and Scheider (1981) believe that "transcending the loss" is the final stage, wherein the person has done the painful grief work, searched for meaning in the loss and grief, grown and matured, and reintegrates into life. Facing a loss and working through grief can be phenomenally challenging. How it is done can make a difference between moving on with one's life or "staying stuck" in one's grief. It is important to remember that grief is not a finite point on the continuum between loss and adjustment; it is a process. For example, grieving older women whose husbands have hospice care and die describe a process of "being aware," "experiencing distress," "supporting," "coping," and finally, "facing new realities" (Jacob, 1996). This is congruent with Worden's (2002) tasks of mourning.

Health professionals use a bereavement model to describe the process of loss and readjustment. In a study of people who had strokes and their caregivers and health professionals, the people with strokes acknowledged the losses and disabilities that disrupted their lives (Alaszewski, Alaszewski, & Potter, 2004). To help return their lives to "normal," they establish goals to progress toward recovery. Health providers tend to use a bereavement model when they disagree with the goals set by their clients, believe them to be unrealistic, and perceive that the clients have become "stuck." A valuable message here is that health providers need to clearly and understandably communicate and develop plans of care that work in tandem with the goals and strategies of the clients.

Someone who goes through the loss and bereavement process may discover a new sense of purpose. Actor and director Christopher Reeve, forever known as *Superman* in the movies, came crashing to the ground when the horse he was riding unsuccessfully attempted a jump over an obstacle on a course. Fracturing his cervical vertebrae, Reeve suddenly became a person with high-level quadriplegia. With his catastrophic injury and celebrity status, Reeve developed a new mission, a new purpose in life. He created a research foundation and became a major spokesman and fundraiser for spinal cord injury.

Although there are "typical" reactions to loss, people's responses do vary. There are no set, predictable sequences of mourning and no specific timeframes. Grief usually lasts six months to a year or longer, but the acute pain of it diminishes slowly over time, commonly within the first few months. However, in our society of instant relief, instant satisfaction, and quick studies, people are often impatient with the "schedule" of the grieving. It is not unusual to hear comments like, "When will they get over it?"; "When will *I* get over it?"; "What's the problem? It's been a year already."; "Put the past behind you." For some people, grief can become chronic and even perpetual.

# Chronic Sorrow

Sadness is a response to loss and is a natural part of the grieving process. There is sadness around acute loss, which can be short-lived or prolonged. There is sadness around chronic conditions. There is also sadness that is lifelong, episodic in nature, or progressive. It may be a response to a chronic or terminal illness. It can affect both the individual with a chronic illness or disability, as well as the family members (Rosenberg, 1998). It can be experienced by the parents of a child who faces permanent problems, which is also the loss of the fantasy of the "perfect" child. It can also be part of a spousal relationship. The "it" is chronic sorrow, the grief experienced from continual loss of milestones of life that are not reached, unrelenting loss of future plans, and lifestyle adaptations based on restrictions (Hainsworth, 1995). It is also characterized by antecedent events that cause the sorrow to recur.

Living with certain conditions carries a high risk for living with chronic sorrow, such as multiple sclerosis (80%; Hainsworth, 1994) and cancer (90%; Eakes, 1993). Over a long period of time, feelings of chronic sorrow occur episodically, triggered by an event that reminds people of the chronicity of their situation. Consider the case study of a woman with multiple sclerosis and her husband that describes chronic sorrow throughout her illness and disability (Hainsworth, Burke, Lindgren, & Eakes, 1993). She endures the progressive loss of bodily functions, the stigma associated with chronic illness, a restricted social life, and loss of future plans. Each functional loss provokes a new episode of sorrow.

Chronic sorrow is also experienced by parents in a lifetime of ongoing losses. For parents of a child with a disability, each failure to achieve a typical milestone triggers a new episode of grief. This "sadness without end" continues to be an enduring focus in the lives of parents, even when they may no longer be the caretakers of their child (Krafft & Krafft, 1998). However, behavior may differ between parents. For example, mothers of children with developmental disabilities tend to lapse into chronic sorrow, while the fathers' behavior leans toward resignation (Mallow & Bechtel, 1999). Activated by health care crises, responses also differ among parents. Affective aspects tend to dominate in mothers, as they feel sadness and grief. In contrast, fathers emphasize cognitive aspects, as they compare social norms in their children with others. It is also interesting to note that children who lose a parent also experience chronic sorrow when the parent is absent at significant life events.

This chronic sorrow, which is the periodic recurrence of permanent, pervasive sadness and other feelings associated with grief related to a loss, can emanate from mental, as well as physical, illness. An excerpt from a mother's journal (personal communication, February 2, 2001), whose daughter has been living with mental health problems, epitomizes chronic sorrow.

> After a while, it becomes obvious that this disability is forever. She is 18 now and is making her own decisions. She is living away from us and has a very unhealthy lifestyle, and she is not safe. Her doctor told me that I had done a wonderful job taking care of her. It doesn't matter. She is not safe, and I can't help her. I can't fix her.
>
> I know that the child I had is gone and that I have to grieve this terrible loss. I miss the smart, funny, warm, caring person she used to be. I don't know who she is now.
>
> I have accepted the permanence of this loss, and I have given up the future. She is lost to us as the child who we knew and the relationship that we had. Her doctor and her therapist tell me that things will get better, but I can't go there. I have to ac-

cept that she is gone and is not coming back as the child we had. That means that anything that we get from this point on is a gift, and not another disappointment.

Chronic sorrow is characterized by lifelong, periodically recurring sadness. Although people differ in their reactions, in one study, 83 percent of people and their spouse caregivers experienced chronic sorrow (Hainsworth, Eakes, & Burke, 1994).

There is a middle-range theory of chronic sorrow, which recognizes the phenomenon as a normal response to loss across the lifespan for people who experience continued differences due to loss (Eakes, Burke, & Hainsworth, 1998). This framework also acknowledges the role of antecedent trigger events. Comparing the reality of one's situation to the "normal" milestones of life can also precipitate the sorrow. A mother's journal continues:

> It was excruciatingly painful for me to walk into her school. It was so painful, I used to get physically ill. I could not participate in the PTA or be a room mother because I could not bear to hear the other mothers talking about all their children's activities and successes, when our daughter wasn't doing any of those things. All my closest friends have family members with serious illness or disabilities.
>
> A couple of months ago, my mother came to visit. She wanted to buy my daughter a birthday present, so we went to [the department store]. She ended up trying on prom dresses, even though she is not going to the prom, and she is not going to graduate on time. She has never been to a single high school dance or football game or any of those things. I had to leave the store and sit in my car and cry. I wasn't crying about the prom. It was the prom that opened the door for everything.

## SUMMARY

This chapter began where the previous chapter on loss ended. In response to loss, there is the universal human phenomenon of grief, a psychological and physiological process that occurs in response to loss in every age group and culture. It is a painful process during which people, hopefully, can understand the meaning of the loss and accept its place in their lives. Reactions to loss are as varied as the people who experience them, but there are common themes.

We explored the types of grief, including anticipatory, acute, chronic, and delayed or suppressed grief. We also described grieving behaviors, emphasizing that the outward behavior of a grieving person can be deceiving.

Following a loss, many variables affect the outcome, including the anguish of the loss, the deprivation experienced by the loss, and the diminution of cognitive capabilities. We also discussed the lifelong, episodic, and progressive sadness characteristic of the phenomenon of chronic sorrow.

Three models of bereavement were presented, the widely known stage theory of Kübler-Ross, the integrative theory of bereavement, and the tasks of mourning. Because grief is also a natural response to a loss of meaning in one's life, adjustment necessitates finding a new or reframing one's purpose and meaning. It may require creating a harmony between one's losses here and now and the possibilities for future opportunities.

In the next chapter, we will study therapeutic responses to loss and grief and how the health care provider may assist in the process of adjustment.

## REFLECTIVE QUESTIONS

1. Of the three models of grieving presented in this chapter, which one feels most valid to you? Explain why.
2. Out of fear of doing or saying the "wrong" thing, people often avoid those who are grieving.
   a. What are some verbal and nonverbal responses or actions that might be supportive or helpful to a person who is grieving?
   b. What responses might be detrimental?
3. What behaviors might you observe in a person who is experiencing grief that are indicative of
   a. denial?
   b. anger?
   c. guilt?
   d. bargaining?
   e. sadness or depression?
   f. anxiety?
   g. diminished problem-solving?
4. Complete this sentence: When I think of myself becoming ill or disabled, I _____.
5. How can you protect yourself from becoming overwhelmed by clients' losses and grief?

## CASE STUDY

*Note:* Because loss, grief, and adjustment are presented on a continuum as a process rather than finite stages in time, there is only one Case Study in Part IV to reflect this. It is, however, told in parts, each with its own set of questions that pertain to the information in the particular chapter. It is suggested that you begin by reading the previous section about Cynthia Osbourne before proceeding.

Throughout this difficult period in Cynthia's life, the physical therapist, physical therapist assistant, and occupational therapist were able to make Cynthia laugh. She credits their supportive, nurturing care in helping her to reach this point in time and "not be crazy." Although Cynthia was the youngest person at the rehabilitation center, she was close in age to the therapy team, who would "break up the day" by dropping in to visit her.

Her young sons were able to visit Cynthia weekly, which also helped keep her "as normal as possible," yet presented other challenges for her. The 10-year-old was strong and took the events in stride. In contrast, the 7-year-old was initially quiet and would not talk to Cynthia or go near her for weeks. Eventually, he was able to climb up on her bed, hug her, and begin asking questions.

Because everything in her life is now different, she has had moments of weeping and sadness. However, she has maintained a positive attitude throughout the hospitalization part of the ordeal. Cynthia and her fiancé were planning a wedding and shopping for a home. She has had to grieve her situation, as well as the loss of her partner.

1. Discuss grieving behavior that Cynthia may be experiencing.
2. a. What phase of grieving might Cynthia now be experiencing in each of the three models described in the text–Stages of Grieving and Dying, Integrative Theory of Bereavement, and Tasks of Mourning.
   b. Provide a rationale for each of your decisions.

**3.** In what ways are the therapeutic team members influencing possible outcomes of Cynthia's grief?

**4.** What other variables may affect the outcome of Cynthia's grief?

## REFERENCES

Alaszewski, A., Alaszewski, H., & Potter, J. (2004). The bereavement model, stroke and rehabilitation: A critical analysis of the use of a psychological model in professional practice. *Disability Rehabilitation, 26* (18), 1067–1078.

Beck, M. N. (1999). *Expecting Adam.* New York: Berkley.

Blanchard, C. G., & Ruckdeschel, J. C. (1986). Psychosocial aspects of cancer in adults: Implications for teaching medical students. *Journal of Cancer Education, 1*(4), 237–248.

Bowlby, J. (1980). *Attachment and loss: Vol. 3. Loss: Sadness and depression.* New York: Basic Books.

Cable, D. G. (1998). Grief in the American culture. In K. Doka & J. Davidson (Eds.), *Living with grief: Who we are, how we grieve* (pp. 61–71). Philadelphia: Hospice Foundation of America.

Caplan, G. (1990). Loss, stress, and mental health. *Community Mental Health Journal, 26*(1), 27–48.

Cerney, M. S., & Buskirk, J. R. (1991). Anger: The hidden part of grief. *Bulletin of the Menninger Clinic, 55*(2), 228–237.

Chapman, K. J., & Pepler, C. (1998). Coping, hope, and anticipatory grief in family members in palliative home care. *Cancer Nursing, 21*(4), 226–234.

Coughlin, R. (1993). *Grieving: A love story.* New York: Random House.

Drench, M. E. (1998). *Red ribbons are not enough: Health caregivers' stories about AIDS.* Wilsonville, OR: BookPartners.

Eakes, G. G. (1993). Chronic sorrow: A response to living with cancer. *Oncology Nursing Forum, 20*(9), 1327–1334.

Eakes, G. G., Burke, M. L., & Hainsworth, M. A. (1998). Middle-range theory of chronic sorrow. *Image Journal of Nursing Scholarship, 30*(2), 179–184.

Frankl, V. E. (1984). *Man's search for meaning: An introduction to logotherapy* (3rd ed.). New York: Simon & Schuster.

Frears, L. H., & Schneider, J. M. (1981). Exploring grief and loss in a wholistic framework. *Personnel and Guidance Journal, 59*(6), 341–345.

Fulton, G., Madden, C., & Minichiello, V. (1996). The social construction of anticipatory grief. *Social Science and Medicine, 43*(9), 1349–1358.

Gilliland, G., & Fleming, S. (1998). A comparison of spousal anticipatory grief and conventional grief. *Death Studies, 22*(6), 541–569.

Gordon, W. A., & Hibbard, M. R. (1997). Poststroke depression: An examination of the literature. *Archives of Physical Medicine and Rehabilitation, 78,* 658–663.

Grealy, L. (1994). *Autobiography of a face.* Boston: Houghton Mifflin.

Hainsworth, M. A. (1994). Living with multiple sclerosis: The experience of chronic sorrow. *Journal of Neuroscience Nursing, 26*(4), 237–240.

Hainsworth, M. A. (1995). Helping spouses with chronic sorrow related to multiple sclerosis. *Journal of Gerontological Nursing, 21*(7), 29–33.

Hainsworth, M. A., Burke, M. L., Lindgren, C. L., & Eakes, G. G. (1993). Chronic sorrow in multiple sclerosis: A case study. *Home Healthcare Nurse, 11*(2), 9–13.

Hainsworth, M. A., Eakes, G. G., & Burke, M. L. (1994). Coping with chronic sorrow. *Issues in Mental Health Nursing, 15*(1), 59–66.

Hermann, N., Black, S. E., Lawrence, J., Szekely, C., & Szalai, J. P. (1998). The Sunnybrook stroke study: A prospective study of depressive symptoms and functional outcomes. *Stroke, 29,* 618–624.

Hirst, M. (1989). Patterns of impairment and disability related to social handicap in young people with cerebral palsy and spina bifida. *Journal of Biosocial Science, 21*(1), 1–12.

Jacob, S. R. (1996). The grief experience of older women whose husbands had hospice care. *Journal of Advanced Nursing, 24*(2), 280–286.

Krafft, S. K., & Krafft, L. J. (1998). Chronic sorrow: Parents' lived experience. *Holistic Nursing Practice, 13*(1), 59–67.

Kübler-Ross, E. (1969). *On death and dying.* New York: Macmillan.

Langer, K. G. (1994). Depression and denial in psychotherapy of persons with disabilities. *American Journal of Psychotherapy, 48*(2), 181–194.

Longman, A. J., Braden, C. J., & Mishel, M. H. (1999). Side effects burden, psychological adjustment, and life quality in women with breast cancer: Pattern of association over time. *Oncology Nursing Forum, 26*(5), 909–915.

Lowes, L., & Lyne, P. (2000). Chronic sorrow in parents of children with newly diagnosed diabetes: A review of the literature and discussion of the implications for nursing practice. *Journal of Advanced Nursing, 32*(1), 41–48.

Maguire, P., Walsh, S., Jeacock, J., & Kingston, R. (1999). Physical and psychological needs of patients dying from colorectal cancer. *Palliative Medicine, 13*(1), 45–50.

Mallow, G. E., & Bechtel, G. A. (1999). Chronic sorrow: The experience of parents with children who are developmentally disabled. *Journal of Psychosocial Nursing and Mental Health Services, 37*(7), 31–35.

Peretz, D. (1980). Reaction to loss. In B. Schoenberg, A. C. Carr, D. Peretz, & A. H. Kutscher (Eds.), *Loss and grief: Psychological management in medical practice* (pp. 20–35). New York: Columbia University Press.

Purtilo, R. (1984). *Health professional/patient interaction* (3rd ed.). Philadelphia: W. B. Saunders Company.

Rosenberg, C. J. (1998). Faculty–student mentoring. A father's chronic sorrow: A daughter's perspective. *Journal of Holistic Nursing, 16*(3), 399–404.

Sanders, C. M. (1989). *Grief: The mourning after.* New York: Wiley.

Sussman, N. (1995). Reactions of patients to the diagnosis and treatment of cancer. *Anticancer Drugs, 6*(Suppl. 1), 4–8.

Svedlund, M., & Axelsson, I. (2000). Acute myocardial infarction in middle-aged women: Narrations from the patients and their partners during rehabilitation. *Intensive Critical Care Nursing, 16*(4), 256–265.

Waltz, M., Badura, B., Pfaff, H., & Schott, T. (1988). Marriage and the psychological consequences of a heart attack: A longitudinal study of adaptation to chronic illness after 3 years. *Social Science and Medicine, 27*(2), 149–158.

White, Y., & Grenyer, B. F. (1999). The biopsychosocial impact of end-stage renal disease: The experience of dialysis patients and their partners. *Journal of Advanced Nursing, 3*(6), 1312–1320.

Worden, J. W. (2002). *Grief counseling and grief therapy* (3rd ed.). New York: Springer.

# 14

# *Adjustment*

When I first looked at Diane sitting in her wheelchair by the edge of the pool, I only saw a woman "crippled" by her condition. (Honestly, that's the word that came to mind; so much for people-first, acceptable language.) Scleroderma had stretched the skin so taut over her tiny frame that I thought it would tear. It pulled with such force that her facial features were distorted into a perpetual smile, and her hands and feet were deformed. She was a 20-year-old woman, though she looked at least 40, and was frozen in place. There was nothing she could functionally do for herself. On Saturday mornings, though, she was transformed as she "swam" in the community pool. As her volunteer pool buddy this week, I gingerly lifted her welded body off the chair and lowered her into the water. Almost inaudibly, she said, "This is what heaven feels like. It's the one time all week that I feel like a human being."

Wearing flotation pads and barely propelling herself with her arms, she was able to mentally let go of her restricting disease and emphasize what she could do and how good it made her feel. Because she could participate in the pool program, Diane valued both the activity and herself. It was one way that she coped with her life.

—*From the journal of Paul Rodriguez, physical therapist student*

Albert Camus, Nobel laureate for literature, said, "In the depth of winter, I finally learned that within me there lay an invincible summer." On the continuum of loss and grief, there is adjustment—an adaptation to new circumstances, awareness, knowledge, and growth. In the early phases of the adjustment period, there can be heightened stress and anxiety, particularly as external support begins to dwindle. Some people may anticipate a progression or recurrence of an illness. Others need to discover how best to adapt to loss of function or chronic symptoms, such as paresthesias or pain. Individuals may need to adjust to changes in relationships with family and friends or deal with employment, financial, and insurance issues. This chapter discusses coping behavior, psychosocial adaptation strategies, and implications for health care professionals.

# Coping Behavior

As we discussed in the two previous chapters, there are many types of personal losses and grief responses. Sometimes we experience a collective grief. The public united in shock and bewilderment at the April 1995 bombing of the Alfred P. Murrah Federal Building in Oklahoma City, which killed 168 people and injured hundreds of others. We joined together in collective horror at the sudden attack on the United States one September morning in 2001, when terrorists hijacked commercial airplanes and used them to crash into and destroy the World Trade Center in New York and part of the Pentagon in Washington, DC, killing thousands of people. The world community faced incomprehensible shock and grief in December 2004, when a devastating earthquake and tsunami suddenly and swiftly killed more than 220,000 people in more than eleven countries.

The passage of time may dull the intensity of emotions, but memories can become embedded in our common psyches. Decades after November 1963, millions of people still remember where they were and what they were doing when they heard that President John F. Kennedy was shot. We gasped in anguish. We wept at the images of the flag-draped coffin, the riderless horse with its boots in the reverse position in the stirrups, and his young son, holding the American flag in one hand and saluting his father with the other. Cable (1998) suggests that these "public deaths and rituals have given us an opportunity to openly express our feelings and perhaps, in our own way, deal with other personal grief" (p. 65).

Most of us are untrained in how to cope with loss and grief. In contemporary society, people create artificial timetables and expect themselves and others to conform to them. We believe that grieving should only last so long. We should resume life's activities and return to the workplace within a prescribed period of time. Try to have another baby. Start dating. While a structured routine fills the often endless hours with activities and thoughts other than mourning, it does not put closure on bereavement. Because the loss and grief experience is distinct for every individual, people have their own unique timetables for responding.

Value judgments are often made about the way people grieve, as if there is a "right" way. Some of those judgments concern social recognition of a loss (Rando, 1984). People assess losses and determine the validity of a loss and subsequent grief. For instance, the loss of a 3-month-old child is considered a valid reason to grieve. On the other hand, not everyone understands the full significance of a miscarriage, stillbirth, or neonatal death. They may not even consider it a "real" loss and, therefore, not support the grieving person.

Other losses that may be trivialized or not validated through social recognition include the death of a pet or of someone in a relationship that is not socially sanctioned, such as a partner in a gay or extramarital relationship (Cable, 1998). The manner of death has an impact on the social support offered to grieving people. Death resulting from suicide or substance abuse may be perceived as a choice, or the individuals may be blamed for their weaknesses. Yet, the loss is real to those left behind, and they still need supportive care. Often they feel isolated and alone because the social stigma attached to their loss prevents "normal" levels of social support. They may also experience negative and hurtful messages about the manner of death.

Illness does not have the same finality as death, and people may use different coping behavior. Many factors contribute to how a person emotionally responds to learning the diagnosis of an illness. These can include:

- Premorbid personality
- Past anger or grief experiences
- Nature of lifestyle changes caused by the illness (i.e., unexpected timing, how far-reaching the changes will be, how long the disruption will last)
- Personal and social support to deal with the stressful situation
- Lifecycle phase (i.e., age, responsibilities, expectations, dreams)
- Experience with prior illness or critical situations
- Level of family functioning (Lewis, 1998).

It may be more difficult to contend with the news of an injury or the diagnosis of an illness than its physical ramifications. The emotional response caused by an illness or injury can be very challenging. Adjustment to disease is a process involving three areas of adaptation: loss and change, illness uncertainty, and suffering (Maunder & Esplen, 1999). In order to optimally adjust to change, the person first needs to accept the loss, grieve the loss, and then learn to adapt to the changes.

## Coping Skills

People who experience loss and subsequent grief use different coping skills to "get through the day." The word "skill" is often paired with "coping," which connotes an active process that can be learned. The purpose of coping behavior is to support people during stressful circumstances by diminishing or eliminating psychological distress and allowing them to function (Folkman & Lazarus, 1986). It is also a step in adapting to the changed circumstances. There is no one strategy for everyone, or a model to be used at all times. Rather, effective coping behavior is situation- and person-specific. To make matters more complex, the word "effective" is a value judgment.

Moos and Billings (1982) propose three models for coping with the stresses of illness. People employ strategies that are appraisal-focused, problem-focused, emotion-focused, or a combination of those approaches. Table 14–1 summarizes coping behavior.

### APPRAISAL-FOCUSED COPING

Appraisal-focused coping deals with the meaning associated with a crisis, enabling a person to understand the posed threat. It is a logical cognitive process that entails assessment and mental practice, definition and reframing, and avoidance or denial. Individuals divide an overpowering situation into smaller manageable parts, rather than absorbing the entire situation at once, which can be incredibly overwhelming (Drench, 2003a, 2003b). They evaluate what is happening in the present and integrate how well they may have handled troublesome situations in the past.

Mental practice, when individuals mentally rehearse possible scenarios, helps prepare them for different courses of actions and evaluate potential outcomes of those actions. When

**Table 14–1   Coping Behavior**

Appraisal-focused coping behavior (focus on meaning)
- Assess and mentally practice
- Define and reframe
- Deny or avoid

Problem-focused coping behavior (focus on action)
- Collect information
- Build support
- Act!
- Develop other measures of satisfaction or success

Emotion-focused coping behavior (focus on feelings)
- Control emotions
- Release emotions
- Accept and surrender

*(Adapted from Moos & Schaefer, 1986)*

facing illness, injury, or other grief, it often helps to find some meaning in what is happening. For some, this meaning comes in the context of spirituality or a belief in divine intervention or purpose.

Appraisal-focused coping involves reframing or redefining circumstances once they are understood. For example, a man diagnosed with cutaneous lymphoma considered himself in a better position than another client with non-Hodgkin's lymphoma. By comparing himself to another, he realized that his situation "wasn't so bad."

In addition, some people reframe the grief experience and perceive it as a gift, enabling them to grow in positive ways. Candy Lightner, founder of Mothers Against Drunk Driving, believes that although death takes something precious away, it can also give something back. She became a crusader for driving while sober after her child was killed by a drunk driver. This tragedy became the motivating factor for her to create an organization that has significantly raised the public's awareness.

After grief work, some people develop greater compassion and awareness that enables them to help themselves and others. Illness can also be a catalyst for changing priorities and values. Some people develop dissatisfaction or a sense of urgency in their lives, while others become empowered to do things that they might otherwise not have contemplated (Johnson & Klein, 1988). They may seek different jobs, homes, or relationships. These changes, however, may be understandably disturbing to family and friends. See Chapter 4 for a discussion of family roles and systems.

Appraisal-focused coping also involves denial or avoidance. People may minimize or deny the severity or existence of a situation in order to protect themselves from fully recognizing the stress. This allows them to unconsciously "stall," providing time for additional coping skills to be developed or called upon. After a young National Hockey League hopeful sustained a substantial eye injury during a game, he initially said he planned to pursue his dream and would play at that level again. A year later, despite the fact that he maintained his overall physical fitness and underwent multiple eye treatments, it became obvious to him that his optimistic outlook would not be realized. He would need to pursue other career goals.

## PROBLEM-FOCUSED COPING

Problem-focused coping emphasizes the practical aspects of a situation. The person garners information and support, learning the facts about the situation, courses of action, and possible consequences. A woman who is diagnosed with breast cancer may use appraisal-focused coping to analyze the situation and psychologically prepare herself for possible outcomes. Using problem-focused coping, she must consider the risks and benefits of a lumpectomy versus a mastectomy and the value of chemotherapy, radiation, or a combination of treatment options. These two coping modes are not necessarily mutually exclusive. In this instance, the woman may have first employed appraisal-focused coping and then became problem-focused to collect information and find support from friends, family, health care providers, support groups, or counseling. She is now ready to face making difficult decisions.

After collecting information and support, problem-focused coping also leads to action, such as scheduling rehabilitation appointments, arranging transportation to the clinic or Meals on Wheels, or structuring the day around care and rest periods (Drench, 2003b). Developing other measures of satisfaction or success is another aspect of problem-focused coping skills. When the challenges of Parkinson's disease reportedly became too significant for actor Michael J. Fox to continue with the demands of a popular television show, he left the work and redirected his energy toward raising awareness and funds for the disease. He also balanced his life to spend more time with his family. By making these changes in his life, he created other avenues of satisfaction and measures of success.

## EMOTION-FOCUSED COPING

In addition to appraisal- and problem-focused coping skills, there are emotion-focused skills, involving the emotions associated with a critical situation. Affective regulation helps people control and modulate their emotions in the face of a crisis. Consider the expectant parents who have wallpapered and equipped a nursery, in preparation for bringing their newborn home. When the infant dies in the hospital, it takes a period of time until they are emotionally ready to dismantle the room and donate the gifts from the baby shower. In effect, they are regulating their affect and emotions by controlling their environment and exposure to stressful activities.

Emotional discharge involves a release of feelings, which may take the form of crying, yelling, joking, overeating, drinking, or other behaviors. Consider 12-year-old Gregory, who suddenly became unruly in school and then started skipping it altogether. He had remained silent for years about the neglect he felt while his parents devoted all their time and attention to his sister with cystic fibrosis.

Resigned acceptance is another part of emotion-focused coping behavior. A person accepts the reality as it is perceived, believing that there is nothing that can change it. This can be a form of surrender. Consider parents who need to remove their 19-year-old son from their home. His refusal to take medication to treat his schizophrenia has resulted in behavior that endangers the safety of the family.

These coping skills may be used individually or in combination. When distress is heightened, people may rely more on emotion-focused behaviors to alter how they perceive the situation (Jean, Paul, & Beatty, 1999). This is not always productive. In clients with multiple sclerosis, for example, depression is correlated with emotion-focused responses (Aikens, Fischer, Namey, & Rudick, 1997; Jean et al., 1999).

It is interesting to note that some generalizations have been drawn regarding how people with specific injuries or illnesses cope with their situations. We just discussed the use of emotional coping by clients with multiple sclerosis. Let us take this one step further. When the Personal Styles Inventory and the Ways of Coping Inventory were used to assess the psychological needs of forty-five people using wheelchairs who participated in a university-based, drop-in physical activity center and outpatient rehabilitation program, people with multiple sclerosis incorporated emotional coping strategies more frequently than those with traumatic brain injury or spinal cord injury (Wheeler et al., 1996). Those with multiple sclerosis also demonstrated introverted, stability-based personality styles. In contrast, people with spinal cord injuries tended to use problem-focused coping strategies and had extroverted and stable personality styles. Those who had sustained traumatic brain injuries had the most limited coping assets of these three groups. The researchers postulated that the individual disease process or condition may have affected a person's ability to adapt and cope with the need to use a wheelchair. The characteristics of the onset and progression of the disease or injury and the premorbid psychological profile may also be mediating factors.

In a medically defined illness, pessimistic health cognitions and heightened anxiety can have adverse psychological consequences on adjustment, including social support systems. In one study, negative thoughts were related to spousal conflict and lower intimate marital attachment in people who had had a heart attack (Waltz, Badura, Pfaff, & Schott, 1988). In contrast, greater intimacy seemed to foster sufficient social support.

Establishing goals and problem-solving strategies to achieve the goals can result in lower psychosocial impairment scores (Elliott, Witty, Herrick, & Hoffman, 1991). The Ways of Coping Checklist—Revised (Vitaliano, Russo, Carr, Maiuro, & Becker, 1985) indicates that there are effective strategies for both problem solving (i.e., developing a plan and implementing it) and finding social support (i.e., networking with others or discussing the circumstances with a person to gather information). Some people thrive on information and problem solving. They feel better when armed with information and knowledge. They are most comfortable when they know what to expect. Others prefer to know little. Health care providers need to carefully assess and respect these two styles.

Not everyone is an active problem solver. Some individuals blame themselves for their own problems, such as the client with critical emphysema who has a long history of smoking. Others exercise "wishful thinking" or denial, like the client who hoped his brain tumor would miraculously disappear. Still other people deny, ignore, or avoid their situation, like a person with high cholesterol, hypertension, and diabetes who continues a sedentary lifestyle and overindulges in high-calorie and high-fat foods.

Because coping strategies do not exist in a vacuum, they interact with other factors. While coping strategies influence therapeutic adjustment, there are issues that first affect coping. For example, in adults with extremity amputations, age as well as the cause and site of the amputation influence their coping responses, which, in turn, influence their adjustment to wearing prostheses (Gallagher & MacLachlan, 1999). In addition, those with more effective coping responses report less phantom limb pain (Pucher, Kickinger, & Frischenschlager, 1999).

Coping behavior is a key element in how people adjust to the changes in their lives and how they regard these changes. Interestingly, some middle-age people with acquired hearing loss perceive their hearing "impairment" as a hearing "handicap" (Hallberg & Carlsson, 1991). These researchers point out that active coping strategies concentrate attention on the problems and may enhance the perception of a handicap. Indeed, McKnight (1994) maintains that the medical model focuses on the "injury, disease, deficiency, problem, need, empty half" rather than on the "able, gifted, skilled, capable, and full part of a person" (p. 25). Some people make their "problem" the central focus of their lives, overshadowing everything and everyone else and disturbing their priorities.

Ann Kaiser Stearns (1984) uses the term "cue points" to evaluate one's own grieving process, to assess the ability to cope with life. "The ability to continue one's work, the ability to sustain good friendships and working relations with others at home or at work, the ability to maintain self-care habits, the ability to safeguard oneself from harm, all of these are positive indicators of personal functioning and of the healing process" (p. 135).

# Psychosocial Adaptation Strategies

Although coping behavior helps reduce or eliminate psychological distress, it is only one part of adapting to changed circumstances. To achieve successful adjustment, there are many psychosocial adaptation strategies that can be employed, including stress management, skill acquisition, peer support, occupational accommodations, cognitive reframing, and others (Drench, 2003b).

Adequate information and resources are necessary to manage a condition or illness and are vital to adjustment. It is necessary to obtain essential equipment, counseling, and personnel, such as homemakers, nurses' aides, and friends (Sebring & Moglia, 1987). Emotional and practical support from friends and health professionals are needed for the caregivers, as well as the affected individuals. This kind of support provides respite to family caregivers who need both time for other aspects of their lives and opportunities for venting their feelings and concerns. Refer to Chapter 4 for a discussion of the needs, roles, and responsibilities of families.

Although some people find it essential to "let go" of what they cannot control, adjustment often has an active connotation, something one needs to "do." Susan Nessim survived cancer as a teenager and founded Cancervive, a national support group that addresses challenges of survivorship. She discovered that being cured of cancer did not mean that she was released from its stigma. "There was more to overcoming this disease than surviving the hardships of treatment. Instead, the end of treatment marked the beginning of a new and unexpected challenge: adapting to life after cancer" (Nessim & Ellis, 1991, p. xix).

The need for positive psychosocial adaptation strategies cannot be underestimated. In a study of long-term survivors of bone sarcoma, treated with a limb salvage procedure or initial amputation, positive coping skills enhanced adjustment in clients with limb-sparing versus those with amputations. They had lower scores on measures of psychopathology, depression, and anxiety and higher scores on the coping variable. More of them married after their diagnosis. In contrast, the people with amputations believed they faced more job and social discrimination, were not employed commensurate with their skills and training regarding type of work and salary, and had more distress. Although the people with amputations had greater mobility than those with the limb-salvage procedures, they saw themselves more as "disabled people" versus "people with disabilities" (Christ, Lane, & Marcove, 1995).

Many people equate disability, loss, and dependence with a life that is not worth living. Yet, even clients with a significantly disabling condition, such as amyotrophic lateral sclerosis (ALS), commonly referred to as Lou Gehrig's disease after the legendary baseball player who faced its challenges, can find beneficial adaptation strategies. Health providers need to understand that even catastrophic physical limitations do not necessarily rob clients of their purpose in living and the potential for a high quality of life. Consider Morrie Schwartz, the professor and mentor who guides his former student through one last private discourse on "The Meaning of Life." Every Tuesday, until his death marks graduation day, Morrie holds a private seminar in his home.

ALS is like a lit candle: It melts your nerves and leaves your body a pile of wax. Often, it begins with the legs and works its way up. You lose control of your thigh muscles, so that you cannot support yourself standing. You lose control of your trunk muscles, so that you cannot sit up straight. By the end, if you are still alive, you are breathing through a tube in a hole in your throat, while your soul, perfectly awake, is imprisoned inside a limp husk, perhaps able to blink, or cluck a tongue, like something from a science fiction movie, the man frozen inside his own flesh. *Do I wither up and disappear, or do I make the best of my time left?* he had asked himself. He would not wither. He would not be ashamed of dying. Instead, he would make death his final project, the center point of his days. He could be research. A human textbook. *Study me in my slow and patient demise. Watch what happens to me. Learn with me* (Albom, 1997, pp. 9–10).

## Cognitive Reframing

Reframing, altering the way one perceives fears and concerns, can be beneficial. Some people use meditation, psychotherapy, relaxation techniques, visualization, guided imagery, or prayer. Changing parts of a lifestyle to regain control over parts of life is another form of action, such as through dietary modifications, exercise, or amount or type of work.

It is important to remember that grieving is a requisite step on the loss-to-adjustment continuum. Promoting grief work and adjustment helps prevent maladaptive behavior, instill positive coping strategies, and create windows of growth (Mallinson, 1999). The person first needs to mourn the loss, whether it be of a person or a function of the body. Then, they need to put it into perspective and integrate it into their lives. To be able to integrate a loss, Kushner (1981) suggests that people need to change the questions they are asking. "In the final analysis, the question of why bad things happen to good people translates itself into some very different questions, no longer asking why something happened, but asking how we will respond, what we intend to do now that it has happened" (p. 147).

Young and McNicoll (1998) found that people with ALS use cognitive reappraisal to consider what aspects of their lives they can control and which they cannot. They reframe their situations in a more positive light and work at developing positive attitudes. Instead of being overwhelmed by all the aspects and potential sequelae of their progressive disease, they try to focus on each day's concerns. Seeking mental stimulation challenges their intellect. A sense of humor helps balance the darker side of the picture, including sadness and frustration. Peer support provides valuable insights, as well as practical suggestions. Interpersonal relationships are critically important and include an expanding network of friends, clergy, health providers, and professional homemakers.

In addition, personal insights and growth, or what Young and McNicoll (1998) call the development of wisdom, can occur. Some people in their study reported that ALS was a positive force in their lives: "One of the biggest blessings I've had in my life has been this illness in that it got me off the track I was on and started me on a different journey which zigzagged for awhile but basically allowed me to find out who I am" (p. 40).

## MEANING OF LIFE

Along the loss–grief–adjustment continuum, people frequently redefine the meaning of their illness, disability, and life. "Being better" means different things to different people. It could indicate an improvement or resolution of the disorder, an adjustment to working around the condition, or an adaptation to living with the problem. In their research of the meaning of recovery in twenty-four people with work-related musculoskeletal disorders of the upper extremity, Beaton, Tarasuk, Katz, Wright, and Bombardier (2001) called this "resolution, readjustment, and redefinition." They found that the concept of "getting better" was influenced by people's perceptions of how justifiable the disorder was, their definition of health and illness, and their coping styles. In short, while individuals' physical conditions (i.e., symptoms, impairments, or function) may not improve, they may consider themselves "better" (Drench, 2003b).

Furthermore, clients may seek meaning in death (Yedidia & MacGregor, 2001) or redefine the meaning of life amidst a new set of circumstances. In a study of ten women newly diagnosed with breast cancer, awareness of the meaning of existential issues was a central phenomenon. These existential issues included varying levels of life expectations, battling against death, life related to future outlook, religious beliefs and doubts, and an enhanced understanding of values in life. A core finding resulting from this research was the significance of the will to live. The investigators suggest that if health professionals increase their awareness of existential issues linked to the will to live, they can better help women and their families cope (Landmark, Strandmark, & Wahl, 2001).

The personal crisis and interruption of work that results from having a life-threatening illness may also endanger an individual's identity regarding wellness and ability. In a small pilot study of three women diagnosed with breast cancer, the main message was that "doing equals living," demonstrating a powerful connection between meaningful occupation and a perception of oneself as healthy and capable. Remaining active or resuming activities may be the catalyst for people to reconstruct the meaning of life, a process of reclaiming control and a sense of normalcy (Vrkljan & Miller-Polgar, 2001).

In addition to meaningful occupational activities, social integration and coping skills are important to the quality of life in people with physical disabilities (Viemero & Krause, 1998). The theme of social integration is also evident in people adjusting to changes associated with aging. In adults ages 65 to 92 who have higher cognitive functioning, relationships with people were described as both giving meaning to life, as well as being a source of strength. These individuals had begun a new activity postretirement, typically having to do with social interests, which gave their lives a sense of meaning. Having enthusiasm for life and connections with others were associated with meaningfulness (Takkinen & Ruoppila, 2001).

Clients frequently redefine the meanings of disability and life. If their perceptions about disability are negative, their expectations tend to be low, which may keep them apart from the world around them. Schlaff (1993) advocates that people with disabilities need to become supporters of current disability rights. Through these actions, they have the opportunity to gain success, self-reflect, and redefine disability. Health professionals can foster their efforts, which are a form of cognitive reframing and may be a positive psychosocial adaptation strategy.

## Emotional and Practical Support

Impairments, limitations, and disabilities affect both the individual and their significant others. They challenge all types of relationships. Some individuals become stronger in the face of adversity, while others do not endure. Sometimes people closely bond in the short term, but eventually falter. Following a motor vehicle accident caused by a drunk driver, a woman took care of her partner who had sustained a traumatic head injury and multiple fractures. She nursed her partner, was an active participant in her rehabilitation, and stayed by her side, in spite of embarrassing disinhibited behavior. A few years later, the person who was injured returned to work and life activities. Having seen her through the catastrophic times, the caregiver ended the relationship.

Support from families and friends has an important impact on adaptation (Drench, 2003b). Researching older adults with age-related vision loss, Reinhardt (1996) found that close relationships yielded higher outcome scores in life satisfaction and adaptation and lower scores in depressive symptoms when compared to the scores of individuals not having close relationships. Interestingly, there were gender differences, too. The relationships meant greater attachment for the women and more "instrumental assistance and social integration" for the men (p. P268).

Health providers can offer suggestions to clients and caregivers on how to organize their schedules, encourage and accept external support from friends, give voice to their emotions and worries, and prioritize their decision making. They can also encourage counseling for people to express their feelings about their situation, such as issues of progressive loss, dependence on others, and perhaps anticipated death (Drench, 2003b). Formal counseling is not always indicated. Sometimes, providing the opportunity to talk about the changes and losses is sufficient to help people feel less isolated and adjust more successfully (Pound, Gompertz, & Ebrahim, 1998).

Focusing on functional adaptation to a changed physical situation is another part of adjustment. This may involve learning or relearning skills using new strategies, such as eating, dressing, bathing, becoming mobile, or driving a car. Outcomes may include improved physical independence as well as enhanced self-esteem (Drench, 2003b).

Clients and families often feel the loss of professional support once they leave a clinical setting or the health care system. They may have been partners in care for a loved one, only to feel adrift once the individual dies. Perhaps they have completed their own course of treatment or rehabilitation. Some agencies and institutions provide follow-up telephone calls and letters for the immediate period following the loss of this professional support. Unfortunately, this is not a universal practice. A significant benefit of this bridge of communication is that it maintains continuity of care. Sensitive discussion can elicit questions and evaluate adjustment responses (Kaunonen, Aalto, Tarkka, & Paunonen, 2000).

Returning to work, when possible, is another adaptation strategy. Losing one's occupational identity can result in anxiety and depression, but resuming work enhances personal control and instills a sense of normalcy (Peteet, 2000). Clinicians can help clients accommodate to the workplace psychologically, emotionally, and physically.

## Counseling

I can't seem to get through to Bill, he's just so angry. He's the star quarterback for his high school team, a big man on campus. At least he was until the thresher accident. He was working on his family's farm, and his right arm got pulled into the grain machine. It tore his arm off above the elbow. I guess if I were him, I'd be angry, too. Even as I sit here and type this, I'm using two hands.
*—From the journal of Walter Johnson, occupational therapy student*

As discussed in Chapter 13, clients and their significant others grieve many kinds of losses. They also experience various responses to their grief, such as sadness, anger, guilt, loss of control, and fear (i.e., of abandonment or pain). Clients often benefit from psychological support from someone who is not part of their primary health care team (Hunter, Robinson, & Neilson, 1993). Counselors, social workers, psychologists, and psychiatrists can help a person address anxieties and fears and guide in the development of constructive coping strategies.

Counseling skills include listening and attending to clients, as well as verbal counseling approaches (Drench, 2003b). Whereas the latter are the purview of specific health disciplines, all health providers play a role in listening and attending to clients. Recognizing what the client needs and wants is part of being effective. Does Mr. Rutkowski need you to listen to his "venting," stay close as he cries, or help him problem solve? If you are unclear about this, you can ask the client.

The purpose of counseling is to enable people to recognize and use their own coping resources. Clients and significant others need the time, opportunity, and permission to grieve (Markus, Murray Parkes, Tomson, & Johnston, 1989). It is often helpful to let them tell what happened and how they feel about it. Health providers can encourage clients to talk about their memories, concerns, and fears. This also places the situation in a very real context. Acknowledging the fears can be a precursor to dealing with them. In addition, "rehabilitation must aim to restore patients' confidence in their bodies. This will not take place if everyone around continues to treat them as if they are made of Dresden china" (Markus et al., 1989, p. 306).

It is important to heed the impact of what you say. Although constructive feedback can be helpful for clients, criticism is not. Consider Mr. Ettington, a 45-year-old man with myasthenia gravis, who repeatedly comes for his appointments with poor grooming and hygiene. He tells the clinician, "I'm just too tired and weak to wash my hair, or myself for that matter." Responding with, "Do you realize what you look like?" or "You could at least brush your hair" or "Don't you care how you look?" would belittle him and miss the opportunity for a therapeutic moment. Instead, the clinician could open a dialogue by saying, "How does that make you feel?" or "Let's think about ways to make this easier for you."

Another part of a healthy, helping relationship is having and demonstrating patience. Consider the 55-year-old woman with a possible diagnosis of bilateral thoracic outlet syndrome complicated by carpal tunnel syndrome in the right wrist and hand. When she tells the doctor that she is depressed by several months of numbness, tingling, and burning in both hands, plus loss of function, he tells her, "That's not my department. I really don't know what to say or who to send you to. I still have the card of a psychiatrist in the file. I could check that." He appeared flustered and impatient with that aspect of the conversation. The client began to cry. He might have responded, "This must be difficult for you to deal with" or "You sound frustrated by the amount of time it's taking to notice an improvement." These types of statements show effective listening, therapeutic responses, and seek to draw out the client. They also enhance the relationship between health care provider and client.

Health care providers facilitate a person's autonomy by helping people express their feelings, educating and supporting them, managing the client's environment, and providing interventions, such as counseling and support groups. The nature of their relationship with the client directly affects all of their work (Drench, 2003b). Providing comprehensive care requires integrating psychosocial issues into every aspect of assessment and treatment. Health care students can better learn the elements of this key skill through client presentations, role-playing, videotapes, and using health care providers as role models (Blanchard & Ruckdeschel, 1986).

Grief counseling can help people work through their issues, prevent or mitigate unresolved grief and destructive feelings of anger and guilt, and facilitate personal growth (Borins, 1995). Professionals can help the clients with anticipatory grief, support the scope of emotions, and support or deconstruct denial. These are beneficial aspects in the continuum of loss, grief, and adjustment (Sebring & Moglia, 1987). Professional counseling can address issues that need to be recognized and worked through if adjustment is to occur. Denial can either be confronted or sustained, depending on the need of the client and assessment of the health care provider (Langer, 1994). Anger can forestall the grieving process and may result in maladaptive behavior, illness, and lack of joy in life (Cerney & Buskirk, 1991). It can also release long-repressed feelings and allow the mourner to move forward in life.

Earlier wisdom held that people with mental retardation did not grieve. The contemporary view not only negates this, it also postulates that bereavement counseling be done with both the individuals and their caregivers. Proactive educational methods assist the person with mental retardation to cope with loss in a healthy manner. In addition, caregivers need to be trained to provide the necessary support (Read, 1996).

Chronic sorrow, as discussed in Chapter 13, is a normal response to loss. Health care providers can respond by increasing people's comfort and promoting positive coping strategies to help them deal with their grief (Eakes, Burke, & Hainsworth, 1998). These include interpersonal, emotional, cognitive, and action-oriented strategies. The cognitive and action strategies are similar to problem solving, a positive coping approach that seeks to change a situation or the manner in which it is perceived (Hainsworth, Eakes, & Burke, 1994; Lindgren, 1996). Part of this is identifying the client's emotional needs, both those articulated and those remaining silent (Hainsworth, Eakes, & Burke, 1994). Only then can positive coping strategies be recognized and supported by clinicians.

Early intervention can foster a person's adjustment. The Support Center for Perinatal and Childhood Death, in Illinois, organized a counseling program for families who have experienced miscarriage, stillbirth, fetal anomalies, and therapeutic abortion for genetic or congenital abnormalities (Weiss, Frischer, & Richman, 1989). Counselors nurture a healthy grieving process and inhibit negative or pathological adaptations. This hospital-based support program manages prenatal, intrapartum, and delivery room loss by also providing counseling services to other family members, including surviving siblings, who might otherwise not identify or resolve their grief.

Grieving for the losses caused by injuries and illnesses can create stress in a person's life, hindering adjustment. Managing stress can be a beneficial tool to facilitate adaptation to changed circumstances. These skills empower the individual to manage impairment, disability, and handicap, as illustrated in one stress management program for people with spinal cord injury (Bertino, 1989). This program presented the contributing factors to stress and taught relaxation techniques, resulting in positive outcomes.

## COUNSELING APPROACHES

Different counseling approaches may be indicated. Although these may not be within your scope of practice, a brief discussion can enhance your understanding of their value for the clients with whom you work.

Potential psychological sequelae of spinal cord injury include changes in mood and altered cognitive function, both negatively affecting a person's adjustment (North, 1999). Exciting research indicates that cognitive-behavioral therapy may facilitate adjustment to spinal cord injury and guard against mood disorders (Craig, Hancock, Chang, & Dickson, 1998; Craig, Hancock, & Dickson, 1999; Craig, Hancock, Dickson, & Chang, 1997).

To address the clinical depression and anxiety commonly seen in elderly people who are chronically ill, a cognitive-behavioral psychotherapy approach has been suggested, based on five points: "resolving practical barriers to participation, accepting depression as a separate and reversible problem, limiting excess disability, counteracting the loss of important social roles and autonomy, and challenging the perception of being a 'burden'" (Rybarczyk et al., 1992).

The type of psychological intervention provided depends on the needs of the client and his or her underlying personality, including how it may have been altered by illness. As discussed earlier in this chapter, clients cope with the idea of using wheelchairs in different ways. In one study, people who had spinal cord injuries, with limited mobility, were anxious about attempting something new and profited from verbal encouragement and support from health professionals (Wheeler et al., 1996). Those with multiple sclerosis who exhibited "socially distancing behavior and an analytical questioning attitude" (p. 356) benefited from a cognitive approach that worked to establish trust. Clients with traumatic brain injuries improved their coping in a supportive, structured environment.

As we discussed in Chapters 12 and 13, people with illnesses and injuries may perceive a loss of personal control. To address that issue, an empowerment model of counseling can help clients take charge of their lives and develop strategies to optimize their control (Gray, Doan, & Church, 1990). This empowerment includes getting all the necessary care, strengthening one's voice in decision making, and helping to change attitudes.

As with cognitive reframing, counseling may also include imagery or relaxation therapy. These latter techniques have been helpful in ameliorating the nausea and vomiting side effects of chemotherapy (Blanchard & Ruckdeschel, 1986).

It is suggested that health care providers refer to the body of literature regarding adjustment for specific disciplines and disease processes to further individualize care. Psychotherapists who work with people with multiple sclerosis, for example, note that clients have higher scores on the Symptom Checklist-90—Revised. This information can assist them in distinguishing which clients may have unsatisfactory coping skills (Jean et al., 1999). Then, counseling interventions, including problem-focused strategies and stress management, can be incorporated to enhance self-efficacy.

## Support Groups

Sharing practical information and "success" stories with others are additional rehabilitation and psychosocial strategies. Learning *how* others cope can open a door of reality and pragmatic tips. Knowing *that* others cope can open a world of possibilities. Sometimes dreams seem like unattainable goals. Consider the dynamic, professional sports careers of three legendary, world-class athletes with diabetes—Ty Cobb (baseball), Arthur Ashe (tennis), and Joe Frazier (boxing). In contemporary times, Lance Armstrong competed and won more than one Tour de France bicycle race after his debilitating treatment for testicular cancer. Achievers, such as these athletes, can inspire others. Sometimes what seems impossible begins to sound plausible when information is shared.

The person needs to move through the grief process in order for adjustment to occur. It is difficult work that can be facilitated and eased by the support of others. Communities, agencies, and health facilities have recognized the benefit of peer support and have organized groups by diagnosis, age group, role (i.e., parents, families, children), and other common denominators.

Careful attention needs to be given to group composition. It can be demoralizing for those with early stages of a progressive disease to partner with those in an advanced stage (Sebring & Moglia, 1987). In addition, helpful discussion is promoted when members are on a "level playing field." Many bereavement support groups focus on people whose partners die. However, most of them target older people, who may have grown children and grandchildren. These people do not share some of the issues of younger widows and widowers who may have young children to now parent alone. In addition, it is more common for an older population to have peers who have also had a spouse die (with husbands frequently predeceasing their wives). Because this is less likely with younger people, they often grieve in isolation. Recently, support groups for young widows and widowers have begun to form.

Sometimes people are so entrenched in their own problems that they may initially think that listening to those of others would add to their heartache. However, once exposed, they realize that sharing information and support in a group environment can help them adapt to their own situations (Bracht, Ardal, Bot, & Cheng, 1998). They find that it is helpful to speak with people who have experienced similar losses, learn about anticipated grieving responses, and create adaptive strategies to deal with their circumstances (Drench, 2003b; Goldstein, Alter, & Axelrod, 1996). It is also comforting to be in a place where you feel like you "belong." Often, it is those who are most involved in the group who experience greater positive change over time (Videka-Sherman, 1982).

Generally, these programs are very beneficial in the course of adjustment. In a study of men with noise-induced hearing loss and their wives, there were early and long-lasting positive effects of peer support (Hallberg & Barrenas, 1994). Short-term benefits included feeling supported by talking with others who were experiencing a similar loss. As wives became more aware of the effects of the hearing impairment, they better understood the problems associated with the hearing disability. There was also a diminution of perceived handicap.

Special issues can arise in group work. Losing a group member through death is a sensitive matter that may have positive growth outcomes (Badger & Knott, 1993). It can also be devastating to face one's own vulnerability. This can be an opportunity to communally grieve a "family" member, in a safe, supported environment, and accept the reality of mortality.

Arrangements can be made for special needs. As discussed in Chapter 4, support groups for clients and family caregivers can meet simultaneously, when everyone is available. Another example of a special arrangement is a bereavement support group program for children who experience the loss of a family member from cancer. The intervention promotes communication about grief and healing, as well as family communication (Mulcahey & Young, 1995). These support groups can also provide a bridge of care between an outpatient cancer care program and a community-based home care agency.

Continuity of care is an important issue. Because individual or group bereavement care aids significant others in dealing with their feelings and lessens their risk of maladaptive grief responses, some settings, such as outpatient cancer centers, have established psychoeducational groups to lend support and provide information (Goldstein, Alter, & Axelrod, 1996). Family support groups help people survive their losses and move on (Amato, 1991).

There are different kinds of psychoeducational group intervention programs that provide support and information. Although there are varying methodologies, they all generally work to optimize adaptive strategies (Brown, Krief, & Belluck, 1995). Groups at the Support Center for Perinatal and Childhood Death, mentioned earlier in this chapter, address perinatal loss, possible subsequent pregnancies, and the unique needs of prenatal decision making to terminate a pregnancy compromised by genetic or congenital abnormalities (Weiss et al., 1989). Another pregnancy can stir the memories of earlier loss, and parents benefit from working with peers and professionals to separate the two events, celebrating a healthy newborn child and reframing the previous child as a memory.

There are other therapeutic approaches used in the group setting. One approach uses expressive art therapy, which allows participants to express their feelings and reflect on their self-perceptions (Ferszt, Heineman, Ferszt, & Romano, 1998). Another employs music therapy, using precomposed music that has importance to the client following a loss (Bright, 1999). The music serves as an additional tool, used in conjunction with verbal processing. Still another approach uses literary resources for adaptation. The premise is that since healing incorporates storytelling of one's experiences, literature can enable the process (Bowman, 1999). Hippocrates, the father of the oath taken by physicians committing themselves to their clients, had asserted, "Healing is a matter of time, but it is sometimes also a matter of opportunity."

## Bereavement Services

Memorial services are one form of ritual that provide the opportunity to publicly remember the person and share the experience. They can also help staff members. One psychiatric liaison nurse coordinated hospital memorial services for each client who died on her unit. She invited the hospital chaplain to officiate and attended every service.

> A big part of my job is dealing with the nursing staff. I need to be a role model for them by attending the memorial services and trying to deal with feelings on work time. Many people here do go to funerals, which concerns me. Some people make AIDS their life and go to the funeral of every client who dies on this unit. It's not healthy. By taking a leadership role in organizing on-the-job memorial services, I'm taking care of business (Drench, 1998, p. 167).

While these bereavement services may occur in some clinical settings, they are uncommon in acute care settings. In unfamiliar surroundings, significant others of clients in acute care may receive informally given aid, but there is often no structured service or follow-up. Health providers who are particularly versed in psychosocial needs (i.e., social workers, psychiatrists, psychologists, nurses, and pastoral counselors) may want to consider bereavement services or provide assessments and referrals for those grieving from sudden loss (Fauri, Ettner, & Kovacs, 2000). This support can provide an early step in tending to the emotional distress and resolution of grief for the survivors.

## Hope

"Hope is the ability to invest our energy and vision in a reality beyond our sight in the present moment, the capacity to yearn for and expect a meaning deeper and an outcome better than the circumstances seem to allow" (Phillips, 1989, p. 31). Although it has a variable impact on despair, somatization, loss of control, and social isolation, hope is not predictive of the anxiety people experience in the face of death (Chapman & Pepler, 1998; Elliott et al., 1991).

Hope plays a central role in healing. Establishing and maintaining hope can be critically important in the adjustment process (Sebring & Moglia, 1987) and is a key role of the health provider (Kim, 1989; Sussman, 1995). However, it is important to provide realistic hope rather than offer false promises. When Mrs. Williams asks if her 3-year-old son, who has lead poisoning from ingesting paint chips in their apartment, will ever be normal again, the clinician has a myriad of possible responses. Rather than tell her, "He'll probably show improvement soon and be okay," the clinician can respond, "We have a lot of work to do together."

Fostering hope begins with the development of an open, trusting, forthright relationship with the client (and family) (Kim, 1989). Recall the elements of effective communication discussed in Chapter 2 (i.e., active listening and conveying a sense of genuine caring) and relationship-building strategies discussed in Chapter 5. The second step in promoting hope is analyzing the client's (and family's) ability to accomplish the tasks of hoping.

Mr. Klements, now 83 years old, had been a world-class athlete and marathon runner who had competed in the Olympics. Although he never won a medal, he was quite proud of his accomplishments and took great satisfaction in showing pictures and sharing stories.

As he got older, he competed in "masters" marathons for many years and did well. Over time, his hip began to bother him and he had to give up running in marathons. However, he continued to compete in shorter 10K competitions for many years. Now recovering from a total hip arthroplasty, he can only walk about 20 feet, using crutches, before having to stop and rest. Surprisingly, he is in great spirits.

He continues to be hopeful that he will progress without difficulty and be able to do "light running" again. He has been setting goals for himself. The first day, he could only transfer from the bed to the chair. By the following day, he could walk as far as the bathroom in his room. Now, he can walk to the lounge on the ward. He hopes, and therefore plans, to be able to complete one, then two, and finally three laps around the ward.

*—From the journal of Anne Marie Geiger, nursing student*

In a seminal study on the process and tasks of hoping (Wright & Shontz, 1968), four cognitive-affective tasks were identified: reality surveillance, encouragement, worry, and mourning. Reality surveillance is a cognitive function that integrates hope with reality, as it is perceived by the individual. Adults need to base their hopes in reality. Conversely, because children rely on adults to be responsible for their welfare, they can verbalize hopes without considering the reality and possibility of future outcomes.

Health care providers can assist clients in evaluating their fact-based reality (Kim, 1989). Through this role, they can acknowledge and confirm that the facts the person believes are indeed realistic (Drench, 2003b). Table 14–2 presents examples of helping clients with fact-based reality.

Whereas reality surveillance, the first task of hoping, is a cognitive function, the other three tasks—encouragement, worry, and mourning—are affective (Wright & Shontz, 1968). Reality surveillance checks and tests reality to see if the hopes are possible. Encouragement is the feeling side of reality surveillance. It helps people know that they do have a basis for hope and, therefore, it is both motivating and comforting. In contrast, worry works in tandem with the cognitive process when it is uncertain. The client takes another look at the perceived reality. The fourth task of hoping, mourning, is accomplished when a hope has to be abandoned. It is a necessary step if the person is going to be able to reevaluate the situation and develop other hopes to replace the one that had to be surrendered.

**TABLE 14–2**   How Health Providers Help Clients with Fact-Based Reality

- Validate or shed accurate light on the patient's/client's beliefs—"I thought that if I could get into that special Eye and Ear Clinic, my macular degeneration could be cured, and I'd see again."
- Guide the patients/clients in assessing their physical, emotional, and interpersonal strengths and weaknesses—"I can no longer use my hands to paint, but I could try mouth-painting."
- Help them make accurate comparisons to complete the evaluation of their assets—"I thought I was the worst one off here, until I met Joe."
- Help the patient/client perceive the positive growth opportunities from the situation—"It's funny to think of this accident as a good thing in my life, but I've slowed down, learned to listen more, and feel good hugging my kids."
- Seek verification of statements with the patient/client—"Your shoulder motion is still very limited. Have you been working with the home exercise program as much as you need to? I want to stress to you why it is so important."
- Equip patients/clients with accurate information and reassure them while they face their challenges and take responsibility for themselves—"I can't bury my head in the sand any longer. I'm ready for the biopsy."
- Practice empathetic communication while helping people face what may lie ahead—"We'll certainly keep working to maintain the strength of Mark's muscles, but with your son's type of muscular dystrophy, we also need to consider other ways to help him be mobile."
- Help the patient/client be optimistic and yet realistic—"Your wound is looking better. With your diabetes, though, we need to continue our close monitoring and dressing changes."
- Provide current information and indicate that newer treatments may be developed—"There are clinical trials being researched, using a combination of newer antiviral medications."
- Help sustain hope by professing its value—"There are no guarantees of what tomorrow will bring. Nothing is written in stone."

*(Adapted from Kim, 1989)*

# Implications for Health Care Providers

Health professionals need to understand the psychosocial impact that illness and injury have on individuals and their significant others. For example, in Leo Tolstoy's classic story of Ivan Ilych (1886/1971), the "client" is alone in dealing with his dying, in the face of his family's code of silence. Instead of discussing death or providing him the opportunity to express himself and confront his mortality, they pretend that Ivan is not dying. Health care providers may also abandon the client to face death or loss alone (Harper, 1977). Their code of silence may even be disguised by meaningless chatter and averted eyes.

People tend to use euphemisms for death, as discussed in Chapter 13, and try to "cheer up" the grieving individual. They steer the conversation away from death and loss or use platitudes, such as "God wanted her by His side," "He lived a full life," and "It's better this way. He's out of pain." This creates a barrier between the professional and the person who is grieving.

People often do not know what to say or are uncomfortable or fearful of sickness and death, so they say nothing or offer meaningless, though well-intended, remarks, such as "I know what you're going through." Since each experience of loss and grief is unique, and the meaning of the loss distinct, no one can really know what another person is feeling. Health care providers are no exception. We process all of our similar personal and professional experiences and offer consolation, but we really cannot understand what another person is feeling at the deepest level.

We may avoid people who are grieving because we are at a loss of what to say or are embarrassed or uncomfortable by their open display of emotions. Perhaps we find ourselves changing the subject or "selling" the idea that keeping busy is the answer to moving through grief and adjustment. It is no wonder that grieving people often try to conceal their emotions or isolate themselves (Cable, 1998). We can acknowledge a loss, show concern, and perhaps open a dialogue by saying, "This must be a difficult time for you. Do you want to talk?" or "How are you doing?"

Just as we try to cheer people, we also attempt to relieve their guilt by offering comfort through trite remarks such as "No one could have been a more dutiful husband. You did everything for her." Feelings of guilt can be a natural part of the grieving process, as discussed in Chapter 13. Health care providers have a role to support bereaved people rather than mitigate their feelings. It is more therapeutic for their adjustment for us to recall the helpful things they did and the attention they gave. As much as we might want to ease their pain, we cannot do the grief work for them.

Clients grieve and adapt in their own manner and time. The intensity of the grief response is often influenced by the significance of the loss to them. Health professionals need to assess how clients perceive the body function, parts, or other issues that are involved in the primary loss, as well as secondary losses (see Chapter 12) (Drench, 2003b). A speech-language pathologist is working with an 8-year-old boy with muscular dystrophy on a swallowing disorder. He had already lost mobility and independence in activities of daily living (primary losses), which restricted his freedom (secondary loss). The swallowing disorder (primary loss) has an impact in his attendance in school and anticipated summer camp experience (secondary losses).

These assessments of loss and its meaning assist health care providers in understanding the client's behavior, which may be attributed to a grief response, such as anger, denial, or despair (Drench, 2003b). This may also cast light on the apparent nonadherence discussed in Chapter 6. Is a client not adherent with treatment because of a lack of future orientation—"I may not improve anyway, so what's the use?" or "I'm not going to live long enough to have this matter." It is important for health care providers to be aware of these issues and work with them within the scope of one's professional boundaries. Consider how an occupational therapist can help a client relate the components of the treatment to activities needed at home or in the workplace, associating treatment with adaptation and adjustment.

We often see clients and families when they are grieving, when their coping behavior and dynamics are sorely challenged. Yet, we label them as "noncompliant" or as "problems" and expect them to work, progress, and follow our wisdom, in short, "get with it." It is critical that we examine our own motivation, patience, and our understanding of the situation. If our tunnel vision only focuses on a specific piece of the puzzle, overlooking the cognitive and affective dimensions of care, we are not providing the most comprehensive care possible.

## Tasks of Mourning

In Chapter 13, we highlighted Worden's (2002) conceptualization of four tasks of mourning, which all need to be achieved to complete the grieving process. There is a role for health professionals to facilitate adjustment each step of the way. In the first task, the person needs to *accept the reality of the loss.* This is more difficult if the loss is unanticipated, such as a sudden amputation of an arm by a grain machine or an unexpected death of a teenager on a basketball court.

People often avoid seeing or touching someone who has died, yet it can be therapeutic to do so. Facing reality often facilitates adjustment. It is also one way to feel closeness and say goodbye. Consider the woman whose baby died *in utero* during the ninth month of pregnancy. After the baby was delivered, the nurses arranged a secluded room so that the parents had the opportunity to hold their son and spend private time with him. They also named him, reinforcing his individuality and connecting with him on a very personal level. At that moment, the parents were able to begin their grief work.

As these nurses illustrated, health care providers can encourage these types of opportunities. People who do not physically face the reality, either at the time of death or later, often have greater difficulty with their grief (Cable, 1998). Seeing the body is one way to begin accepting the reality of the loss. This is especially useful if the death has been sudden and unexpected. Another way to help people accept the reality of the loss is to use plain and direct language, such as "died" or "dead." Using euphemisms may reinforce denial or foster confusion. Consider the 4-year-old girl who was told that she had "lost" her grandfather. She searched the house and yard trying to find him. Over the ensuing weeks, she looked for him everywhere she went.

In Worden's (2002) second task of mourning, the grieving person needs to *experience the pain associated with grief.* The person may be unable to participate in his or her normal patterns of activity. There may be considerable preoccupation with what has been lost. As discussed in Chapter 13, there may be intense feelings such as anger or guilt. In a situation of death, those remaining may feel like they have no purpose in life. Disaster survivors may feel that part of them is gone, such as when a hurricane or tornado demolishes their neighborhood. If the individual is part of a society that does not encourage people to express their feelings and emotions around the loss, there may be a temptation to lightly touch upon or even skip this mourning task. Although initial brief denial can comfort and shield the person, avoiding the pain can later be manifested in depression or other psychiatric problems.

Assisting with grief work and adjustment, health care providers can encourage sharing of memories of who or what once was. They can support outward expressions of grief, such as crying or yelling, as a healthy, warranted response to the loss. It is important to be aware that confronting the pain associated with grief can take many forms. Consider the siblings whose idea it was to "play funeral" with their 6-year-old brother who was dying of leukemia. The children gave the role of funeral director to their social worker. She was able to honestly answer their questions and let them express their feelings in a safe environment. By dealing with their grief in the "here and now," they will be less likely to have adjustment problems later. Compare this example to a home where little if anything is said about dying, and the children use their imagination in place of real information. This can be far more scary.

Worden's (2002) third task of mourning is *adjusting to circumstances created by the loss.* This could mean adjusting to life without a right arm or assuming roles in life that were once fulfilled by the person who died. Health care providers can encourage this adjustment at a pace that is comfortable for the individual. Their role also includes nurturing the people, fortifying their strength, and reinforcing positive growth. A new sense of self, including one's perceived worth and esteem, may be a healthy by-product of this task.

The fourth task of mourning in this model is *emotionally relocating the deceased and progressing with life.* Relocating does not connote erasing the person and the corresponding memories from one's life. Rather, it means giving those memories a different emotional role so that the individual may resume life's activities, that is, to go on despite the loss. In a study of the relationship of continuing attachment and adjustment, bereaved spouses used mock interviews plus role-play with their dead spouses (Field, Nichols, Holen, & Horowitz, 1999). Those who used their spouse's possessions for comfort revealed distress, which was predictive of grief symptoms that did not significantly diminish over time. However, continuing attachment through tender memories was associated with less distress. The form of the attachment can influence the effectiveness of an adaptation strategy. Health professionals can encourage people to express their memories rather than forget them.

## Helping Clients Adjust

Health care providers need to assist clients with processing their grief. This help can include discussing grief, being supportive, and arranging resources, such as grief counseling (Drench, 2003b). Acknowledging the values and preferences of clients and families, clear communication, and shared decision making are also elements of quality therapeutic intervention to ease adjustment (Alaszewski, Alaszewski, & Potter, 2004; Steinhauser et al., 2000). It also entails being alert to changes in clients. Since grief and depression may appear similar, it is important to recognize the differences or make referrals to those who can identify problems. For example, someone who is grieving generally does not have an altered self-esteem, but someone with depression may.

Mood disorders or pathological signs of grief, such as suicidal ideation, are also red flags of warning for all health care providers to recognize and act upon. If acute grief reactions are present after several months, there may be major depression, which can require psychiatric treatment (Krigger, McNeely, & Lippmann, 1997). Untreated depression in people following cerebrovascular accidents impairs functional recovery (Hermann, Black, Lawrence,

Szekely, & Szalai, 1998) and is predictive of an increased risk of death in the acute stage of recovery from strokes (Morris, Robinson, Andrzejewski, Samuels, & Price, 1993).

Social support for the grieving person entails practical assistance, as well as comfort and empathy. It is empathy that allows people to share and understand the meaning of the inner thoughts and feelings of others. A key concept is "sharing." In the empathetic experience, a person *shares* the thoughts and feelings while maintaining a professional distance, not becoming so involved in the other's world that one gets lost in it. Although this facilitates adjustment, many professionals do not know how to therapeutically use empathy or are uncomfortable with the concept. Through their caring and empathetic presence, health care providers can help people regain control of their lives (Eakes, 1993; Hainsworth, 1994). Sometimes just being present in silence is sufficiently beneficial and may be more important than trying to think of the "right" thing to say.

Grieving can be exceptionally difficult when there is a definite loss, but the individuals have the opportunity to deal with its finality and the meaning of the void in their lives. However, when the loss is "ambiguous," such as that experienced with dementia and terminal illness, people need to "let go" at the same time they are trying to maintain a connection.

Because dementia manifests in many losses *during* life, family caregivers have a long process of repeatedly grieving. *If* they are ever going to be able to conclude their grieving and progress with their own lives, it can only be done after the person with dementia dies (Liken & Collins, 1993). Health care providers can assist significant others by their empathetic "presence" and coaching, which encourage people to express their feelings and perceptions and collaborate in problem solving (Cutillo-Schmitter, 1996). This in turn helps them identify and manage personal, client, and other family issues. They "provide hope that a disease can be managed by making the unfamiliar familiar" (p. 32).

Health professionals need to provide support, coping strategies, and information. They can recognize the clients' concerns, feelings, and fears, such as those of recurrence of disease, disfigurement, disability (see Table 13–1 for others), and foster conversations to bring these issues to the surface (Drench, 2003b; Sussman, 1995). They can also teach clients and families about their conditions and recovery and help them understand current and potential future emotions and responses (Drench, 2003b; Svedlund & Axelsson, 2000). If there is impending death, health professionals can also assist the family through anticipatory grief, resolving unfinished matters, and "letting go" (Krohn, 1998). Part of the health care providers' role is to "transform desolation into consolation" (Soderberg, Gilje, & Norberg, 1999).

Health care providers employ varying strategies to help their clients adjust to the changes in their lives. Some health practitioners endorse confronting clients with spinal cord injury with the consequences of their injury in stages (Trieschmann, 1988). Others support the research that indicates that people with spinal cord injury, as well as those without injuries, rely on optimism to protect themselves from monumental stress (Frank et al., 1987; Taylor, 1983). While it is important to be honest, it is wise to regard how much truth clients are ready to hear (Drench, 2003b). Consider the physician who sat and discussed the following day's treatment with his client, knowing that the man was probably going to die within a few hours. He was responding to what he believed the client wanted or needed to cope with his situation.

Still other health professionals promote a melded approach, accepting wishful thinking or unrealistic optimism as a possible adjustment strategy, only if combined with problem-focused coping and getting support or information from other people (Moore & Patterson, 1993). Film director and actor Christopher Reeve had an equestrian accident that resulted in a high-level cervical spinal cord injury with dependence on a ventilator. While he maintained that he would walk again, he was active in rehabilitation to be able to breathe more independently, be mobile in an electric wheelchair, and improve or maintain the condition of his muscles. This mixed strategy leads to adaptation, whereas unrealistic optimism alone, without action, would not be adaptive (Moore, Bombardier, Brown, & Patterson, 1994). The intervention of health care providers is critically important. Even with beneficial changes in people with spinal cord injury, there may be a reduced level of well-being over the long term (Krause, 1997).

The individualized interventions of health care providers can positively influence the physical, mental, and emotional health and adjustment of others (Lev & McCorkle, 1998; White & Grenyer, 1999). Nursing interventions for women with breast cancer have reduced the perceived severity of the disease so that the women can more successfully adjust and enhance their quality of life (Longman, Braden, & Mishel, 1999).

Individualized interventions may sometimes be unorthodox, but they can have a significant impact on the well-being of the client. One client with terminal cancer knitted sweaters for her two children to remind them of her love after she died. Another debilitated client could not eat very much, except for grilled-cheese sandwiches. The nurses began to cancel some of his food trays and prepare several grilled-cheese sandwiches for him during each shift as part of their care plan (Drench, 1998). At times, although the therapeutic opportunity may be missed, the lesson can still be learned, as in the case of a nurse who was caring for a dying woman.

> She had a little girl whom she hadn't been able to spend much time with. I went in one day and she said, "My little girl, I wanted to make her a Cinderella." I knew right away that she wanted to buy her a party dress and dress her all up. She was feeling really bad that she hadn't. It was too late, and it didn't happen. The next time there was a woman here and a child involved, I made sure that things like that happened (Drench, 1998, p. 136).

Certain health concerns require significant changes in lifestyle, and health care providers can work with clients and families to improve adaptation and quality of life. For example, nurses, therapists, social workers, and vocational rehabilitation counselors can work together to emphasize goals, mood, and finance with people with spinal cord injuries (Dunnum, 1990). These efforts target financial resources, create realistic goal-setting congruent with physical ability, and provide referrals, including to counseling or support groups. Thoughtful listening to problems, concerns, and feelings by health care providers and support groups may also improve client's affect.

Emotional rollercoasters do not elude health care providers, especially those working with frequent losses. Although there may be a temptation to share problems with clients, this adds to their burdens and is not client-centered care. Consider when Mr. Russo said, "Are you okay? You look run down." The clinician responded, "I've picked up this cold that's going around. Because so many staff members are out sick, we're covering their patients, too." A different message might have been delivered if the response had been, "I have a cold, but I'm fine for your treatment today."

Similar to clients and their families, health care providers can also benefit from support groups to weather the emotional toll of professional losses and prevent burnout (Amato, 1991). A designated liaison can be helpful to the staff, such as a psychiatric nurse (Drench, 1998) or psychiatrist. This consultant can meet weekly with staff groups to discuss and clarify psychological issues that are inherent in working with certain client populations. In addition, the psychiatric consultant can attend client care meetings and advise staff members on the functional and organic psychiatric problems of clients, such as depression (Shanfield, 1983).

## SUMMARY

This chapter addressed the third part of the loss–grief–adjustment continuum, highlighting coping behavior, psychosocial adaptation strategies, and the implications for health care providers.

To cope with the stresses of an illness, some people use strategies that are appraisal-focused, problem-focused, emotion-focused, or a combination of these approaches. These strategies are key elements in how people adjust to the changes in their lives and are influenced by many factors.

The need for positive psychosocial adaptation strategies cannot be underestimated. These strategies incorporate counseling, health care personnel, and emotional and practical support for the caregivers, as well as the affected individuals. Some of the other adaptation strategies discussed include sharing practical information, returning to work or other life activities, bereavement services, stress management, support groups, and hope.

Listening actively and compassionately, inviting feelings to be expressed, and facilitating an understanding of the situation are parts of the helping relationship. Encouraging individual expressions of grief and honoring culturally appropriate rituals are also vitally important.

In addition, health care providers assist the person in accepting a new reality, finding relevant coping strategies, connecting with a support system, and following through with the identified ways to cope (Hoff, 1989).

Health care providers can offer information and education to clients and caregivers and help them articulate their emotions and worries. This includes discussing grief, remaining supportive, arranging resources, and being alert to changes in the clients. In addition to providing practical assistance, it helps to establish empathetic presence and comfort. We explored strategies for health care providers to facilitate adaptation, emphasizing that their interventions can positively influence the physical, mental, and emotional health and adjustment of others. By helping people express their feelings, educating and supporting clients, and adapting the client's environment, health care providers facilitate a person's autonomy and clarify positive indicators of the healing process.

## REFLECTIVE QUESTIONS

1. As a response to illness or injury, what adaptations and adjustments would be most difficult for you to make?
2. Everyone needs support to cope with losses.
   a. What kind of supportive responses might *you* find most helpful?
   b. What kind of supportive responses might *you* find least helpful?
3. a. How can you determine what types of support to offer to clients?
   b. What kind of feedback could you use to determine if you are being effective?
4. In this chapter, we discussed being "present in silence" as a demonstration of empathy. Describe a situation when this might be beneficial.
5. When working with a terminally ill client, how can you communicate realistic expectations while maintaining the client's hope?

# CASE STUDY

Note: Because loss, grief, and adjustment are presented on a continuum as a process rather than finite stages in time, there is only one Case Study in Part IV to reflect this. It is, however, told in parts, each with its own set of questions that pertain to the information in the particular chapter. It is suggested that you begin by reading the previous two sections about Cynthia Osbourne before proceeding.

Six weeks after entering the rehabilitation hospital, Cynthia returned to her own state, to the home of her parents. She's struggling to reclaim her life. No longer able to bicycle or play pickup basketball with the children, her vision is sufficiently improving, enabling her to resume reading, another area of enjoyment for her.

She is hopeful that recent surgery on her hands will enable her to return to work as a ward secretary at a hospital. The therapists are assisting Cynthia in identifying strategies and resources that will help her overcome her difficulties. As much as she would like to return to her "old self," her physicians have told her "to forget that person," a thought that she rejects. She rejoices at small improvements in walking, although she is beginning to accept that things will never be "perfect." She is also hopeful that she may be able to do more in the future. In the meantime, her low endurance and limited flexibility remain factors, and she continues to descend stairs in a backwards position. Every time she plays with her children, doing what she is able, she rejoices in her small pleasures.

1. What factors might be contributing to how Cynthia is coping with her situation?
2. Discuss in what ways Cynthia is using or has used appraisal-focused, problem-focused, and/or emotion-focused coping behavior.
3. a. Discuss psychosocial adaptation strategies that Cynthia employed and their effect on her.
   b. Identify other possible psychosocial adaptation strategies that you believe would have been or still might be useful to Cynthia and provide a rationale for your beliefs.
4. a. What role is hope playing in Cynthia's life?
   b. How might the therapeutic team members help Cynthia be realistic yet hopeful?

# REFERENCES

Aikens, J. E., Fischer, J. S., Namey, M., & Rudick, R. A. (1997). A replicated prospective investigation of life stress, coping, and depressive symptoms in multiple sclerosis. *Journal of Behavioral Medicine, 20*(5), 433–445.

Alaszewski, A., Alaszewski, H., & Potter, J. (2004). The bereavement model, stroke and rehabilitation: A critical analysis of the use of a psychological model in professional practice. *Disability Rehabilitation, 26* (18), 1067–1078.

Albom, M. (1997). *Tuesdays with Morrie.* New York: Doubleday.

Amato, C. A. (1991). Malignant glioma: Coping with a devastating illness. *Journal of Neuroscience Nursing, 23*(1), 20–22.

Badger, J. M., & Knott, J. E. (1993). Death of a support group member: A practical guide to helping other members cope. *Journal of Cardiovascular Nursing, 7*(3), 63–72.

Beaton, D. E., Tarasuk, V., Katz, J. N., Wright, J. G., & Bombardier, C. (2001). "Are you better?" A qualitative study of the meaning of recovery. *Arthritis and Rheumatology, 45*(3), 270–279.

Bertino, L. S. (1989). Stress management with SCI clients. *Rehabilitation Nursing, 14*(3), 127–129.

Blanchard, C. G., & Ruckdeschel, J. C. (1986). Psychosocial aspects of cancer in adults: Implications for teaching medical students. *Journal of Cancer Education, 1*(4), 237–248.

Borins, M. (1995). Grief counseling. *Canadian Family Physician, 41,* 1207–1211.

Bowman, T. (1999). Literary resources for bereavement. *Hospital Journal, 14*(1), 39–54.

Bracht, M., Ardal, F., Bot, A., & Cheng, C. M. (1998). Initiation and maintenance of a hospital-based parent group for parents of premature infants: Key factors for success. *Neonatal Network, 17*(3), 33–37.

Bright, R. (1999). Music therapy in grief resolution. *Bulletin of the Menninger Clinic, 63*(4), 481–498.

Brown, D. G., Krief, K., & Belluck, F. (1995). A model for group intervention with the chronically ill: Cystic fibrosis and the family. *Social Work in Health Care, 21*(1), 81–94.

Cable, D. G. (1998). Grief in the American culture. In K. Doka & J. Davidson (Eds.), *Living with grief: Who we are, how we grieve* (pp. 61–71). Philadelphia: Hospice Foundation of America.

Cerney, M. S., & Buskirk, J. R. (1991). Anger: The hidden part of grief. *Bulletin of the Menninger Clinic, 55*(2), 228–237.

Chapman, K. J., & Pepler, C. (1998). Coping, hope, and anticipatory grief in family members in palliative home care. *Cancer Nursing, 21*(4), 226–234.

Christ, G. H., Lane, J. M., & Marcove, R. (1995). Psychosocial adaptation of long-term survivors of bone sarcoma. *Journal of Psychosocial Oncology, 13*(4), 1–21.

Craig, A. R., Hancock, K., Chang, E., & Dickson, H. (1998). Immunizing against depression and anxiety after spinal cord injury. *Archives of Physical Medicine and Rehabilitation, 79,* 375–377.

Craig, A. R., Hancock, K., & Dickson, H. (1999). Improving the long-term adjustment of spinal cord-injured persons. *Spinal Cord, 37,* 345–350.

Craig, A. R., Hancock, K., Dickson, H., & Chang, E. (1997). Long-term psychological outcomes in spinal cord-injured persons: Results of a controlled trial using cognitive behavior therapy. *Archives of Physical Medicine and Rehabilitation, 78,* 33–38.

Cutillo-Schmitter, T. A. (1996). Managing ambiguous loss in dementia and terminal illness. *Journal of Gerontology Nursing, 22*(5), 32–39.

Drench, M. E. (1998). *Red ribbons are not enough: Health caregivers' stories about AIDS.* Wilsonville, OR: BookPartners.

Drench, M. E. (2003a). Loss, grief, and adjustment: A primer for physical therapy, Part I. *PT Magazine, 11* (6), 50–52, 54–61.

Drench, M. E. (2003b). Loss, grief, and adjustment: A primer for physical therapy, Part II. *PT Magazine, 11* (7), 58–70.

Dunnum, L. (1990). Life satisfaction and spinal cord injury: The patient perspective. *Journal of Neuroscience Nursing, 22*(1), 43–46.

Eakes, G. G. (1993). Chronic sorrow: A response to living with cancer. *Oncology Nursing Forum, 20*(9), 1327–1334.

Eakes, G. G., Burke, M. L., & Hainsworth, M. A. (1998). Middle-range theory of chronic sorrow. *Image Journal of Nursing Scholarship, 30*(2), 179–184.

Elliott, T. R., Witty, T. E., Herrick, S., & Hoffman, J. T. (1991). Negotiating reality after physical loss: Hope, depression, and disability. *Journal of Personality and Social Psychology, 61*(4), 608–613.

Fauri, D. P., Ettner, B., & Kovacs, P. J. (2000). Bereavement services in acute care settings. *Death Studies, 24*(1), 51–64.

Ferszt, G. G., Heineman, L., Ferszt, E. J., & Romano, S. (1998). Transformation through grieving: Art and the bereaved. *Holistic Nurse Practitioner, 13*(1), 68–75.

Field, N. P., Nichols, C., Holen, A., & Horowitz, M. J. (1999). The relation of continuing attachment to adjustment in conjugal bereavement. *Journal of Consulting Clinical Psychology, 67*(2), 212–218.

Folkman, S., & Lazarus, R. S. (1986). Stress processes and depressive symptomatology. *Journal of Abnormal Psychology, 95,* 107–113.

Frank, R. G., Umlauf, R. L., Wonderlich, S. A., Askanazi, G. S., Buckelew, S. P., & Elliott, T. R. (1987). Differences in coping styles among persons with spinal cord injury: A cluster-analytic approach. *Journal of Consulting and Clinical Psychology, 55,* 727–731.

Gallagher, P., & MacLachlan, M. (1999). Psychological adjustment and coping in adults with prosthetic limbs. *Behavioral Medicine, 25*(3), 117–124.

Goldstein, J., Alter, C. L., & Axelrod, R. (1996). A psychoeducational bereavement-support group for families provided in an outpatient cancer center. *Journal of Cancer Education, 11*(4), 233–237.

Gray, R. E., Doan, B. D., & Church, K. (1990). Empowerment and persons with cancer: Politics in cancer medicine. *Journal of Palliative Care, 6*(2), 33–45.

Hainsworth, M. A. (1994). Living with multiple sclerosis: The experience of chronic sorrow. *Journal of Neuroscience Nursing, 26*(4), 237–240.

Hainsworth, M. A., Eakes, G. G., & Burke, M. L. (1994). Coping with chronic sorrow. *Issues in Mental Health Nursing, 15*(1), 59–66.

Hallberg, L. R., & Barrenas, M. L. (1994). Group rehabilitation of middle-aged males with noise-induced hearing loss and their spouses: Evaluation of short- and long-term effects. *British Journal of Audiology, 28*(2), 71–79.

Hallberg, L. R., & Carlsson, S. G. (1991). Hearing impairment, coping, and perceived hearing handicap in middle-aged subjects with acquired hearing loss. *British Journal of Audiology, 25*(5), 323–330.

Harper, B. (1977). *Death: The coping mechanism of the health professional.* Greenville, SC: Southeastern University Press.

Hermann, N., Black, S. E., Lawrence, J., Szekely, C., & Szalai, J. P. (1998). The Sunnybrook stroke study: A prospective study of depressive symptoms and functional outcomes. *Stroke, 29,* 618–624.

Hoff, L. A. (1989). *People in crisis: Understanding and helping* (3rd ed.). Redwood City, CA: Addison-Wesley.

Hunter, M. D., Robinson, I. C., & Neilson, S. (1993). The functional and psychological status of patients with amyotrophic lateral sclerosis: Some implications for rehabilitation. *Disability and Rehabilitation, 15*(3), 119–126.

Jean, V. M., Paul, R. H., & Beatty, W. W. (1999). Psychological and neuropsychological predictors of coping patterns by patients with multiple sclerosis. *Journal of Clinical Psychology, 55*(1), 21–26.

Johnson, J. L., & Klein, L. (1988). *I can cope: Staying healthy with cancer.* Minneapolis, MN: DCI Publishing.

Kaunonen, M., Aalto, P., Tarkka, M. T., & Paunonen, M. (2000). Oncology ward nurses' perspectives of family grief and a supportive telephone call after the death of a significant other. *Cancer Nursing, 23*(4), 314–324.

Kim, T. S. (1989). Hope as a mode of coping in amyotrophic lateral sclerosis. *Journal of Neuroscience Nursing, 21*(6), 342–347.

Krause, J. S. (1997). Adjustment after spinal cord injury: A 9 year longitudinal study. *Archives of Physical Medicine and Rehabilitation, 78,* 651–657.

Krigger, K. W., McNeely, J. D., & Lippmann, S. B. (1997). Dying, death, and grief: Helping patients and their families through the process. *Postgraduate Medicine, 101*(3), 263–270.

Krohn, B. (1998). When death is near: Helping families cope. *Geriatric Nursing, 19*(5), 276–278.

Kushner, H. S. (1981). *When bad things happen to good people*. New York: Avon Books.

Landmark, B. T., Strandmark, M., & Wahl, A. K. (2001). Living with newly diagnosed breast cancer: The meaning of existential issues. A qualitative study of 10 women with newly diagnosed breast cancer, based on grounded theory. *Cancer Nursing, 24*(3), 220–226.

Langer, K. G. (1994). Depression and denial in psychotherapy of persons with disabilities. *American Journal of Psychotherapy, 48*(2), 181–194.

Lev, E. L., & McCorkle, R. (1998). Loss, grief, and bereavement in family members of cancer patients. *Seminars in Oncology Nursing, 14*(2), 145–151.

Lewis, K. S. (1998). Emotional adjustment to a chronic illness. *Lippincott's Primary Care Practitioner, 2*(1), 38–51.

Liken, M. A., & Collins, C. E. (1993). Grieving: Facilitating the process for dementia caregivers. *Journal of Psychosocial Nursing and Mental Health Services, 31*(1), 21–26.

Lindgren, C. L. (1996). Chronic sorrow in persons with Parkinson's and their spouses. *Scholarly Inquiry for Nursing Practice, 10*(4), 351–366.

Longman, A. J., Braden, C. J., & Mishel, M. H. (1999). Side effects burden, psychological adjustment, and life quality in women with breast cancer: Pattern of association over time. *Oncology Nursing Forum, 26*(5), 909–915.

Mallinson, R. K. (1999). Grief work of HIV-positive persons and their survivors. *Nursing Clinics of North America, 34*(1), 163–177.

Markus, A. C., Murray Parkes, C., Tomson, P., & Johnston, M. (1989). *Psychological problems in general practice*. Oxford, UK: Oxford University Press.

Maunder, R., & Esplen, M. J. (1999). Facilitating adjustment to inflammatory bowel disease: A model of psychosocial intervention in non-psychiatric patients. *Psychotherapy and Psychosomatics, 68*(5), 230–240.

McKnight, J. (1994). Two tools for well-being: Health systems and communities. *American Journal of Preventive Medicine, 10* (3 Suppl.), 23–26.

Moore, A. D., Bombardier, C. H., Brown, P. B., & Patterson, D. R. (1994). Coping and emotional attributions following spinal cord injury. *International Journal of Rehabilitation Research, 17*, 39–48.

Moore, A. D., & Patterson, D. R. (1993). Psychological intervention with spinal cord-injured patients: Promoting control out of dependence. *SCI Psychosocial Process, 6*, 18–24.

Moos, R., & Billings, A. (1982). Conceptualizing and measuring coping resources and process. In L. Goldberger & S. Breznitz (Eds.), *Handbook of stress: Theoretical and clinical aspects* (pp. 212–230). New York: Macmillan.

Moos, R. H., & Schaefer, J. A. (1986). Life transitions and crises: A conceptual overview. In R. H. Moos (Ed.), *Coping with life crises: An integrated approach* (pp. 3–28). New York: Plenum Press.

Morris, P. L., Robinson, R. G., Andrzejewski, P., Samuels, J., & Price, T. R. (1993). Association of depression with 10-year poststroke mortality. *American Journal of Psychiatry, 150*(1), 124–129.

Mulcahey, A. L., & Young, M. A. (1995). A bereavement support group for children: Fostering communication about grief and healing. *Cancer Practitioner, 3*(3), 150–156.

Nessim, S., & Ellis, J. (1991). *Cancervive: The challenge of life after cancer*. Boston: Houghton Mifflin.

North, N. T. (1999). The psychological effects of spinal cord injury: A review. *Spinal Cord, 37*, 671–679.

Peteet, J. R. (2000). Cancer and the meaning of work. *General Hospital Psychiatry, 22*(3), 200–205.

Phillips, J. (1989). Sustaining our hope. In J. B. Meisenhelder & C. L. LaCharite (Eds.), *Comfort in caring: Nursing the person with HIV infection* (pp. 31–40). Boston: Scott, Foresman.

Pound, P., Gompertz, P., & Ebrahim, S. (1998). A patient-centered study of the consequences of stroke. *Clinical Rehabilitation, 12*(4), 338–347.

Pucher, I., Kickinger, W., & Frischenschlager, O. (1999). Coping with amputation and phantom limb pain. *Journal of Psychosomatic Research, 46*(4), 379–383.

Rando, T. A. (1984). *Grief, dying, and death.* Champaign, IL: Research Press.

Read, S. (1996). Helping people with learning disabilities to grieve. *British Journal of Nursing, 5*(2), 91–95.

Reinhardt, J. P. (1996). The importance of friendship and family support in adaptation to chronic vision impairment. *Journal of Gerontology: Biological, Psychological Sciences, Social Sciences, 51*(5), P268–P278.

Rybarczyk, B., Gallagher-Thompson, D., Rodman, J., Zeiss, A., Gantz, F. E., & Yesavage, J. (1992). Applying cognitive-behavioral psychotherapy to the chronically ill elderly: Treatment issues and case illustration. *International Psychogeriatrics, 4*(1), 127–140.

Schlaff, C. (1993). From dependency to self-advocacy: Redefining disability. *American Journal of Occupational Therapy, 47*(10), 943–948.

Sebring, D. L., & Moglia, P. (1987). Amyotrophic lateral sclerosis: Psychosocial interventions for patients and their families. *Health and Social Work, 12*(2), 113–119.

Shanfield, S. B. (1983). Some observations of a psychiatric consultant to a hospice. *Hillside Journal of Clinical Psychiatry, 5*(1), 31–42.

Soderberg, A., Gilje, F., & Norberg, A. (1999). Transforming desolation into consolation: The meaning of being in situations of ethical difficulty in intensive care. *Nursing Ethics, 6*(5), 357–373.

Stearns, A. K. (1984). *Living through personal crisis.* New York: Ballantine Books.

Steinhauser, K. E., Christakis, N. A., Clipp, E. C., McNeilly, M., McIntyre, L., & Tulsky, J. A. (2000). Factors considered important at the end of life by patients, family, physicians, and other care providers. *Journal of the American Medical Association, 284*(19), 2476–2482.

Sussman, N. (1995). Reactions of patients to the diagnosis and treatment of cancer. *Anticancer Drugs, 6* (Suppl. 1), 4–8.

Svedlund, M., & Axelsson, I. (2000). Acute myocardial infarction in middle-aged women: Narrations from the patients and their partners during rehabilitation. *Intensive Critical Care Nursing, 16*(4), 256–265.

Takkinen, S., & Ruoppila, I. (2001). Meaning in life in three samples of elderly persons with high cognitive functioning. *International Journal of Aging and Human Development, 53*(1), 51–73.

Taylor, S. E. (1983). Adjustment to threatening events: A theory of cognitive adaptation. *American Psychologist, 38,* 1161–1173.

Tolstoy, L. (1971). *The death of Ivan Ilych and other short stories* (L. Maude & A. Maude, Trans.). London, UK: Oxford University Press. (Original work published 1886)

Trieschmann, M. E. (1988). *Spinal cord injuries: Psychological, social, and vocational rehabilitation* (2nd ed.). New York: Demos Publications.

Videka-Sherman, L. (1982). Effects of participation in a self-help group for bereaved parents: Compassionate friends. *Preventive Human Services, 1*(3), 69–77.

Viemero, V., & Krause, C. (1998). Quality of life in individuals with physical disabilities. *Psychotherapy and Psychosomatics, 67*(6), 317–322.

Vitaliano, P., Russo, J., Carr, J. Maiuro, R., & Becker, S. (1985). The ways of coping checklist: Revision and psychometric properties. *Multivariate Behavioral Research, 20,* 3–26.

Vrkljan, B. H., & Miller-Polgar, J. (2001). Meaning of occupational engagement in life-threatening illness: A qualitative pilot project. *Canadian Journal of Occupational Therapy, 68*(4), 237–246.

Waltz, M., Badura, B., Pfaff, H., & Schott, T. (1988). Marriage and the psychological consequences of a heart attack: A longitudinal study of adaptation to chronic illness after 3 years. *Social Science and Medicine, 27*(2), 149–158.

Weiss, L., Frischer, L., & Richman, J. (1989). Parental adjustment to intrapartum and delivery room loss: The role of a hospital-based support program. *Clinical Perinatology, 16*(4), 1009–1019.

Wheeler, G., Krausher, K., Cumming, C., Jung, V., Steadward, R., & Cumming, D. (1996). Personal styles and ways of coping in individuals who use wheelchairs. *Spinal Cord, 34*(6), 351–357.

White, Y., & Grenyer, B. F. (1999). The biopsychosocial impact of end-stage renal disease: The experience of dialysis patients and their partners. *Journal of Advanced Nursing, 30*(6), 1312–1320.

Worden, J. W. (2002). *Grief counseling and grief therapy* (3rd ed.). New York: Springer.

Wright, B. A., & Shontz, F. C. (1968). Process and tasks in hoping. *Rehabilitation Literature, 29*, 322–331.

Yedidia, M. J., & MacGregor, B. (2001). Confronting the prospect of dying: Reports of terminally ill patients. *Journal of Pain Symptom Management, 22*(4), 807–819.

Young, J. M., & McNicoll, P. (1998). Against all odds: Positive life experiences of people with advanced amyotrophic lateral sclerosis. *Health and Social Work, 23*(1), 35–43.

## ADDITIONAL READINGS FOR PART IV

Armstrong, L., & Jenkins, S. (2000). *It's not about the bike.* New York: Berkley Books.

Bowlby, J. (1980). *Loss: Sadness and depression. Vol. 3: Attachment and loss.* New York: Basic Books.

Cole, H. A. (1991). *Helpmates: Support in times of critical illness.* Louisville, KY: Westminster/John Knox Press.

Cousins, N. (1983). *The healing heart.* New York: Avon Books.

Dubus, A. (1997). *Meditations from a moveable chair.* New York: Vintage Books.

Felder, L. (1990). *When a loved one is ill: How to take better care of your loved one, your family, and yourself.* New York: New American Library.

Frank, A. (1991). *At the will of the body.* Boston: Houghton Mifflin.

Hockenberry, J. (1995). *Moving violations.* New York: Hyperion.

Kluger-Bell, K. (1998). *Unspeakable losses: Healing from miscarriage, abortion, and other pregnancy loss.* New York: W.W. Norton.

Kübler-Ross, E. (1981). *On living with death and dying.* New York: Macmillan.

Kübler-Ross, E. (1982). *Working it through.* New York: Macmillan.

Kübler-Ross, E. (1983). *On children and death.* New York: Macmillan.

LeShan, L. (1989). *Cancer as a turning point: A handbook for people with cancer, their families, and health professionals.* New York: E.P. Dutton.

Levin, R. F. (1987). *Heartmates: A survival guide for the cardiac spouse.* New York: Pocket Books.

Little, D. W. (1985). *Home care for the dying: A reassuring, comprehensive guide to physical and emotional care.* Garden City, NY: Doubleday.

Mairs, N. (1996). *Waist high in the world.* Boston: Beacon Press.

McDermott, J. (2000). *Babyface.* Bethesda, MD: Woodbine House.

Moffatt, B. C. (1986). *When someone you love has AIDS: A book of hope for family and friends.* New York: Plume.

Monette, P. (1988). *Borrowed time: An AIDS memoir.* New York: Harcourt Brace Jovanovich.

Peabody, B. (1986). *The screaming room: A mother's journal of her son's struggle with AIDS—A true story of love, dedication, and courage.* New York: Avon Books.

Register, C. (1987). *Living with chronic illness: Days of patience and passion.* New York: Bantam Books.

Remen, R. N. (1996). *Kitchen table wisdom: Stories that heal.* New York: Riverhead Books.

Robinson, F. M., West, D., & Woodworth, D., Jr. (1995). *Coping plus dimensions of disability.* Westport, CT: Praeger.

Segal, J. (1984). *Living beyond fear: A course for coping with the emotional aspects of life-threatening illness for patients, families, and health care professionals.* North Hollywood, CA: Newcastle.

Stepanek, M. J. T. (2001). *Journey through heartsongs.* Alexandria, VA: VSP Books.

# Part V

# *Responses to Illness and Disability that Complicate Care*

Very few people respond to illness or disability in ways that are simple or predictable. There are many factors that complicate a client's circumstances, symptoms, and recovery, such as psychiatric disorders, destructive behaviors, and chronic illness, which are described in Part V. In order to be able to provide effective care for all clients, health care providers must be knowledgeable about these conditions and prepared to assess their impact.

Chronic illness and disabilities affect 90 million Americans. For many clients, medical conditions that begin as acute health problems develop into chronic pain. In addition, unremitting pain is the leading cause of disability in the United States. Chapter 15 discusses the impact of these conditions on clients and their need for lifelong medical care and supportive services. Strategies to evaluate symptom magnification, or malingering, are provided.

Over the course of a lifetime, one in five Americans will develop a psychiatric condition. Chapter 16 explores how these problems significantly interfere with the ability to work, have satisfying relationships, or enjoy life. In addition, psychiatric conditions can be life-threatening. Unfortunately, many psychiatric disorders mask themselves as physical symptoms, such as neck or back pain, stomach distress, or cardiac problems. Clients may undergo unnecessary pain, medical tests, or procedures because the true nature of the disorder is not recognized and effective treatments not implemented.

Chapter 17 explores destructive behaviors, including substance abuse and eating disorders. Because many individuals who have these diagnoses have experienced some form of abuse, this chapter begins with an explanation of family violence and its possible outcomes. Substance abuse is both a common cause and result of family violence. It is also the most frequently occurring form of psychiatric disorder. Over time, the consequences of substance abuse affect all organ systems, leading to serious chronic illness, disability, or death. Eating disorders and destructive behaviors, such as cutting, can also lead to other medical disorders, significant physical harm, or death. Therefore, it is important for health care providers to be able to recognize clients who are engaging in these practices and make appropriate referrals.

# 15

# *Chronic Illness*

The Chronic Pain Clinic is a very difficult place to work. All of the clients are there because no one else has been able to "fix" their problems. Many clients have been sick for years. All of them are in severe distress. It is especially hard for me to work with Alejandro, a very proud man who emigrated from Guatemala when he was in his teens. Working his way through college washing dishes in a restaurant, he became a certified public accountant and landed a really good job in an accounting firm. Everything was going well until five years ago, when his car was rear-ended and he sustained a severe whiplash injury. Ever since the accident, he's had headaches and pain in his neck, radiating down his right arm. Because of the pain, he can't concentrate or sit at a desk longer than an hour. He had to give up his job and is collecting disability payments. His wife now works to help support their family of three children, but this doesn't feel "right" to Alejandro. In addition to his physical pain, he feels like a failure as a husband, a provider, and man. I hope that we'll be able to help him.

—*From the journal of Melissa Chan, occupational therapy student*

The goal of the health care system is to treat disease and maintain good health. We perform physical examinations and tests to detect signs of disease; prescribe medication, surgery, or therapy when a problem is detected; and often expect that the client's problem will be cured. However, many people receive treatment for illnesses, survive devastating accidents, or develop chronic disorders that must be managed rather than abated. For these clients, medical problems become a way of life. Some lose hope of ever feeling "well" again.

In this chapter, we discuss what happens when health problems become chronic. We explore the effects of chronic illness, chronic pain, and permanent disability on clients' function and psychosocial well-being. Strategies for supporting clients' long-term needs and improving their quality of life are suggested.

# Chronic Health Problems

Our current health care system was developed to identify and treat acute diseases; it was never designed to support the needs of clients whose lives are affected by chronic disease or disabling conditions (Curtin & Lubkin, 1998). Health care professionals have been trained to provide focused short-term interventions that are effective in eliminating health problems. Both clients and professionals often expect medical problems to be cured so the client can return to his or her premorbid state without ongoing difficulties. However, the explosion of scientific discoveries and advances in medical care that occurred in the past century has enabled many clients with previously fatal conditions to live for many years. The goal of treatment for chronic diseases must be to decrease suffering, diminish disability, and reduce the frequency and severity of symptoms or exacerbations (Kleinman, 1988).

While the focus of health care has changed significantly, the focus of the health care delivery system and insurance industry has not (Hoffman, Rice, & Sung, 1996). Ten percent of Americans consume 72 percent of our health care dollars (Haas, 1995). A major cause of the current crisis in providing and financing health care is linked to the failure to change the health care paradigm. Many health plans exclude clients with preexisting conditions, set arbitrary limits for types and costs of services they provide, and put more restrictive caps on psychiatric illnesses than on medical diagnoses (Batavia, 1993). Rehabilitation services have been given low levels of reimbursement (Neff & Anderson, 1995). Policies force many clients and families to forgo needed health care visits or avoid filling expensive prescriptions due to their inability to pay. The end result is that clients become ill from preventable conditions and health care costs escalate. It has been estimated that every dollar invested in rehabilitation will save between $11 and $30 of future health care expenditures (Aitchison, 1993).

Consider the case of Emma Brown, who lives in a large industrialized city. She is a single mother who provides the sole support for her two young sons. Although her job cleaning rooms in an upscale hotel pays a good hourly wage, she has only a modest health insurance plan and a limited number of paid sick and vacation days. Emma has asthma, which is exacerbated by her exposure to the cleaning products she uses at work, the poor air quality in her city, and environmental factors in her neighborhood. She does not want to take time off from work for doctor visits. Because she must pay 50 percent of her expensive prescriptions, she uses them only when she "needs to" rather than routinely, as she has been instructed. As a result, she has frequent asthmatic episodes that are treated in the local hospital's emergency room. Although she misses time from work and loses wages, her insurance plan covers these treatments fully.

Chronic health conditions include both chronic diseases and permanent impairments (Hoffman et al., 1996). One definition states that it is "the irreversible presence, accumulation, or latency of disease states or impairments that involve the total human environment for supportive and self-care, maintenance of function, and prevention of further disability"

(Curtin & Lubkin, 1998, p. 6). Other definitions simply state that chronic diseases are conditions that last more than three months. For the most part, people live with, rather than die from, these chronic conditions (Verbrugge & Jette, 1994). Furthermore, while chronic conditions may cause disruption or difficulties, the majority of clients with chronic health care problems are not disabled and live "normal" lives (Hoffman et al., 1996).

Chronic conditions take many forms and affect all age groups. Disease-specific characteristics are discussed in Chapter 10, but it is important to this discussion to briefly note some specific characteristics that may affect clients' responses to their medical problems. Some conditions are constant with little change in acuity or severity, such as an amputation resulting from an automobile accident, or a congenital hearing loss secondary to a nonprogressive condition. Other disorders, such as asthma, diabetes, and arthritis, may have acute exacerbations. Management of these conditions may involve considerable client time, energy, and lifestyle modifications. Still other diagnoses may be terminal, such as some forms of cancer, or progressive, like multiple sclerosis. They can result in significant loss and grief for the client and his or her family.

## Incidence

Chronic health conditions are common, with over 90 million Americans affected by one problem, and 39 million living with more than one. This accounts for 45 percent of people living outside of institutions or long-term care facilities. Although these conditions occur in all age groups, the incidence rises significantly with age. The incidence of people who have at least one chronic health condition is

- one in four children under 18,
- one in three adults between 18 and 44,
- two out of three adults between 44 and 65.

Rates of chronic disease are highest for the elderly, with 88 percent having at least one chronic health condition (Hoffman et al., 1996).

Clients with severe mental illness are more likely to have chronic medical conditions than the general population (Dixon, Goldberg, Lehman, & McNary, 2001). Increased rates of cardiovascular disease, lung, kidney, and digestive disorders, and cancer have been found in people with mental illness. Mental illness also affects the outcome of physical disorders with increased duration, severity, and morbidity and mortality rates for clients with both mental and physical disorders (van Hemert, Hengeveld, Bolk, Rooijmans, & van den Broucke, 1993). In addition, there is a strong connection between self-perceptions of physical health, mental health, and overall health status (Dixon et al., 2001).

## Chronic Health Conditions and Income

Chronic medical conditions are linked to poverty, with a well-established connection between low income and poor health. Lynch, Kaplan, and Shema (1997) retrospectively evaluated the records of clients from 1965 to 1994. They found that clients who were in a low income bracket were more likely to have chronic health problems than clients who earned more than double the income limit for the poverty level. There was a significant relationship between sustained economic hardship and ability to function in the physical, psychological, and cognitive arenas. This is important because those who had low income for a prolonged time had the highest incidence of health-related problems. Rates of depression were particularly high in the study sample who had a low income. It would be anticipated that poor health may lead to an inability to work and a lower income; however, study data did not support that poor health caused the economic hardship (Lynch et al., 1997).

It is not surprising that poor health is linked to reduced income. People with low incomes are more likely to be exposed to conditions that would cause health problems or psychological distress. Inadequate housing or homelessness, lack of access to health care, poor nutrition, extended exposure to environmental pollutants, and increased exposure to infectious diseases all amplify risk of disease. Psychosocial stressors, such as exposure to violence and drugs, single-parent households, and overburdened social support systems, also may contribute to the development of psychological difficulties (Lynch et al., 1997; Philipp & Black, 1998).

## Cost of Chronic Health Conditions

Chronic health conditions are costly in many ways. There are the direct costs of medical care, including doctors' visits, hospitalizations, prescriptions, surgery, therapies, supportive personnel, and aids and devices. These direct costs account for 75 percent of health care expenditures, not including institutional or nursing home care (Hoffman et al., 1996).

Indirect costs are more difficult to calculate. These costs include lost wages, decreased productivity, and an inability to manage household responsibilities or childcare. They are associated with many types of disorders, even those that do not produce obvious disability. For example, 18 percent of the general population has some form of musculoskeletal disorder. These disorders can cause significant pain, which may result in an inability to perform household chores or perform activities of daily living. People with musculoskeletal disorders are less likely to be employed than individuals without these conditions (Yelin, Trupin, & Sebesta, 1998).

Disease or feeling ill contributes to work-loss days, with resultant loss of productivity. However, many people go to work when they are not feeling well and "cut back" or curtail their performance. In one survey, 17.5 percent of workers reported at least one work-loss day in the past month, and 22 percent reported at least one "cut back" day. This accounts for an estimated 1.5 work-impairment days *per capita, per month.* The most prevalent disorder leading to work-impairment days was cancer, primarily due to fatigue, followed by depression, asthma, arthritis, and high blood pressure (Kessler, Greenberg, Mickelson, Meneades, & Wong, 2001).

Consider Cindy, who works for a large university that arranged flexible hours and specialized computer equipment to accommodate the rheumatoid arthritic changes in her hands. When she is feeling well, she is able to work a full day, performing her responsibilities competently and efficiently. Many days, however, she does not feel well or has pain and cannot work to her full potential. When she experiences pain, she is unable to care for her two children as she would like, and her husband bears the extra burden. Although Cindy would like to be able to coach the soccer team or be a Cub Scout leader, her condition is unpredictable. She often feels badly about all the people she has "failed."

Chronic conditions present significant costs to the individual, family, employer, general public, and public agencies that pay for services. Better management of health care resources and services could promote improved health and prevent secondary disability. Currently, employers pay for some health promotion services, such as influenza vaccinations and employee assistance programs. Expansion of employer and public programs to help individuals manage chronic physical and mental health disorders might improve quality of life for clients and families at a reduced overall cost.

# Disease versus Illness

As discussed in Chapter 7, historically some health care providers have been concerned with disease, which is seen as a biological process gone awry, an alteration in the structure or function of the body. Clients, on the other hand, are also concerned with how the experience of illness and disruption affects their lives (Curtin & Lubkin, 1998). Arthur Kleinman (1988) describes this frame of reference in his classic text, *The Illness Narratives*. "By invoking the term illness, I mean to conjure up the innately human experience of symptoms and suffering. Illness refers to how the sick person and members of the family or wider social network perceive, live with, and respond to symptoms and disability" (p. 3). For clients, illness is far more than just a cluster of symptoms or a treatment protocol.

The illness experience is the sum total of all life experiences that result from having a disease or injury. This includes the client's and family's belief system about what the disease means to them and how they choose to cope with its practical problems (Kleinman, 1988). Illness does not occur in a vacuum, but rather in a system of social, cultural, and spiritual values. There is substantial research that indicates that psychological and social factors affect clients' physical improvement or decline. Thoughts and emotions are entwined with physiological processes. The onset of depression or anxiety or loss of significant social support can lead to symptom exacerbation or amplification. Conversely, a strengthened support system, an increased sense of self-efficacy, or a renewal of hope are often associated with symptom remission.

People live complex lives that are affected in multiple ways by the chronicity of some health conditions. An expanded scope of reference is important for each client. Neglecting to consider the personal and lifestyle factors that are important to clients can limit their quality of life.

Richard Galli speaks of the dilemma he faced in choosing life or death for his son. In his autobiographical book, *Rescuing Jeffrey*, he describes the first ten days after his 17-year-old son sustained a high cervical spinal cord injury in a diving accident. He writes,

> I began to understand, at last, why I was so distraught over Jeffrey's paralysis. It was not just action he would lack. It was the spiritual fulfillment that comes from action. Our limbs are connected to our souls as well as to our brain. To bow a head; to kneel; to raise the Eucharist. But there are these as well. To swing a five iron smoothly and with grace. To roll a ball down an echoing lane. To scoop a grounder, twist, and toss to second (Galli, 2000, p. 142).

Our society and physical world are designed for people who are healthy and fit. Without realizing it, we frequently place barriers to independence in the path of people with limitations and impairments, often rendering them unable to do the things they want and would otherwise be able to do (Verbrugge & Jette, 1994). Social prejudice and stigma, lack of flexible jobs and work schedules, and architectural obstacles all create barriers. The goal of medical treatment and rehabilitation is to restore clients' abilities to live the lifestyles they choose. "It is the restoration of the power of living well, living meaningfully, that rehabilitation essentially seeks" (Jennings, 1993, p. 402). It is our responsibility to find the meaning of living well for each of our clients and to collaborate with them to attain that goal.

Disease and physical impairments can be diagnosed and assessed using clinical signs, medical symptoms, and degree of variation from normative values. In contrast, illness is unique to each individual, and each client will have his or her own experiences. The presence of illness is assessed by looking at the client's presentation of *illness behaviors*. Illness behaviors are "observable and potentially measurable actions and conduct which express and communicate the individual's own perception of disturbed health" (Waddell, 1991, p. 663). These behaviors may be adaptive, by signaling the need for intervention, or maladaptive, out of proportion to the level of pathology or dysfunction (Waddell, 1991).

Illness behaviors take many forms, such as verbalizing distress or hopelessness, insomnia, fatigue, lying down, sighing, grimacing, moaning, and irritability. Many of these behaviors are the same symptoms of depression, discussed in Chapter 16. There may also be comorbid physical and psychiatric illness.

# Chronic Pain

Everyone experiences pain. Physical pain can result from a fall on the stairs or the onset of severe abdominal pain that signals acute illness. Emotional pain follows a death, loss of a job, or beginning of a psychiatric or physical disorder. It serves a positive, protective function, indicating significant changes or injuries that demand attention and may require medical care (Simon, 1989).

Pain has been defined as localized physical suffering associated with bodily disorder (disease or injury) or acute mental or emotional distress (Simon, 1989). Acute pain is caused by a noxious peripheral stimulus or tissue damage. The amount of discomfort or distress is typically in direct proportion to the level of injury or disease (Waddell, 1991). Conversely, chronic pain may have no obvious physical relationship to current pathology. For some clients, an acute medical event becomes a chronic often unremitting condition. Pain specialists estimate that 97 million Americans suffer from chronic pain, the leading cause of disability (Jackson, 2000).

## Progression from Acute to Chronic Pain

For a small percentage of clients, acute pain will develop into a subacute or chronic condition. A common response to pain is to become passive and physically inactive. This leads to weakness, tight muscles, and deconditioning, which can result in more pain when the client attempts to resume activity. Pain may also be accompanied by insomnia, fatigue, loss of appetite, and disturbances in family or social life. Anger, depression, and anxiety are frequently seen in clients with chronic pain. This emotional distress is often somaticized, turned into physical distress, which triggers a cycle of more physical pain, leading to more emotional distress. It is difficult to determine the cause-and-effect importance of the physical and emotional symptoms (Simon, 1989). In addition, prolonged absence from work and social roles is detrimental to physical, social, and mental well-being (McGrail, Lohman, & Gorman,

2001). While physical impairments may have subsided, the client may genuinely feel too ill to return to work or assume other life responsibilities.

It has been proposed that chronic and acute pain are entirely different disorders (Morris, 1991). Pain is arbitrarily classified as chronic when it is present for longer than six months. It is often linked with disability, chronic illness behavior, emotional distress, and depression (Waddell, 1991). While acute pain has a direct relationship to pathology and impairment, chronic pain, chronic disability, and chronic illness behavior may be dissociated from the original source, with little evidence of the original physical condition.

Chronic pain progressively becomes a self-sustaining condition or "pain syndrome," which is resistant to traditional medical treatment (Waddell, 1987). The initial response to pain is triggered by a nociceptive stimulus. Pain messages pass upward through the spinal cord to the thalamus, where they are interpreted, and terminate at the cortex, where pain is perceived. It is hypothesized that the memory of the pain is retained in the cortex where neurons become sensitized to future stimuli. In the absence of noxious stimuli, small, nonnoxious events can trigger the reactivation of the cycle. This can elicit the pain–tension–fear cycle (Simon, 1989).

Nonmalignant musculoskeletal pain is one of the leading causes for consultation to primary care providers, missed work days, and lost wages. Neck, back, and shoulder pain account for many of these complaints (Karjalainen et al., 2001). Low back pain has been well studied and presents a model for explaining the progression from acute to chronic pain. Approximately 80 to 90 percent of clients with low back pain improve, regardless of treatment; the remainder develop chronic pain (Greenberg & Bello, 1996; Waddell, 1987). The decision to seek health care for low back pain appears dependent on the client's perception and interpretation of the pain. These may be enhanced by the presence of anxiety or emotional distress. The physician is likely to base treatment aggressiveness on the extent of the expressed level of distress and illness behavior (Waddell, 1987). The level of initial emotional response to acute pain may indicate a predisposition for it to become chronic (Waddell, 1987). Other premorbid risk factors for the onset of chronic pain include personal or family history of disability, dysfunctional family dynamics or abuse, history of substance abuse, and comorbid medical conditions (McGrail et al., 2001).

Prolonged pain causes difficulties in physical, psychological, and social areas of function. It is estimated that half of all clients with chronic pain also have depression (Kleinman, 1988). Manifestations of chronic pain may be frequent complaints, irritability, and inability to participate in "normal" activities. This can exhaust family and friends, driving the client into social isolation. The most difficult aspect of chronic pain may be that, after a time, other people no longer believe the pain is real. The paradox is that clients with chronic pain are not well, but they are not sick either (Morris, 1991).

Consider Elizabeth, a postal worker who injured her back as a result of carrying large sacks of mail. Long before her back injury, she was anxious about her health and frequently sought medical care for her various complaints. Since childhood, she responded to minor symptoms of disease with exaggerated illness behavior and excessive absences from school and work. In the eight years following her back injury, she has been placed on bedrest several times, received physical therapy, consumed large amounts of nonsteroidal pain medications, and for the past three years has been taking steroids. Yet, she is still disabled by her pain and only works sporadically. She is unable to participate in family social activities, go out with her friends, or fully enjoy the company of her husband. Her life revolves around the pain and her attempts to find relief.

## Pain and the Mind–Body Connection

Perhaps nowhere in medicine are the mind and body more closely linked than in chronic pain. It is neither practical nor reasonable to distinguish mental from physical suffering, what Morris (1991) cautioned as "the myth of two pains." In Chapter 8, we discussed the connection between the mind and the body. The sympathetic nervous system responds to physical pain with emotional distress. Pain creates fear that releases catecholamines and stress hormones that can disrupt bodily functions, causing muscle tension and more pain. In Chapter 16, we explored the physical symptoms that arise from various psychiatric disorders. The linkages are powerful, and pain cannot be distinctly dichotomized into physical and psychological realms. Physical and psychological pain are both regulated through central nervous system mechanisms at several levels, leading to the pain–stress–fear cycle (Yocum, Castro, & Cornett, 2000).

What matters most about pain may well be the personal and social meaning that we attach to it. Religion, gender, age, socioeconomic status, past experiences, and psychological traits all converge to affect our perception and response to pain. Our pain is shaped by our culture, which also legitimizes or stigmatizes it (Morris, 1991). For example, the person who has pain as a result of bone cancer is generally afforded sympathy and care. In contrast, the person with perhaps equally severe pain secondary to a migraine headache may be perceived as exaggerating pain for secondary gain; after all, it is "*just* a headache."

Today, most health care providers subscribe to the gate control theory of pain, developed by Melzack and Wall (1965). Their model is useful because it explains how the direct physical stimuli causing pain impulses are affected by ascending and descending neurological input at the level of the spinal cord. It also acknowledges the role of emotional and cognitive factors in mediating the perception of pain. This theory provides the framework for a holistic approach to medical care, which is frequently employed in centers that treat clients with chronic pain (Karjalainen et al., 2001). The model stresses the importance of human illness rather than disease (Waddell, 1987). It also enables clinicians to add psychological, behavioral, and educational interventions to physical rehabilitation techniques (Karjalainen et al., 2001).

# Permanent Disability

I have been working with a wonderful client who recently sustained a spinal cord injury, resulting in paraplegia at the mid-thoracic area. George is a skilled carpenter who did beautiful finish work on the insides of homes. He took great pride in his work. Now that he is unable to walk and has some weakness in his trunk, he cannot perform the work he loved to do. He also has no source of income other than disability payments. We have been thinking about ways he can make reasonable accommodations at work for his impairments, but there really don't seem to be any. In addition to all his other challenges, George will now have to find a new line of work.

—*From the journal of Ann Nichols, rehabilitation counseling student*

## Health Care Needs of People with Disabilities

Earlier in this chapter, we discussed clients who have chronic health care problems but are not disabled, as well as clients with chronic pain who may be disabled. Both of these groups of clients have problems that may not be visible. You could sit next to them in class or sing with them in the choir and never realize that a problem exists. However, there are individuals whose impairments are obvious, such as the person who is blind and uses a cane, the person undergoing chemotherapy for cancer who has lost hair, or the individual who uses a wheelchair for mobility.

As medical care extends the lives of people with serious diseases or disabling conditions, the number of people with disabilities is increasing rapidly (Batavia, 1993). Tiny premature babies, people with AIDS, and survivors of high spinal cord injuries are living with their conditions rather than dying from them.

In Chapters 12 through 14, we discuss the issues of loss, grief, and adaptation that clients face when they become severely ill or disabled. However, once clients leave the hospital or rehabilitation setting, they must *live with* the effects of the disability. This influences their ability to work and earn an income, pursue hobbies and spiritual activities, engage in family and community life, and receive health care services. These multiple complex needs of clients and families challenge our health care and social service system (Sutton & DeJong, 1998).

The existence of a disability presents substantial challenges in achieving access to primary and secondary health care, as well as to preventive services. Physical barriers may prevent a person with a disability from receiving appropriate care. Health providers may not be aware of the specialized needs that accompany disabling conditions, and both health maintenance and promotion services may be unavailable (Sutton & DeJong, 1998). People with disabilities may have no insurance, have to pay high rates for insurance, or need to be in a very low income level to be eligible for public insurance (Batavia, 1993).

Gans, Mann, and Becker (1993) have summarized several specialized health care needs of people with disabilities. Despite the enactment of the Americans with Disabilities Act (ADA) (Public Law 101–336), many public buildings, including hospitals, medical facilities, and doctors' offices, are not physically accessible to people with disabilities. Medical office staff may not be knowledgeable about how to physically handle a client who lacks mobility. They may not know how to transfer a client on or off an examination table, assist with dressing, or gather a urine sample from someone who lacks voluntary bladder control. Examination tables may be too high or too narrow to accommodate a wheelchair transfer. The scale may not be accessible to someone who cannot stand independently, and the bathroom may not accommodate a wheelchair.

Time may also be a barrier to medical office visits. It may take the client who has a disability longer to change into and out of clothing and to move around the office environment. Extra staff time may be needed to assist the person, and the examination itself may take longer to perform. Transportation to the medical office may be unreliable, and the client may arrive late and disrupt the client "flow" (Gans et al., 1993).

Finding providers who understand their specialized needs can be a challenge for people with disabilities. Internists, pediatricians, family practitioners, or gynecologists may be very competent in their specialty area but lack information about the specialized medical needs of people with disabilities (Gans et al., 1993). People with multiple medical conditions may take a "cocktail" of medications, with potentially dangerous drug interactions. There may be an increased susceptibility to secondary medical conditions. For example, 67 to 100 percent of people with spinal cord injuries have at least one bladder infection (Sutton & DeJong, 1998). Proper monitoring and care could prevent some of these complications. The functional impact of small changes in health status can be significant for someone with a chronic disability. A fractured wrist due to a fall is an inconvenience to someone who can walk independently. For someone who uses a wheelchair, it may mean the inability to transfer independently and propel the wheelchair until the fracture heals, resulting in immobility and dependence.

Finally, preventive and health maintenance services may not be available for people with disabilities. Osteoporosis, arthritis, balance disorders, obesity, and depression have an increased prevalence in people with disabling conditions (Rimmer, 1999). Although it is important for people with mobility impairments to maintain cardiovascular fitness, there are few health and fitness centers accessible and affordable for them (Rimmer, 1999). Routine mammograms, Pap smears, and other cancer screening tests may not be readily available for these same reasons. Clients with disabilities need access to hearing, vision, and dental examinations, yet these health professionals often practice in offices that do not accommodate people in wheelchairs. Access to counseling for personal, marital, or substance abuse problems, stress management, weight management, and smoking cessation programs may also be needed (Gans et al., 1993; Rimmer, 1999).

Daniel Callahan (1993) believes that an ethic of caring should drive our health care system: "Caring means nonabandonment of the sick, rehabilitative care for the injured and disabled, as well as whatever nursing care is needed to relieve immediate pain and suffering" (p. 104). A caring health system would also provide the social and economic support to ensure living a life with dignity. Unfortunately, we are still far from that goal. Collaboration between health care consumers with disabilities and health care providers is needed to improve access and care (Sutton & DeJong, 1998).

## Return-to-Work Issues

Fewer than 40 percent of people with disabilities are employed, and only 25 percent work full-time (Batavia, 1993). There are significant social, emotional, physical, and financial barriers to entering the workforce. As discussed in Chapter 1, stigma and discrimination are also barriers to including people with disabilities as full members of society. The ADA was passed in 1990 and went into effect in 1992 as a remedy for some of these discriminatory practices. It provides comprehensive civil rights protection to people with disabilities in the areas of employment, transportation, telecommunications, and government services (Public Law 101–336).

The language of the law was intentionally designed to be vague to allow for interpretation on an individual basis (Rothstein, 1995). Under the ADA, an individual is considered disabled if he or she has a physical or mental impairment that substantially limits one or more of the major life activities. Until the passage of this legislation, people with disabilities had little protection against discrimination on the basis of disability. Now, Title I of the ADA states that employers may not discriminate against otherwise qualified applicants on the basis of disability. However, implementation of the ADA has been difficult.

A key feature of this legislation provides that the employee must be able to perform *essential functions* of the job with *reasonable accommodations*. An accommodation is any modification to the work site or job responsibilities. This may include physical adaptations to the workplace, retraining the employee for a new job, changing work location, or allowing flexible hours (Seigel & Gaylord-Ross, 1991). The question of what constitutes a reasonable accommodation will vary at each work site. For example, it might be reasonable for a large corporation to purchase computer modifications or programs to help an employee with a disability, but it might not be reasonable for a small "mom-and-pop" operation. It may also not be feasible for the company's only receptionist to have flexible hours.

Research indicates that most accommodations are not unduly costly. Twenty-eight percent of accommodations cost less than $1,000, and 69 percent are achieved at no cost. This includes flexible work schedules, moving the employee to a more quiet work environment, or changing the duties of the job (Rothstein, 1995). "Reasonable accommodations facilitate participation in meaningful occupations and enable the integration of persons with disabilities into the mainstream of society with maximal functional independence" (American Occupational Therapy Association, 2000, p. 625).

Difficulty obtaining health insurance prevents many people with disabilities from working (Batavia, 1993). Most public health insurance coverage that is available for people with disabilities, such as Medicaid, requires that the individual also have a low income. Paid employment may raise income too high to be eligible for this public insurance. Many private insurance plans restrict coverage for people with preexisting conditions or charge extremely high premiums. Other employers may offer no insurance options at all. The ADA has the potential to improve insurance coverage for people with disabilities. By preventing discrimination in hiring, access to insurance coverage becomes available to all people whose employers offer it. However, Section 501 of the ADA contains contradictory language that can be interpreted to mean that people with disabilities and disabling conditions can be treated differently than people without these conditions when offering insurance benefits (Batavia, 1993).

Work also plays an important role in our culture. While some individuals work without pay as homemakers, parents, or caregivers, others engage in satisfying volunteer activities. Most people, however, define work as a job that pays wages. Unemployment following a disability is a significant financial stressor for the client and his or her family (Krause, Sternberg, Maides, & Lottes, 1998). In addition, employment serves as a primary marker for successful rehabilitation outcomes (Krause & Anson, 1996). Research indicates that people with disabilities who are employed feel better about their quality of life and that employment status is directly related to prolonged survival (Hess, Ripley, McKinley, & Tewksbury, 2000).

Several factors have been identified that are important for successful post-disability employment. Approximately 60 percent of spinal cord injuries occur in people between the ages of 16 and 30, prime years for gaining an education, attaining work skills, and establishing a work history. However, research indicates that only 10 to 50 percent of people with spinal cord injuries are able to return to work following their injury (Hess et al., 2000). Many factors affect this return rate, including the level of lesion and residual motor function, race, age, marital status, and education (Hess et al., 2000; Krause & Anson, 1996; Krause et al., 1998). Clients who sustain incomplete lesions or lower level lesions typically have higher levels of motor function and are more likely to be employed.

Education is an extremely important variable for employment. Clients who have less than a high school education have the lowest employment rates. Completion of college is predictive of the highest level of employment success, with 72 percent of college graduates being employed following their injury (Krause & Anson, 1996). Other factors that are positively associated with employment are being white, married, and younger at the time of injury.

Levels of impairment and functional skills are also predictive of rehabilitation outcome for other injuries. For clients with traumatic brain injuries, burns, and fractures, level of post-injury rehabilitation is correlated with severity of injury (Horn, Yoels, & Bartolucci, 2000; Wehman et al., 1993). In this diverse group of clients, other factors are also important for rehabilitation outcomes. Socioeconomic status, pre-injury employment, and family support, particularly if the client was married, are associated with higher levels of post-injury function. Access to private insurance, which enhances the availability of funds for services, including rehabilitation and vocational counseling, is also coupled with higher levels of function. It appears that medical personnel are more likely to refer clients for rehabilitation who are white, married, employed, and have health insurance (Horn et al., 2000).

Finally, depression is significantly linked to high rates of disability and unemployment (Broadhead, Blazer, George, & Tse, 1990). An indirect measure of depression is suicidality. Clients whose injuries occur as a result of intentional self-harm have a lower rate of referral to rehabilitation services, and therefore, a lower rate of successful employment (Horn et al., 2000). Depression, phobias, and substance abuse are also highly correlated with disability. The presence of any of these conditions greatly elevates the probability of unemployment in persons with comorbid physical and psychiatric illnesses.

# Malingering

Perhaps no subject raises as much emotion in the field of rehabilitation than clients who malinger. We live in a culture with a strong work ethic and expect people will "put their nose to the grindstone" and "pull themselves up by their bootstraps." When medical professionals encounter clients who appear to be using their disability for secondary gain or not working to their potential, they may feel exploited and angry. Yet, many clients who become disabled as a result of chronic pain or other impairments have no visible signs of pathology. So how is one to know when a disability is real and when it is being feigned?

Malingering is the deliberate production of false or grossly exaggerated physical or psychological symptoms for the purpose of external reward. These incentives may include avoiding work, obtaining financial compensation, obtaining prescription drugs, or avoiding jail or military service. It is not considered a psychiatric disorder but rather an abnormal condition that may warrant intervention from a mental health provider (American Psychiatric Association, 2000).

Symptoms of malingering typically fall into one of two types. Clients may deliberately exaggerate or magnify symptoms, especially those that are difficult to measure or quantify, such as pain, stiffness, dizziness, weakness, or poor memory. In addition, clients may intentionally perform poorly on diagnostic tests or fabricate impairments, such as blindness, numbness, or amnesia (Iverson & Binder, 2000). Malingering may be suspected when there is litigation surrounding the claim of disability, a marked discrepancy or inconsistency between physical findings (impairments) and level of disability, a significant lack of cooperation by the client, or the presence of an antisocial personality disorder (Ben-Avi, Rabin, Melamed, Kreiner, & Ribak, 1998).

Malingering presents significant diagnostic and ethical dilemmas for the health care provider. An unsympathetic health professional who underestimates pain and suffering and fails to provide appropriate treatment may cause both physical and emotional harm (Morris, 1991). This violates the ethical principle of nonmaleficence. Conversely, failing to fully investigate a fraudulent claim constitutes abuse of the reimbursement system. The health care provider faces difficult diagnostic choices. Although it is beyond the scope of this chapter to discuss all tests available for properly investigating potential malingering, we will highlight salient points.

Some health care providers erroneously assume that clients who make worker's compensation claims are more likely to be seeking external gain and, perhaps, are malingering. In a study comparing injured workers who were pursuing litigation to those who were not, this assumption was not supported (Tait, Chibnall, & Richardson, 1990). Results indicated that *both* clients who were litigating and those who were not experienced significant levels of pain and dysfunction. Interestingly, clients with attorneys demonstrated lower levels of depression and anxiety than those without attorneys. The researchers interpreted litigation to be a positive coping response and not evidence of malingering.

Detecting sincerity of effort is a key diagnostic criterion for differentiating clients who are malingering from those who are not. This is not an easy task to accomplish. Tests and assessments are readily available, but most are unreliable or lack validity. In addition, while the test may indeed measure sincerity of effort correctly, the interpretation may be inaccurate. Clients may fail to fully cooperate with medical examinations because of fear, pain, failure to understand directions, and failure to understand the importance of effort (Lechner, Bradbury, & Bradley, 1998). Other clients may have a diminished mental capacity to connect their behavior with the desired outcome (Iverson & Binder, 2000). In addition, psychiatric conditions, such as conversion disorder, somatoform disorders, hypochondriasis, or depression, may be misdiagnosed as malingering.

Waddell, McCulloch, Kummel, and Venner (1980) developed eight test items to be used in the assessment of clients with low back pain to identify the presence of psychosocial factors that may have an impact on a client's recovery. These findings were known as nonorganic signs. The identification of nonorganic signs was designed to be used only as a screening tool for clients who might benefit from psychological intervention and indicated the need for referral to a mental health professional. After many years of use, the eight nonorganic signs have been shown to be valid as a clinical measure of distress and illness behavior. However, these signs have often been misused by health care providers as a diagnostic test for malingering. As a result of this misinterpretation, Main and Waddell (1998) have renamed their test items *behavioral signs,* rather than nonorganic signs, to help clarify their significance.

Exaggerated symptoms are often cited as a sign of malingering. Pain behavior that is "out of proportion" to impairment is typically noted. However, pain behavior is influenced by a number of factors, including culture, environment, race, ethnicity, verbal reinforcement, and relationship with one's spouse (Edwards, Doleys, Fillingim, & Lowery, 2001; Kleinman, 1988; Lechner et al., 1998; Morris, 1991). In order to accurately diagnose malingering, there must be compelling, unambiguous evidence that the client is exaggerating or fabricating symptoms. Note that clients may exaggerate symptoms or demonstrate poor effort without intending to malinger. The client must also be mentally and psychologically competent. This is an area where significant diagnostic skill is warranted, and a team of professionals may be needed.

# Conversion Disorder

Although this chapter addresses chronic illness, we need to clarify our discussion of malingering by introducing conversion disorder, another client problem that is not usually chronic in nature. While clients who malinger feign illness or disability for personal gain, clients with conversion disorder develop symptoms of physical illness that have no obvious biological cause. The client believes the symptoms and the illness are real. There are significant diagnostic challenges with conversion disorder, and a thorough neurological and medical examination must be conducted to rule out physical disorders, such as multiple sclerosis. To further complicate establishing a diagnosis, certain symptoms of conversion disorder may reflect cultural mores about socially acceptable ways to express illness. The clinician must, therefore, assess whether symptoms can be explained in a cultural/social context (American Psychiatric Association, 2000).

> Frank is a 23-year-old Marine who presents with apparent paraplegia. He was referred to physical therapy with a diagnosis of conversion disorder, and we're supposed to rehabilitate him. When I took his history, he told me that his legs were completely paralyzed and that he could not move them at all. However, when I transferred him from the wheelchair to the examination table, he supported his weight on his legs. He could not extend his knee or do a straight leg raise, but he tightened his thigh in the strongest quadriceps setting exercise I have ever seen. He doesn't seem to have a clue that this makes no sense.
>
> —*From the journal of Dan Wu, physical therapist student*

It is difficult to accurately determine the prevalence of conversion disorder, but it is believed to occur in about 3 percent of clients seen in outpatient mental health clinics (American Psychiatric Association, 2000). Clients often present with "pseudoneurologic" symptoms that are sensory or motor in nature, such as loss of sensation or paralysis. Professionals who subscribe to psychodynamic treatment theories propose that conversion disorder develops when unresolved psychological conflicts are "converted" into physical symptoms to keep them out of conscious awareness (Kleinman, 1988). This disorder is more common in women than men and is generally seen in clients who are young adults through middle age (Iverson & Binder, 2000).

An important diagnostic feature of conversion disorder is *la belle indifference,* that is, the client seems not to be concerned about the symptoms. In conversion disorder, symptoms do not match known physical conditions. For example, loss of sensation may follow a "gloved hand" pattern, rather than the normal dermatomal distribution. Paralysis may only be seen during certain movements or in certain positions. The onset of conversion disorder is usually acute but may be progressive. Clients who are hospitalized with conversion disorder typically recover within two weeks (American Psychiatric Association, 2000).

# Therapeutic Interventions

In Chapter 14, we discussed adaptation to terminal illness and long-term health problems or disabilities. Strategies were recommended for appropriate therapeutic responses to support clients in their journey from loss to adjustment. These responses are also applicable for clients with chronic illness. Clients and care providers may need to work together for a significant period of time, perhaps for many years. The client's condition may change, and other treatment options may become available or needed. In the case of permanent disability, the goals of rehabilitation must be to restore the client's sense of wholeness and integrity and preserve the ability to live a meaningful life (Jennings, 1993).

As discussed in Chapters 5 and 7, the client–practitioner relationship is the foundation upon which healing is built. The health care provider's ability to ask questions, listen, and interpret the client's illness experiences (refer to Chapter 2) is a powerful medical intervention. Clients with chronic illness have complex problems and histories, and multiple treatment strategies are often necessitated. It is imperative that health care providers consider prior treatments, clients' beliefs, and medical and personal priorities.

Kleinman (1988) suggests several strategies to aid health professionals, beginning with a form of history-taking known as a mini-ethnography or life history. This helps the practitioner understand how the illness has shaped and affected the client's life. The clinician is also able to realize how social supports, coping failures, and life events have shaped the client's illness experience. Interpretation of this information can lead to the development of an illness problem list, which could include financial burdens, school or work problems, relationship difficulties, and challenges in performing activities of daily living. Like the traditional medical problem list, the illness problem list can be documented in the client's medical record so that appropriate therapeutic interventions can be implemented.

As part of the mini-ethnography, health professionals can elicit the clients' and families' ideas, thoughts, and concerns about the illness (Kleinman, 1988). You might ask,

- "What do you think is wrong?"
- "What caused it?"
- "What do you want me to do?"
- "What is the chief way this illness or treatment has affected your life?"
- "What do you fear most about this illness or treatment?" (p. 239)

Their responses to these queries provide information enabling us to start with aspects of the client's illness that are most troubling to them. We can also consider the kinds of interventions that might be most valuable to the client. In addition, by discussing the client's fears, we can try to ease distress and begin the healing process.

The next recommended step in Kleinman's (1988) approach is the presentation of the health care provider's model of the illness and treatment. Typically, this is done using information derived from the traditional biomedical model, with simplified, scientific explanations of disease or impairments. In this phase, we are translating from the client's language and illness model to our own. We need to negotiate as collaborators and partners in their care.

Health care professionals may be able to help prevent the progression from pain and acute problems to disability. Successful disability prevention relies on appropriate diagnosis and management of the illness and its symptoms, as well as on open communication and trust between the client and health care provider. For example, a client who asks for documentation of a disability to avoid returning to work may actually be communicating difficulty coping with other life demands. Sensitive listening and counseling may identify a manageable condition, such as family problems, anxiety, depression, or substance abuse. Careful client education and instruction can convey the message that pain and other problems need not become disabling and may be self-limiting conditions. If pain cannot be eliminated, the health care provider can work with the client, employer, and family to adjust work and home demands or make reasonable accommodations for the residual impairments (McGrail et al., 2001).

## SUMMARY

In this chapter, we explained the effects of chronic illness. Some conditions allow the client to live a "normal" life with minimal disruption. Others, like chronic pain, may affect every waking moment and cause the client significant distress. Certain conditions result in functional limitations and, ultimately, permanent disabilities, requiring accommodations in lifestyle, work, physical environments, and relationships. Health care needs of clients with chronic infirmities may be more complex than for those with acute conditions and require different types of interventions.

In our various educational programs, health care providers spend many years learning the scientific or biomedical basis for client care, as well as anatomy, physiology, pathology, pharmacology, and multiple therapeutic interventions. However, the biopsychosocial model teaches the art of medicine and acknowledges the importance of listening, responding, caring, empathy, and compassion. It provides a humanistic basis for treatment. Integrating the knowledge of our shared humanity into our scientific practices can significantly improve the effectiveness of our care.

## REFLECTIVE QUESTIONS

1. Kleinman has suggested that health care professionals take a mini-ethnography of their clients' illness experiences. Write a mini-ethnography of your health and illness experiences. Include how your life affects your health and how your health affects your life.
2. Consider your own experiences interacting with your health care providers.
   a. Describe how you were treated. Was a biomedical, biopsychosocial, or other model used?
   b. What impact did this have on your outcome?
3. a. What are your personal health care beliefs?
   b. How have your personal health care beliefs been shaped by your social, family, religious, and cultural values?
4. There is a strong link between low income and poor health. Describe strategies that could minimize this problem . . .
   a. on a personal level.

   b. at the government level.

   c. in the workplace.

5. Think about activities in which you participate on a regular basis (i.e., school, work, social, recreational).

   a. What barriers exist that might prevent a person with a disability from participating?

   b. How could these barriers be eliminated?

## CASE STUDY

John Mahoney is a 47-year-old seventh grade science teacher who sustained a traumatic brain injury when his car was hit by an intoxicated driver. He has seizures, impulsive behavior, impaired judgment, and short-term memory loss. As a divorced father of four children, he shares joint custody with his former wife.

1. What barriers exist for John to return to work, family, social, and recreational activities?

2. What kinds of support and services exist to help John return to gainful employment?

3. a. What barriers exist for John to receive good health care and maintain overall health and fitness levels once he has reentered the community?

   b. What can be done to promote John's optimal care after discharge?

4. What are the direct and indirect costs of John's chronic disability?

## REFERENCES

Aitchison, K. W. (1993). Rehabilitation at the crossroads. *American Journal of Physical Medicine and Rehabilitation, 72*(6), 405–407.

American Occupational Therapy Association. (2000). Occupational therapy and the Americans with Disabilities Act. *American Journal of Occupational Therapy, 54*(6), 622–625.

American Psychiatric Association. (2000). *Diagnostic and statistical manual IV—TR*. Washington, DC: Author.

Americans with Disabilities Act of 1990, Pub. L. No. 101–336, *U. S. Code* § (1990).

Batavia, A. I. (1993, Spring). Health care reform and people with disabilities. *Health Affairs*, 41–57.

Ben-Avi, I., Rabin, S., Melamed, S., Kreiner, H., & Ribak, J. (1998). Malingering assessment in behavioral toxicology: What, why, and how. *American Journal of Industrial Medicine, 34*, 325–330.

Broadhead, W. E., Blazer, D. G., George, L. K., & Tse, C. K. (1990). Depression, disability days, and days lost from work in a prospective epidemiologic survey. *Journal of the American Medical Association, 264*, 2524–2528.

Callahan, D. (1993). Allocating health care resources. *American Journal of Physical and Rehabilitation Medicine, 72*, 101–104.

Curtin, M., & Lubkin, I. (1998). What is chronicity? In I. M. Lubkin & P. D. Larsen (Eds.), *Chronic illness* (pp. 3–25). Sudbury, MA: Jones and Bartlett.

Dixon, L., Goldberg, R., Lehman, A., & McNary, S. (2001). The impact of health status on work, symptoms, and functional outcomes in severe mental illness. *Journal of Nervous and Mental Disease, 189*(1), 17–23.

Edwards, R. R., Doleys, D. M., Fillingim, R. B., & Lowery, D. (2001). Ethnic differences in pain toler-ance: Clinical implications in a chronic pain population. *Psychosomatic Medicine, 63*, 316–323.

Galli, R. (2000). *Rescuing Jeffrey.* Chapel Hill, NC: Algonquin Books.

Gans, B. M., Mann, N. R., & Becker, B. F. (1993). Delivery of health care to the physically challenged. *Archives of Physical Medicine and Rehabilitation, 74*, S15–S19.

Greenberg, S. N., & Bello, R. P. (1996). The work hardening program and subsequent return to work of a client with low back pain. *Journal of Sports Physical Therapy, 24*(1), 37–45.

Haas, J. (1995). Ethical issues in physical medicine and rehabilitation. *Journal of Physical Medicine and Rehabilitation, 74*(1), S54–S58.

Hess, D. W., Ripley, D. L., McKinley, W. O., & Tewksbury, M. (2000). Predictors for return to work after spinal cord injury: A 3 year multicenter analysis. *Archives of Physical Medicine and Rehabilita-tion, 81*, 359–362.

Hoffman, C., Rice, D., & Sung, H. Y. (1996). Persons with chronic conditions. *Journal of the Ameri-can Medical Association, 276*, 1473–1479.

Horn, W., Yoels, W., & Bartolucci, A. (2000). Factors associated with patients' participation in rehabil-itation services: A comparative injury analysis 12 months post-discharge. *Disability and Rehabilita-tion, 22*(8), 358–362.

Iverson, G. L., & Binder, L. M. (2000). Detecting exaggeration and malingering in neuropsychological assessment. *Journal of Head Trauma and Rehabilitation, 15*(2), 829–858.

Jennings, B. (1993). Healing the self: The moral meaning of relationships in rehabilitation. *American Journal of Physical Medicine and Rehabilitation, 72*, 401–404.

Karjalainen, K., Melmivivaara, A., Tuldar, M., Roine, R., Jauhiainen, M., Hurri, H., & Koes, B. (2001). Multidisciplinary biopsychosocial rehabilitation for subacute low back pain in working-age adults. *Spine, 26*, 262–269.

Kessler, R. C., Greenberg, P. E., Mickelson, K. D., Meneades, L. M., & Wong, P. S. (2001). The ef-fects of chronic medical conditions on work loss and work cutback. *Journal of Occupational and Environmental Medicine, 43*, 218–225.

Kleinman, A. (1988). *The illness narratives.* New York: Basic Books.

Krause, J. S., & Anson, S. A. (1996). Employment after spinal cord injury: Relation to selected partici-pant characteristics. *Archives of Physical Medicine and Rehabilitation, 77*, 737–743.

Krause, J. S., Sternberg, M., Maides, J., & Lottes, S. (1998). Employment after spinal cord injury: Dif-ferences related to geographic region, gender, and race. *Archives of Physical Medicine and Rehabil-itation, 79*, 615–624.

Lechner, D. E., Bradbury, S. A., & Bradley, L. A. (1998). Detecting sincerity of effort: A summary of methods and approaches. *Physical Therapy, 78*, 867–888.

Lynch, J. W., Kaplan, G. A., & Shema, S. J. (1997). Cumulative impact of sustained economic hardship on physical, cognitive, psychological, and social functioning. *Massachusetts Medical Society, 337*(26), 1889–1895.

Main, C. J., & Waddell, G. (1998). Behavioral responses: A reappraisal of the interpretation of nonor-ganic signs. *Spine, 23*(21), 2367–2371.

McGrail, M. P., Lohman, W., & Gorman, R. (2001). Disability prevention principles in the primary care office. *American Family Physician, 63*(4), 679–684.

Melzack, R., & Wall, P. (1965). Pain mechanisms: A new theory. *Science, 150*, 971–979.

Morris, D. B. (1991). *The culture of pain.* Berkeley: University of California Press.

Neff, J. M., & Anderson, G. (1995). Protecting children with chronic illness in a competitive market-place. *Journal of the American Medical Association, 274*, 1866–1869.

Philipp, T., & Black, L. (1998). Financial impact. In I. M. Lubkin & P. D. Larsen (Eds.), *Chronic illness* (pp. 501–527). Sudbury, MA: Jones and Bartlett.

Rimmer, J. (1999). Health promotion for people with disabilities: The emerging paradigm shift from disability prevention to prevention of secondary conditions. *Physical Therapy, 79*(5), 495–502.

Rothstein, L. F. (1995). *Disability law*. Charlottesville, VA: LRP Publications.

Seigel, S., & Gaylord-Ross, R. (1991). Factors associated with employment success among youths with learning disabilities. *Journal of Learning Disabilities, 24*(1), 39–47.

Simon, J. (1989). A multidisciplinary approach to chronic pain. *Rehabilitation Nursing, 14*(1), 23–28.

Sutton, J. P., & DeJong, G. (1998). Managed care and people with disabilities: Framing the issues. *Archives of Physical Medicine and Rehabilitation, 79*, 1312–1316.

Tait, R. C., Chibnall, J. T., & Richardson, W. (1990). Litigation and employment status: Effects on patients with chronic pain. *Pain, 43*, 37–46.

van Hemert, A. M., Hengeveld, M. W., Bolk, J. H., Rooijmans, H. G., & van den Broucke, J. P. (1993). Psychiatric disorder in relation to medical illness among patients of a general medical outpatient clinic. *Psychological Medicine, 23*, 167–173.

Verbrugge, L. M., & Jette, A. M. (1994). The disablement process. *Social Science and Medicine, 38*(1), 1–14.

Waddell, G. (1987). A new clinical model for the treatment of low back pain. *Spine, 12*(7), 632–644.

Waddell, G. (1991). Occupational low-back pain, illness behavior, and disability. *Spine, 16*(6), 663–664.

Waddell, G., McCulloch, J. A., Kummel, E., & Venner, R. M. (1980). Nonorganic physical signs in low back pain. *Spine, 5*, 117–125.

Wehman, P., Sherron, P., Kregel, J., Kreutzer, J., Tran, S., & Chu, D. (1993). Return to work for persons following severe traumatic brain injury. *American Journal of Physical Medicine and Rehabilitation, 72*, 355–362.

Yelin, E. H., Trupin, L. S., & Sebesta, D. S. (1998). Transitions in employment and disability among persons ages 51–61 with musculoskeletal and nonmusculoskeletal conditions in the U.S. *Arthritis and Rheumatism, 42*(4), 769–779.

Yocum, D. F., Castro, W., & Cornett, L. (2000). Exercise, education, and behavioral modification as alternative therapy for pain and stress in rheumatic disease. *Rheumatic Disease Clinics of North America, 26*(1), 145–159.

# 16

# *Psychiatric Disorders*

I'm feeling so frustrated! I've been working with a client who I just can't seem to motivate, no matter what I do. Brian is an 18-year-old college student who had a terrible car accident three weeks ago. He was driving his car when he lost control and hit a tree. Fortunately, he was alone, so no one else was hurt, but he sustained injuries to his internal organs. He's coming to occupational therapy as an outpatient, but he just doesn't follow through on his exercises at home. He's not getting any stronger. I'm worried about him. He says that he's not sleeping well, and he looks like he's losing weight. Some days, he doesn't shave or shower before he comes to therapy. I think he wears the same clothes several days in a row. If it were me, I'd be working really hard so I could go back to school and hang out with my friends, but he just doesn't seem to care about any of that.

*—From the journal of Judy Goldstein, occupational therapy student*

Health care providers divide illness into two broad but distinct categories. Medical or physical illnesses affect the body and its organs. Mental or psychiatric disorders affect the mind or emotions. This simplistic division of illness creates misconceptions about mental illness. As we saw in Chapter 8, the mind and body function as a unified whole. Some mental illnesses, such as depression, have been proven to affect multiple organ systems, including the endocrine, cardiovascular, and immune systems (Insel & Charney, 2003). In addition, separating disorders of the body and mind does not acknowledge the effects that co-occurrence of medical and psychiatric illnesses have on the client's course of illness and recovery.

"Mental illness can be defined as a disturbance in an individual's thinking, emotions, behaviors, and physiology" (Glod, 1998, p. 9). It negatively affects mood and feelings, cognition, social interactions, and life-sustaining functions, such as eating, sleeping, focus and attention, and monitoring the environment for safety. There are times when we all experience some of the symptoms of various mental illnesses. For example, some of us may be "compulsive" about keeping our home and workspaces neat. Others may act impulsively or use poor judgment. However, in order for symptoms to reach a level of pathology, they must significantly impair the individual's ability to function effectively at work and social settings, consistent with cultural norms.

Currently close to 400 psychiatric conditions are included in the *Diagnostic and Statistical Manual IV-TR* (American Psychiatric Association, 2000). This text focuses on the description, diagnostic criteria, epidemiologic factors, and other information used as the standard of care for diagnosing and treating psychiatric disorders.

While each condition has distinct symptoms and creates unique challenges, all cause distress to the affected individual and his or her family and friends. It is important to recognize and diagnose these conditions because they can be treated. With appropriate care, many clients can manage their illness and enjoy an improved quality of life.

In this chapter, we will discuss mood disorders (depression and bipolar disorder) and anxiety disorders, including posttraumatic stress disorder. While schizophrenia can cause dramatic and disturbing symptoms of psychosis, the incidence of this disorder is only seen in 1 percent of the population and will not be discussed.

Serious psychiatric disorders present an array of symptoms that range from very mild to sufficiently severe to warrant hospitalization for safety. They have a complex interaction with medical disorders and can negatively affect the outcome of treatment or rehabilitation, resulting in increased morbidity and mortality (Koenig, 1998). Our goal in discussing these challenging conditions is to provide an awareness of important diagnostic features so that you may recognize symptoms that may explain the client's failure to make progress in treatment and warrant further diagnosis or referral to another provider.

The etiology of mental illness is complex and poorly understood. In the distant past, people who were seriously ill were believed to be possessed by demons or cursed by gods. In the not so distant past, inadequate parenting was believed to be the cause. Current research indicates that there are complex interactions between inherited genetic vulnerabilities and environmental triggers (Glod, 1998). It is now widely accepted that depression is a disease of the brain that can be triggered by environmental or social factors (National Institute of Mental Health, 2004).

An abnormal variation of a gene that controls the production of a serotonin transporter has been identified. One study followed 847 people for a period of five years, asking them to record adverse life stresses, such as a breakup of a relationship, loss of a job, loss of a loved one, or prolonged illness. Among the people who experienced four or more life stresses, 17 percent with two normal transporter genes developed depression, while 43 percent with two abnormal variations became depressed (Caspi et al., 2003).

Recent brain imaging studies with people diagnosed with depression revealed abnormalities that affect the regulation of neurotransmitters and various hormones (Insel & Charney, 2003). Abnormal gene variations have also been linked to anxiety (Hariri et al., 2002).

Medical illnesses frequently are comorbid, occur together, with psychiatric disorders. Although psychiatric illnesses are common, they are frequently undiagnosed (Katon, 1984). Physical diseases can usually be diagnosed with standardized measures, which indicate specific normal or abnormal test values. We can assess blood sugar levels, blood pressure, hematocrit values, strength, and pulmonary function. However, mood, emotional state, and level of arousal are subjective determinations. These assessments depend on the client's truthfulness, ability to communicate, and cooperation, as well as the skill of the mental health professional. Is someone "lazy" or depressed? What is the difference between high energy levels, enthusiasm, and mania? It is all a matter of degree.

Currently, one in ten Americans has a mental disorder, and over the course of a lifetime, one in five will develop a mental illness ("Surgeon General's Call to Action," 1999). Stigma and shame associated with mental illness often inhibit a client from disclosing a mental health diagnosis to the primary care provider, or the client may not disclose suspicious symptoms, even when they cause significant distress.

In addition, many primary care providers and nonmental health professionals do not screen for psychiatric disorders as a routine component of the physical examination (Katon, 1984). For example, despite evidence that there is a high correlation of low back pain and depression that results in a poor treatment outcome, many clients are not screened for depression. A study of physical therapists in Australia, who are able to treat clients without physician referral, revealed that they did not recognize the presence of depressive symptoms, even when the symptoms were more distinctive (Haggman, Maher, & Refshauge, 2004). When the researchers screened for depressive symptoms, 40 percent of the clients tested positive, with 23 percent having severe or extremely severe depression.

Only half of the individuals with psychiatric disorders seek care for their illness, and half of those who do seek care are never referred to a mental health professional. Although depression is a common psychiatric disorder with effective interventions, one study revealed that fewer than 50 percent of people with depression consulted their physicians (Kessler et al., 2003). Of those who sought care, only 42 percent received adequate care.

Medical disorders can mask the presence of psychiatric disorders, and psychiatric disorders can create symptoms that are not attributable to a medical condition or amplify symptoms of existing conditions (Katon, 1984; Schubert, Yokley, Sloan, & Gottesman, 1995). Many clients with psychiatric disorders seek care for physical complaints, such as headaches, chronic low back pain, gastrointestinal distress, insomnia, shortness of breath, or fatigue (Katon, 1984). A study of clients who visited a medical clinic with medically unexplained symptoms found that 42 percent had an undiagnosed psychiatric condition (Speckens, van Hemert, Bolk, Rooijmans, & Hengeveld, 1996).

It is important for health care providers to keep in mind that the occurrence of mental illness is significantly higher in people who are receiving medical care or rehabilitation services than in the general population (Silverstone, 1996). As many as one-third of clients with a medical condition may also have a psychiatric disorder (Everett, Dennis, & Ricketts, 1995; Silverstone, 1996). In addition, many clients seek care for somatic symptoms when the underlying cause is actually a psychiatric disorder (Friedman, 1997). The presence of a severe mental illness can complicate coexisting medical conditions and increase mortality rates. Clients with severe mental illness have higher rates of diabetes, cardiovascular, pulmonary, and renal diseases and have more intense forms of these disorders (Dixon, Goldberg, Lehman, & McNary, 2001).

Having a psychiatric disorder with a physical condition can complicate the care of both conditions. People with mental illness are more likely to engage in high-risk behaviors (Everett at al., 1995), which can lead to accidents, injuries, and unsafe sex. In a study of youth in juvenile detention, more than 70 percent of the girls and 65 percent of the boys had one or more psychiatric disorders. They were also significantly more likely to have substance abuse disorders (Abram, Teplin, McClelland, & Dulcan, 2003).

The presence of psychiatric disorders increases the utilization of health care services for clients with medical conditions. With comorbid conditions, the physical illness tends to have a longer duration, greater severity, and a higher level of disability. Morbidity for clients with a myocardial infarction with depression is three to four times higher than patients without depression. Medical costs for elderly clients with depression have been found to be 43 to 51 percent higher than for those without depression. Clients with congestive heart failure who are depressed have more severe functional impairments. There is also increased time lost from work (Kessler & Frank, 1997; Sampson, Benson, Beck, Price, & Nimmer, 1999; Steer, Cavalieri, Leonard, & Beck, 1999). These adverse outcomes may be partly due to clients with mental illness being three times more likely not to adhere to medical interventions and recommendations (DiMatteo, Lepper, & Groghan, 2000).

Physical disorders can also complicate the treatment of psychiatric conditions. Unfortunately, many clients with psychiatric disorders have physical diagnoses that are overlooked by the examining physician. In addition, clients with comorbid physical and mental illnesses are likely to have longer lengths of stay in psychiatric hospitals (Schubert et al., 1995). Treating all the factors that affect clients' health is important.

Another confounding factor in the assessment and treatment of people with mental illness is that many disorders are episodic. There may be significant periods of remission with high levels of function followed by periods of exacerbation. Personal stress and challenging life events may precipitate or trigger a recurrence of symptoms. This reinforces a belief that the individual is not really "ill" but rather is using the symptoms to avoid work or other responsibilities. For many health care providers, it is easier to feel empathy for a client with arthritis who has swollen and, apparently, painful joints than a client with severe depression, with "invisible" pain. It is even more difficult to feel empathy toward a client who refuses your care or screams at you to get out of the room.

When evaluating and treating clients with medical symptoms, it is important to be constantly aware of the possibility that mental illness may also be present. Having a low threshold of suspicion for psychiatric disorders may help health care professionals identify conditions that could complicate the course of medical treatment. Recognizing symptoms that suggest mental health problems will enable health care providers to make referrals to appropriate practitioners, improve the outcome of interventions, and, perhaps, prevent a suicide. Just as with physical illness, appropriate assessment, diagnosis, and intervention are crucial to a good outcome.

# Depression

In the journal entry at the beginning of this chapter, Brian might have major depression. For many years, we knew that depression was common in the clients treated in medical and rehabilitation settings. We assumed that the depression was a result of their physical condition or injury. After all, who would not be depressed following a spinal cord injury or heart attack? However, we now know that depression may be present premorbidly, that is, before the current injury. In addition, secondary to the depression, the clients may have behaved in ways that put them at risk for self-injury.

Depression is not synonymous with sadness or grief. As we discussed in Chapter 13, grieving is the normal, but variable, response to a loss. It can be the loss of a loved one, loss of something that is of significant importance to the individual such as a job or home, or loss of function due to illness or injury. Grief is a normal part of the mourning process, and the individual who is grieving may demonstrate profound sadness and hopelessness. This is often painful for friends or health care providers to witness (Weisman, 1998).

Someone who is experiencing "normal" grief, though, does not express a sense of worthlessness, severe guilt, or a desire to die. These are signs of depression. As health care providers, our response to those who are grieving is to listen compassionately and validate their feelings, without trying to mitigate their distress or "cheer them up." Over time, the mourning process usually ends, and the individual will hopefully be able to integrate the experience and resume all previous life activities.

Psychiatrists use the terms "clinical depression," "major depressive disorder (MDD)," or "unipolar depression" to diagnose someone who demonstrates severe depressive symptoms over a prolonged period of time. Major depression affects 10 percent of the general population and 17 percent of all adults (American Psychiatric Association, 1994). Women are twice as likely to be diagnosed with depression as men. It is a life-threatening illness and should be taken seriously. One in five clients with MDD dies by suicide, the eighth leading cause of death in the United States. For every successful suicide, there are eight to ten unsuccessful attempts. Failed suicide attempts account for 10 percent of general hospital admissions (Weisman, 1998).

It can be difficult for people who have never experienced major depression to understand or have empathy for those affected by this illness. We all have had "the blues" or felt sad or unhappy at some points in our lives. However, the number and severity of symptoms that are experienced by people with MDD distinguishes it from the milder mood swings that are common to us all. MDD causes role impairment in many aspects of the client's life, including work and social responsibilities, thinking, and self-care.

In one study, during a twelve-month period, 96 percent of people with depression reported significant role impairments, and on average, reported missing 35 days from work (Kessler et al., 2003). Although many clients attend work while depressed, they perform at suboptimal levels, resulting in lost productive time. Reduced concentration, needing to repeat a job, working more slowly, making errors, and feeling fatigue contribute to this decreased work performance (Stewart, Ricci, Chee, Hahn, & Morganstein, 2003). The burden of illness is magnified by the frequent comorbidity of other psychiatric disorders, commonly anxiety and substance abuse (Kessler et al., 2003).

> When you are in it, there is no empathy, no intellect, no imagination, no compassion, no humanity, no hope. It isn't possible to roll over in bed because the capacity to plan and execute the required steps is too difficult to master, and the physical skills are too hard to complete (Karp, 1996, p. 24).

According to the *Diagnostic and Statistical Manual of Mental Disorders*, "The essential feature of a major depressive episode is a period of at least two weeks during which there is either a depressed mood or the loss of interest and pleasure in nearly all activities. In children and adolescents, the mood may be irritable rather than sad" (American Psychiatric Association, 1994, p. 320). The diagnosis of depression is dependent on the presence of at least four additional symptoms listed in Table 16–1. It is interesting to note that being able to articulate a depressed mood is not an essential feature of the diagnosis of depression.

Table 16-1   Depression

| | |
|---|---|
| *Cognitive* | Helpless, hopeless, worthless<br>Decreased motivation<br>"Life is not worth living"<br>Suicidal thoughts<br>Impaired memory and concentration |
| *Physiologic* | Changes in appetite (increase or decrease)<br>Changes in sleeping (increase or decrease)<br>General feeling of malaise<br>Joint aches and pains<br>Slowed movements |
| *Mood/Emotion* | Sad, depressed<br>Flat affect<br>Feelings of guilt<br>Lack of joy or pleasure<br>Feeling bored or disinterested<br>World looks gray or empty |
| *Behavioral* | Social withdrawal<br>Isolation<br>Giving up previously pleasurable activities<br>Irritability<br>Appears to lack motivation<br>Angry or hostile |
| *Appraisal Problem* | Unable to access strategies to perform necessary daily tasks<br>Unable to make a decision and follow-through<br>Unable to accurately assess self-worth |

Social withdrawal, isolating behaviors, and loss of interest in previously pleasurable activities are equally as significant as a depressed mood. Many clients with depression describe feeling "empty" or lonely, even in the presence of loved ones. Children or adolescents may lack the language and cognitive experience to identify depression and often describe feeling "bored." For example, one depressed child described himself as feeling "hollow." This social withdrawal and loss of interest may be striking to friends and family members. However, lack of information about the symptoms of depression often prevents them from recognizing the importance of the behavior and knowing how to help or make referrals. Table 16–1 lists the key points of depression.

People who are experiencing an episode of major depression have an array of other symptoms in addition to a depressed mood, isolating behaviors, or loss of interest. Some clients act angry or irritable. Psychomotor agitation, such as restlessness, pacing, or undirected energy, is also common. Rather than sadness, irritability or anger may be expressed. Some clients with depression are short-tempered or verbally abusive. Others report loss of energy, fatigue, and a feeling of heaviness in the limbs. Clients sometimes describe feeling like they are moving through molasses or have heavy weights attached to their arms or legs. Many people with depression "self-medicate" with drugs or alcohol, which exacerbates the effects of depression.

There are significant cognitive changes associated with depression, such as poor ability to concentrate and loss of memory. In addition, there is a triad of behavioral signs that are a hallmark of depression. These signs include feeling worthless or unworthy, feeling negative or pessimistic about the future, and being unable to make a decision or a plan of action. Another way to describe this is feeling helpless, hopeless, and worthless. This may even be misinterpreted as poor motivation, like Brian's behavior, described in the opening journal entry of this chapter.

In addition to mood and cognition, depression also affects neurovegetative functions. There are usually changes in eating and sleeping patterns, with affected individuals doing too much or too little. Additional physical symptoms of depression include fatigue and physical complaints, such as headaches or backaches. Greater than 90 percent of clients with depression manifest physical symptoms (Stewart et al., 2003). Generally, the more severe the depression, the greater the number and intensity of symptoms. In addition, individuals with depression often "look" depressed, with a slouched posture, unkempt appearance, and slowed movements.

These disturbing symptoms interfere with the ability to function at school, work, or in social settings. Some people who are able to perform well, despite feeling depressed, report that it requires enormous energy. Consider Mr. Barrows, who attended a local outpatient department for treatment of an orthopedic disorder. He was also being treated by a psychiatrist for MDD. Mr. Barrows's physical therapist observed him as he entered the clinic to determine how he was feeling. On days when he was feeling well, he was immaculate, dressed in a clean shirt and tie, with neatly groomed hair. There was a spring in his step, and he cheerfully greeted the staff. On days when his mood was low, his appearance was sloppy, and he would wear rumpled clothing. He slowly entered the clinic, looking downward, and did not greet anyone. The perceptive clinician altered her interactions according to his mood. For example, on days when he was "low," she spoke more quietly and modified her expectations of the therapy session.

It is equally important to "tune in" when interviewing clients or taking a history. Changes in lifestyle or function may indicate depression. A study of physical therapists who treat outpatients with low back pain found that they are able to identify clients who are experiencing a depressive episode by asking two simple questions. The questions they ask are: "During the past month, have you been bothered by feeling down, depressed, or hopeless?" and "During the past month, have you been bothered by little interest or pleasure in doing things?" (Haggman et al., 2004). It only takes a little extra time to add these two questions when taking a client's history, and the answers may have a significant impact on the outcome of care.

If left untreated, depression can be life-threatening. In the adolescent or young adult population, risk-taking behaviors and a lack of concern for personal safety can be problematic. Listen carefully to clients with suicidal thoughts and let them know that you are concerned. Often, talking about their problems helps them feel better (Purtilo, 1999). When clients describe severe feelings of hopelessness, ask if they have ever considered suicide. If the answer is yes, ask if they have a plan. If the client has intention, a plan, and the means to commit suicide, an immediate referral to a mental health professional is mandated. You may need to make this referral without the client's consent.

Consider Linda, a young mother with a 3-week-old baby. She was attending a parenting skills class for first-time mothers. She told Doris, the nurse/instructor, that she was crying all the time. Doris followed up on this after class, and Linda admitted that she was so sad that she wanted to die. In fact, she had a plan. Her husband was out of town on a business trip, and she was estranged from her family. She was alone. Doris immediately contacted Linda's doctor, who arranged for a psychiatric evaluation that day.

## Dysthymia

Dysthymia, low or depressed mood, can last for two or more years (American Psychiatric Association, 1994). The distinguishing feature between dysthymia and MDD is the degree and number of symptoms. The client has too few symptoms to qualify for a diagnosis of depression, and the severity of the symptoms is not as great. Neurovegetative symptoms, such as changes in eating and sleeping patterns and physical discomfort, are either absent or are present to a lesser degree.

This condition is chronic and may be described as a "depressed personality." Even though the condition does not cause severe distress, clients are affected by the symptoms and do not experience life as fully as they might otherwise. In some cases, dysthymia may progress to MDD.

# Bipolar Spectrum Disorder

While 10 to 17 percent of the population experiences depressive illness, bipolar disorder occurs in only 1 to 2 percent of the population (Akiskal, 1996). In this disorder, symptoms are episodic. There are intervals of depression and mania, interspersed with periods of remission when clients may be symptom-free. It is a more complex disorder than depression alone, causes extreme emotional discomfort, and carries a higher morbidity and mortality rate. One in four individuals with bipolar disorder attempts suicide (Zornber & Pope, 1993). More than 50 percent of individuals with bipolar disorder abuse drugs or alcohol while ill in an effort to mitigate their symptoms ("Expert Consensus Treatment Guidelines for Bipolar Disorder," 1996).

Although the onset of depression can occur at any age, bipolar illness typically begins in young adults. Recent studies indicate that approximately 20 percent of clients with bipolar illness have their first episode between the ages of 15 and 19 (American Academy of Child and Adolescent Psychiatry [AACAP] Official Action, 1997). Children with bipolar illness have a different clinical picture than adults, making diagnosis much more challenging. Irritability, explosive anger, agitation, antisocial activity, and extreme risk-taking behaviors are the most typical signs of bipolar disorder in children and adolescents. The rate of substance abuse among adolescents is extremely high (Akiskal, 1995). Furthermore, the course of the disease in adolescents tends to be chronic rather than episodic, as in adults.

Interestingly, there is significant overlap between children with attention-deficit/hyperactivity disorder (ADHD) and bipolar disorder. Twenty percent of individuals with ADHD develop bipolar disorder, while 98 percent of people with adolescent-onset bipolar disorder have ADHD (Wozniak et al., 1995). The behavior of children with ADHD and bipolar disorder is characterized by violent, aggressive, "affective storms."

During an episode of mania, a client may be either manic or hypomanic. "A manic episode is defined by a distinct period during which there is an abnormally and persistently elevated, expansive, or irritable mood" (American Psychiatric Association, 1994, p. 346). This elevated mood must last for at least one week or be severe enough to warrant hospitalization. Many people interpret an "elevated" mood to be one of extreme happiness or euphoria. In fact, mania is often anything but a happy event. Someone who is "going high," or moving into a manic state, may have a period of elation or happiness, but this quickly progresses to a state of expansive thinking and poor judgment. The behavior of a client in a manic state is often "out of control."

Hypomania is an elevated mood that is not high enough, severe enough, or does not demonstrate sufficient symptoms to be true mania. The level of severity is comparable to dysthymia, part of the depressive disorders. Some clients pass through a state of hypomania on their way to mania, while others do not progress beyond it.

In addition to the elevated or irritable mood, an individual must demonstrate at least three additional symptoms to be considered manic (American Psychiatric Association, 1994). These may include feelings of inflated importance or grandiosity. For example, a college student with grandiose ideas thought that she could fly. She decided to soar out her dormitory window to a better place. Fortunately, she believed that she would need to take her clothes with her. Thinking the clothing could also fly, she threw it out the window first. Someone on the ground noticed this and called for help—a call that saved her life. Other examples of grandiose ideas include making impossible business plans or thinking of oneself as an extremely powerful and important person, such as one with special religious powers. Refer to Table 16–2 for a summary of key aspects of mania.

While in a manic state, clients commonly feel invincible and believe that no harm can come to them. This poor judgment, combined with hyperactivity or psychomotor agitation, can lead to dangerous ideas and serious risk-taking behaviors without concern for personal

**TABLE 16–2** Mania

| | |
|---|---|
| *Cognitive* | Grandiose thinking—I can do anything! |
| | Invulnerability—Nothing can hurt me! |
| | Decreased ability to assess risks—physical, social, financial |
| | Significant lack of concern for safety |
| | In advanced stages, thoughts are chaotic and disorganized |
| *Physiologic* | Decreased need for sleep |
| | Extremely high energy levels |
| | Loss of perceived need to eat or drink |
| *Mood/Emotion* | Elevated, expansive mood |
| | Feeling "high"—I can accomplish anything! |
| | Agitated, irritable, angry |
| *Behavioral* | May be hostile, aggressive, or belligerent |
| | Rapid, incessant talking |
| | Disregard for needs of others |
| | Creative, flight of ideas |
| | Engages in dangerous behaviors, without regard to safety |
| | Hypersexuality |
| | "Out of control" |
| *Appraisal Problem* | Lacks safety awareness—frequently engages in extremely high-risk behaviors |

safety. For example, people may drive recklessly, get into arguments or fistfights, walk down the middle of a highway, or commit crimes.

Mania also affects the quality and style of speech. Clients may exhibit "pressured speech" (American Psychiatric Association, 1994), talking incessantly about topics of interest only to themselves. It is often impossible to interrupt or redirect them. In addition, their social interactions may be domineering, intrusive, and demanding, "like a bulldozer," as one mother described her daughter. The manic individual often experiences racing thoughts with an uncontrolled flight of ideas. Many of these thoughts are disordered and irrational.

Like depression, mania also causes changes in neurovegetative functions. There is increased energy, with a decreased need for sleep, and a loss of appetite. However, many clients who are in a hypomanic state enjoy this "high" and have productive, creative energy. This productive state may not last. If the hypomania escalates into a full manic episode, judgment and cognitive ability deteriorate.

# Anxiety Disorders

Mrs. Doyle complains all the time. Nothing is ever right for her. I'm treating her for neck and upper back pain, but no matter what I suggest, she has a reason why she can't do it. Every time I touch her, she winces and jumps a foot into the air. She acts like I'm attacking her in some way. I'm only trying to help! She's not getting any better, and I know that the number of visits allowed by her insurance company will soon run out. She told me that she has had two emergency room visits in the last three months because she thought she was having a heart attack. Her heart was pounding, she was sweating profusely, and she was short of breath. When she got there, they couldn't find anything wrong with her. I don't know what to try next.
—*From the journal of Jennifer Kite, physical therapist student*

Feelings of anxiety are not uncommon. They may range from mild, like when facing a difficult test in school, to intense, such as planning a wedding, making a career change, or ending a relationship. These anxious feelings do not usually impair our ability to function or make us give up activities we enjoy. However, some people experience feelings of anxiety that are out of proportion to the intensity of the situational threat or persist longer than is typical. These individuals are experiencing some form of anxiety disorder. Nine percent of Americans are currently affected by anxiety disorders, with a lifetime incidence of 15 percent (Sussman, 1993).

The term *anxiety* comes from the Latin word *angere,* which means to choke or strangle (Buehl, Hesson, & Dimyen, 1993). This is probably because many clients who have feelings of anxiety experience intense sensations of physical distress, including feeling that they cannot breathe or are choking. Anxiety is a diagnostic term, covering a broad range of psychiatric disorders that share the common feature of feeling fearful. Here we discuss symptoms common to anxiety disorders as well as describe several specific disorders. In general, all anxiety disorders are characterized by symptoms that can be grouped into three categories: disorders of thought, physical sensations, and avoidance behaviors.

Several cognitive manifestations have been documented with anxiety disorders (American Psychiatric Association, 1994; Noyes, Roth, & Burrows, 1990). Clients may report irrational beliefs about themselves or their environment. They may have a negative self-concept and self-perception and pessimistically interpret information. Many individuals with anxiety overestimate the risk involved in their daily lives and are hypervigilant for environmental stimuli or cues. Refer to Table 16–3 for a summary of key aspects of anxiety disorders.

Clients with anxiety often fear losing control, feel that the worst is going to happen, or report feeling terrified. These thoughts have been termed "catastrophization." For example, every headache "becomes" a brain tumor, every joint pain is arthritis, and any social *faux pas* threatens social standing. Clients with anxiety disorders describe being unable to relax or feel calm.

Physical symptoms often accompany anxiety, such as increased heart rate, sweating, and hyperventilation (Glod, 1998). Clients report restlessness, fatigue, poor memory or concentration, irritability, and disturbed sleep (AACAP, 1997). In addition, many clients report somatic sensations for which there is no apparent cause, such as headaches, backaches, stomachaches, nausea, or feeling dizzy, shaky, or faint. Many overutilize the health care system and frequently seek emergency room evaluations for symptoms that have no physical basis (Stern, Herman, & Slavin, 1998).

These cognitive and physical symptoms are unpleasant and troublesome to the client. Therefore, in an attempt to eliminate situations that trigger their anxiety, they tend to exhibit avoidance behaviors. Since anxiety causes overstimulation of the sympathetic nervous system, we typically see fight-or-flight behaviors, as described in Chapter 8. Clients may rigidly structure their schedules or environment to eliminate fear-producing stimuli or unexpected situations.

**TABLE 16–3**    Anxiety Disorders

| | |
|---|---|
| *Cognitive* | Irrational fears, worry, apprehension<br>Impaired memory and concentration |
| *Physiologic* | Somatization—aches, pains, discomforts, without a physical cause<br>Increased sympathetic arousal—increased heart rate, blood pressure, palpitations, sweating, shortness of breath, increased muscle tension<br>Nausea, gastrointestinal distress, dizziness, parasthesias |
| *Mood/Emotion* | "Anxious" thoughts and feelings, terror<br>Irrational fears<br>May be constant (generalized anxiety disorder) or transient (panic disorder, social or other phobias) |
| *Behavioral* | Very emotionally "needy"<br>Very demanding behavior<br>Constantly asking for reassurance and guidance<br>May repeatedly request help when making simple decisions<br>May exhibit rigid and controlling behaviors<br>Avoids anxiety-producing situations—may be noncompliant<br>Restless, pacing movements, unable to sit still |
| *Appraisal Problem* | Catastrophization—every molehill becomes a mountain<br>Somatization—amplification of somatic symptoms |

## Generalized Anxiety Disorder

Symptoms of anxiety may be present all the time or may be episodic in nature. Generalized anxiety disorder (GAD) is characterized by a persistently high level of tension, with pervasive feelings of anxiety and apprehension, loss of appetite, difficulty concentrating, restlessness, sleep disturbances, and feelings of overarousal.

Some health providers refer to clients with anxiety as "the worried well." In addition, these clients may stress the resources of the health care provider by making frequent demands for information and assurances that all is well. They may emotionally cling to the provider for support and guidance, repeatedly asking the same questions. These clients may be rigid or manipulative and have difficulty adjusting to the demands of the health care setting because they fear losing control.

## Social and Other Phobias

Many individuals with anxiety also have specific phobias that trigger the symptoms to appear or worsen. A phobia is an intense fear of an event, object, person, or situation. The fear, which occurs whenever the triggering event is present, is intense and not under voluntary control (American Psychiatric Association, 1994). Social phobias include the fear of public speaking or performing one's job in front of others. Some clients fear behaving in a socially awkward manner and causing embarrassment to themselves or their families. Others avoid leaving their homes or familiar settings. Many clients take elaborate steps to avoid an anxiety-producing situation, such as refusing to drive over a bridge or avoiding contact with a dog.

## Panic Disorder

A panic attack is defined as a sudden intense feeling of anxiety. Literally a sympathetic nervous system cascade, it may be so overwhelming in its intensity that the person feels that he or she is going insane or will die. To establish a diagnosis, the individual must experience at least four of the following symptoms during the episode (American Psychiatric Association, 1994):

- Pounding heart
- Sweating
- Trembling
- Choking or smothering sensations
- Chest pain
- Nausea
- Dizziness
- Depersonalization
- Fear of losing control
- Fear of dying
- Numbness or tingling
- Hot or cold flashes

Clients are diagnosed with panic disorder when they have frequent panic attacks that cause them significant concern. Cassano and Savino (1993) described a clinical spectrum of symptoms and difficulties that occur under the umbrella of panic disorder. Clients may experience anticipatory anxiety, caused by the fear of having a panic attack, as well as specific phobias, related to places or events where panic attacks occurred. Catastrophization of physical symptoms, described earlier, can occur.

Although it is of brief duration, usually lasting no more than 10 minutes, the severe intensity of the panic attack can be alarming. While the episode itself is brief, the social and emotional sequelae can be disabling. In the extreme, a client may become homebound (Cassano & Savino, 1993). Consider a middle-age woman who did not visit her grandchildren because she would need to drive on the highway to an unfamiliar, larger city two hours away. She was also not comfortable having them visit her because her home was "too small," and they disrupted her routines. Furthermore, she was always "sick" with vague ailments, which made it even more difficult to tolerate visits. Sadly, she and her grandchildren were unable to develop a relationship.

Health care providers can support the needs of clients with anxiety disorders by understanding the cognitive, physical, and behavioral symptoms they present. Avoiding unnecessary tests and procedures could save health care dollars. Clients would also be spared the discomfort and inconvenience of these procedures. Most importantly, if anxiety is properly diagnosed and treated, clients may experience a reduction of their troubling symptoms and have an improved quality of life.

## Posttraumatic Stress Disorder

Posttraumatic stress disorder (PTSD) is another anxiety disorder. It is unique because it only occurs after clients have experienced a traumatic event that is perceived by the clients to put themselves or a loved one at risk for death or serious injury (American Psychiatric Association, 1994). A diagnosis of PTSD in adults is based on the presence of a cluster of symptoms: reexperiencing the traumatic event, hyperarousal and hypervigilant behaviors, and avoidance of stimuli that trigger memories of the event (deVries et al., 1999). In contrast, children may express their emotions as agitation or disorganized behavior.

There are many types of events that may cause this disorder, including rape, domestic violence, war experiences, torture, and surviving a natural disaster. Exposure alone to a traumatic event is not sufficient to trigger PTSD. The exposed individual must respond to the event with extreme fear and helplessness. Studies of survivors of motor vehicle accidents and their loved ones demonstrate that a person does not need to be injured to develop PTSD; simply experiencing the fear of death or injury is sufficient cause (deVries et al., 1999; Jeavons, Greenwood, & deHorne, 2000). As many as 50 percent of motor vehicle accident survivors develop PTSD. Half still manifest symptoms one year after the accident.

Medical procedures, prolonged illness and disability, and sudden onset of medical crises may also trigger PTSD (Alonzo, 2000). This may be especially important for clients with cancer, human immunodeficiency virus (HIV), and cardiac conditions that require extensive invasive procedures and involve the threat of dying (Rourke, Stuber, Hobbie, & Kazak, 1999). The symptoms of PTSD involve avoiding situations that trigger memories of traumatic events. Consider what may happen when the triggering event is a medical procedure or setting. Clients may be unable to adhere to medical treatment plans or prescribed medication and may miss appointments (Alonzo, 2000). PTSD can have a significant impact on the client's symptoms and response to medical care.

The incidence of the disorder is variable, with estimates of its frequency ranging from 7 to 9 percent. PTSD is more prevalent in areas where there is war and political upheaval. Among individuals who have been exposed to violence, as many as 51 percent may develop the disorder (Sampson et al., 1999). Most of these clients will not present to their primary care provider with symptoms of PTSD but have complaints about symptoms in other areas. Furthermore, individuals who have been abused or traumatized as children are more likely to develop this disorder after a traumatic event they experience as an adult (Glod, 1998). Six months after the traumatizing event, 50 percent of survivors still experience symptoms of the disorder (American Psychiatric Association, 1994).

Many mental health practitioners feel PTSD is underdiagnosed due to medical practitioners' failure to question their clients about prior exposure to abuse or trauma. Zimmerman and Mattia (1999) found that 80 percent of clients with PTSD were undiagnosed in general emergency room screenings.

There are three clusters of symptoms that must be present for a diagnosis of PTSD to be made (refer to Table 16–4 for a summary of key aspects of PTSD). One cluster of symptoms involves persistent reexperiencing of the traumatic event. This can happen in a number of ways. Some clients have intrusive, disturbing thoughts of the event, perhaps in dreams or flashbacks. Seemingly innocuous cues or events may trigger these thoughts. The health care professional may unknowingly trigger these reactions by being in an environment where medical equipment and procedures occur. People who have experienced torture may have

**TABLE 16–4**  Posttraumatic Stress Disorder (PTSD)

| | |
|---|---|
| *Cognitive* | Painful reexperiencing of traumatic event(s) |
| | Flashbacks |
| | Intrusive thoughts or memories |
| | May have amnesia for the event |
| *Physiologic* | Hypervigilance |
| | Hyperresponsiveness to stimuli |
| | Increased levels of sympathetic nervous system arousal |
| | Increased startle reactions |
| | Insomnia |
| *Mood/Emotion* | Emotional numbing |
| | Flat affect |
| | Feeling disconnected from reality—dissociation |
| *Behavioral* | Persistent avoidance of emotionally charged people, places, and events |
| | Persistent avoidance of triggers for memories of traumatic event(s) |
| | Irritability |
| | Self-injurious behavior |
| | Poor impulse control |
| *Appraisal Problem* | Faulty judgment of current environment for safety, based on memories of past traumatic event(s) |
| | Hypersensitivity to danger cues |

flashbacks triggered by the presence of medical equipment or having a body part restrained. For example, being confined to a small space, having traumatized body parts examined (i.e., a gynecological examination for a woman who has been sexually abused), and undergoing uncomfortable procedures may be unbearable to clients with this disorder. Even gentle physical contact may not be tolerated.

A second cluster of symptoms includes avoidance behaviors, such as avoiding physical or emotional stimuli associated with the traumatic event. Clients may refuse to talk about the event or discuss related situations. Survivors typically avoid activities, places, or people that can trigger memories of the event. For example, a student who has been sexually assaulted at school may be unable to return to school. These avoidance behaviors can severely limit the client's ability to function and enjoy life.

Another form of avoidance behavior is to become emotionally detached or to dissociate from the distressing event (American Psychiatric Association, 1994). This interferes with the client's ability to develop relationships with others. The person's emotional affect is often flat. The client may dissociate or experience an altered mental state. In a popular series of children's books, the main character, Harry Potter, dissociates while he experiences flashbacks of watching the murder of his parents.

> An intense cold swept over them all. Harry felt his own breath catch in his chest. The cold went deeper than his skin. It was inside his chest; it was inside his very heart. Harry's eyes rolled up into his head. He couldn't see. He was drowning in cold. There was a rushing in his ears as though of water. He was being dragged downward, the roaring growing louder. And then, from far away, he heard screaming, terrible, terrified, pleading screams. He wanted to help whoever it was, to move his arms, but couldn't—a thick white fog was swirling around him, inside him (Rowling, 1999, pp. 83–84).

The third cluster of symptoms arises from a persistent state of hypervigilance (Glod, 1998). This is a consequence of the sympathetic nervous system being chronically overaroused as it constantly monitors the environment for danger and triggers the alarm at the earliest sign of threat. There is a hyperactive startle response and difficulty focusing, paying attention, sleeping, and eating. There also may be irritability and outbursts of anger.

For a diagnosis of PTSD to be made, these symptoms must last for at least one month. Many would argue that the symptoms of PTSD are a normal response to an overwhelming situation. However, it becomes pathological when the stimulus (danger) has passed and the response continues. The personality and coping style of the client, the strength of the individual, the nature of the trauma, and the past experiences of the client are contributing factors in the development of this disorder (Everett et al., 1995).

There is a range of symptoms associated with PTSD and other anxiety disorders that are significant for health care providers. The overactivity of the sympathetic nervous system can lead to dysfunction of the cardiopulmonary system, manifested in hyperventilation, shortness of breath, and increased blood pressure and heart rate. Increased muscle tension may result in back and neck problems or other joint pain, as well as fatigue and an increased susceptibility to injury. Clients may also experience gastrointestinal distress, dizziness, and headaches. Proper diagnosis of the cause of these complaints is necessary for appropriate and effective treatment.

# Implications for Health Care Professionals

Each health care discipline has its own role to play in providing care for clients who have physical and psychiatric disorders. It is beyond the scope of this text to address each individually, but there are strategies that may be useful to all disciplines. It is common for new psychiatric residents to be told, "When interviewing clients, you should listen to the music, not the song." The implication is that while the clients may appear to be speaking coherently, their actions and demeanor may not "make sense." Impaired judgment, slovenly appearance, risky behavior, off-putting comments, and general social incompetence carry a powerful message.

Confidentiality is an ethic that we are obligated to observe with all our clients. There is, however, an exception to this rule. If you believe that clients present a risk to themselves or to the safety of others, confidentiality must be broken and appropriate authorities informed. The ethics of nonmaleficence (to do no harm) and beneficence (to provide the best possible care) supercede the client's right to confidentiality. Of course, this information is given only on a "need-to-know" basis and is not shared with others (Purtilo, 1999).

Remember that clients with mental health disorders usually present with neurovegetative symptoms, such as changes in eating or sleeping patterns, altered states of arousal, hyperventilation, cardiovascular changes, and changes in muscle tone. When we perform our assessments, we need to ask about these functions. We must focus our evaluations and interventions on determining the scope of the client's problems and treating the symptoms for which we are responsible. We need to develop mechanisms to refer clients to the appropriate professionals when necessary. If we feel comfortable asking follow-up questions and making referrals, the client may also feel comfortable.

Clients with psychiatric disorders may present with altered levels of sensory perception (Everett et al., 1995). It is our responsibility to assess how the client responds to us and to the environment. Then we must individualize our approach. This may mean lowering the level of sensory stimulation by providing a calm, quiet treatment environment with a structured, nonhurried approach. Other clients may respond better to increasing the level of stimulation or making the activities more exciting. It is imperative that we always ask the client's permission before initiating physical contact and continue to seek approval as we proceed.

We must establish a therapeutic relationship built on trust and create an environment in which the client feels safe. This may take longer to do than you or your administration would like, but it is time well spent. Any client who comes for a health care visit may have a mental health problem that he or she may not disclose. Therefore, it is crucial to proceed cautiously with all clients. Respect clients' responses to your questions and work within their tolerance. Using nonthreatening postures, as discussed in Chapter 2, also helps establish trust.

Aerobic and nonaerobic activities can be beneficial for the treatment of clients with depression and anxiety (Byrne & Byrne, 1993; Martinson, 1987). Health care providers can incorporate physical activity into their recommended treatment regime. Exercise that is enjoyable and goal-oriented for the client is most effective (Everett et al., 1995). Walking, hanging up the laundry, performing household chores, or joining an activity group may all be useful. Ask your clients what they enjoy and follow their lead. Nurses, social workers, nutritionists, and others may find this strategy a beneficial addition to incorporate into their plans of care.

Finally, we must not forget to take care of our own mental health needs. Working with clients who are physically or mentally ill can be stressful, and the behavior of clients with mental illness can be challenging. In order to provide the best quality care, we must be calm, focused, and able to cope with unexpected and difficult events. Practicing what we preach in terms of taking care of ourselves will set a healthy example for our clients and help us be more competent and effective care providers.

## SUMMARY

This chapter explored several common psychiatric diagnoses: depression, bipolar spectrum disorder, and anxiety disorders, including posttraumatic stress disorder. Diagnostic features of these disorders were described, as well as the effects of these symptoms on coexisting physical disorders. In addition, strategies for health care professionals to use when treating clients with psychiatric disorders were presented. We need to recognize and address every presenting symptom and provide treatment or referral as appropriate.

## REFLECTIVE QUESTIONS

1. a. What has been your personal experience with the mental illnesses described in this chapter?
   b. Do you or anyone you are close to have any of these illnesses?
   c. What symptoms have you observed or experienced?
   d. How did these symptoms affect the person's ability to function? How did they affect interpersonal relationships?
   e. What are your feelings about these experiences (positive or negative)? Did you feel scared, embarrassed, or safe? Why?
2. a. What have been your experiences with clients who have a diagnosis of mental health?
   b. What symptoms have you observed?
   c. How did these symptoms affect the client's ability to function?
   d. How did these symptoms affect the client's ability to participate in medical interventions/therapy? To achieve goals?
   e. What are your feelings about these experiences (positive or negative)? Did you feel scared, frustrated, or safe? Why?
3. a. Do you think that people with a mental illness should be integrated into the community? Why or why not?
   b. Do you think that people with a mental illness should receive more or fewer support services? Why or why not?
   c. What forms of treatment do you think are most effective for people with mental illness? Why?
4. a. What do you think is the role of your profession in treating people with mental illness who come to you for care?
   b. What techniques or strategies can you use to provide the best possible care to meet all of the client's needs?
   c. When do you think you will need to refer the client to someone else or seek an outside consultation? To whom might you refer the client or consult?

5. When working with people with mental illness:
    a. What stress management strategies might you use for yourself?
    b. How will you keep yourself calm when dealing with challenging behavior?
    c. What professional supports or information might you need? Where can you find them?

## CASE STUDY

Mr. Richards is a 68-year-old man with a history of cardiac disease. Recently discharged from the hospital following coronary artery bypass graft surgery, he now comes to your facility as an outpatient. He is having increasing difficulty following directions, staying focused and concentrating, and remembering what to do. His progress has been very slow. Mr. Richards lives alone since his wife died two years ago, but his sister comes to his home every day to help. Although he says that he is very lonely, he has given up going to church and playing cards with friends. He also says that he does not see the point of working hard with his postsurgical exercise regime because he will not be using the skills the health professionals are trying to help him learn.

1. Mr. Richards' social withdrawal, isolating behaviors, and loss of interest in activities that were previously enjoyable raise warning flags of a depressed mood, among other possibilities.
    a. What questions need to be asked to clarify the situation?
    b. How can these questions be phrased to avoid offending or embarrassing Mr. Richards?
2. What impact might these symptoms have on his progress in cardiac rehabilitation?
3. a. What is the most appropriate plan of action to address Mr. Richards' symptoms?
    b. What referrals might be helpful?
    c. How can this plan be discussed with Mr. Richards to ensure his collaboration?
4. How can the cardiac rehabilitation plan of care be adjusted to accommodate these challenges?

## REFERENCES

Abram, K. M., Teplin, L. A., McClelland, G. M., & Dulcan, M. K. (2003). Comorbid psychiatric disorders in youth in juvenile detention. *Archives of General Psychiatry, 60* (11), 1097–1108.

Akiskal, H. (1996). The prevalent clinical spectrum of bipolar disorders: Beyond DSM-IV. *Journal of Clinical Psychopharmacology, 16*(2, Suppl.), 4s–14s.

Alonzo, A. (2000). The experience of chronic illness and post-traumatic stress disorder: The consequences of cumulative adversity. *Social Science and Medicine, 50,* 1475–1484.

American Academy of Child and Adolescent Psychiatry (AACAP) Official Action. (1997). Practice parameters for the assessment and treatment of children and adolescents with bipolar disorders. *Journal of the American Academy of Child and Adolescent Psychiatry, 36*(10, Suppl.), 157s–176s.

American Psychiatric Association. (1994). *Diagnostic and statistical manual of mental disorders* (4th ed.). Washington, DC: Author.

American Psychiatric Association. (2000). *Diagnostic and statistical manual IV—text revision* (4th ed.). Washington, DC: Author.

Buehl, D., Hesson, K., & Dimyen, S. (1993). Anxiety and somatic awareness. In K. Craig & K. Dobson (Eds.), *Anxiety and depression in adults and children* (pp. 265–284). London: Sage.

Byrne, A., & Byrne, D. G. (1993). The effect of exercise on depression, anxiety, and other mood states: A review. *Journal of Psychosomatic Research, 37*(6), 565–574.

Caspi, A., Sugden, K., Moffitt, T. E., Taylor, A., Craig, I. W., Harrington, H., McClay, J., Mill, J., Martin, J., Braithwaite, A., & Poulton, R. (2003). Influence of life stress on depression: Moderation by a polymorphism in the 5-HTT gene. *Science, 301* (5631), 386–389.

Cassano, G. B., & Savino, M. (1993). Symptomatology of panic disorder: An attempt to define the panic-agoraphobic spectrum phenomenology. In K. Craig & K. Dobson (Eds.), *Anxiety and depression in adults and children* (pp. 185–211). London: Sage.

deVries, A., Kassam-Adams, N., Cnaan, A., Sherman-Slate, E., Gallagher, P., & Winston, F. (1999). Looking beyond the physical injury: Post-traumatic stress disorder in children and parents after pediatric traffic injury. *Pediatrics, 104*(6), 1293–1299.

DiMatteo, M. R., Lepper, H. S., & Groghan, T. W. (2000). Depression is a risk factor for noncompliance with medical treatment: Meta-analysis of the effects of anxiety and depression on patient adherence. *Archives of Internal Medicine, 160* (14), 2101–2106.

Dixon, L., Goldberg, R., Lehman, A., & McNary, S. (2001). The impact of health status on work, symptoms and functional outcomes in severe mental illness. *Journal of Nervous Mental Disease, 189* (1), 17–23.

Everett, T., Dennis, M., & Ricketts, E. (1995). *Physiotherapy in mental health*. London: Butterworth-Heinemann.

Expert consensus treatment guidelines for bipolar disorder: A guide for patients and families. (1996). *Journal of Clinical Psychiatry, 57*(Suppl. 12A), 1–8.

Friedman, M. (1997). Post-traumatic stress disorder. *Journal of Clinical Psychiatry, 58*(Suppl. 9), 33–36.

Glod, C. (1998). *Contemporary psychiatric-mental health nursing*. Philadelphia: F. A. Davis.

Haggman, S., Maher, C. G., & Refshauge, K. M. (2004). Screening for symptoms of depression by physical therapists managing low back pain. *Physical Therapy, 84* (12), 1157–1166.

Hariri, A. R., Mattay, V. S., Tessitore, A., Kolachana, B., Fera, F., Goldman, D., Egan, M. F., & Weinberger, D. R. (2002). Serotonin transporter genetic variation and the response of the human amygdala. *Science, 297* (5580), 400–403.

Insel, T. R., & Charney, D. S. (2003). Research on major depression: Strategies and priorities. *Journal of the American Medical Association, 289* (23), 3167–3168.

Jeavons, S., Greenwood, K., & deHorne, D. (2000). Accident cognitions and subsequent psychological trauma. *Journal of Traumatic Stress, 13*(23), 359–365.

Karp, D. (1996). *Speaking of sadness*. New York: Oxford University Press.

Katon, W. (1984). Depression: Relationship to somatization and chronic medical illness. *Journal of Clinical Psychiatry, 45*(3), 4–11.

Kessler, R. C., Berglund, P., Demler, O., Jin, R., Koretz, D., Merikangas, K. R., Rush, A. J., Walters, E. E., & Wang, P. S. (2003). The epidemiology of major depressive disorder: Results from the National Comorbidity Survey Replication. *Journal of the American Medical Association, 289* (23), 3095–3105.

Kessler, R., & Frank, R. (1997). The impact of psychiatric disorders on work loss days. *Psychological Medicine, 27*, 861–873.

Koenig, H. G. (1998). Depression in hospitalized older patients with congestive heart failure. *General Hospital Psychiatry, 20* (1), 29–43.

Martinson, E. W. (1987). The role of exercise in the treatment of depression. *Stress Medicine, 3*, 93–100.

National Institute of Mental Health. (2004). Depression research at the National Institute of Mental Health. In *National Institute of Mental Health*. [Online]. Available: http://www.nimh/nih.gov/publicat/depresfact.cfm. Date accessed: 6/6/05.

Noyes, R., Roth, M., & Burrows, G. D. (Eds.). (1990). *A handbook of anxiety* (4th ed.). New York: Elsevier.

Purtilo, R. (1999). *Ethical dimensions in the health professions* (3rd ed.). Philadelphia: W. B. Saunders.

Rourke, M. T., Stuber, M. L., Hobbie, W. L., & Kazak, A. (1999). Post-traumatic stress disorder: Understanding the psychological impact of surviving childhood cancer into young adulthood. *Journal of Oncology Nursing, 16*(3), 126–135.

Rowling, J. K. (1999). *Harry Potter and the prisoner of Azkaban.* New York: Scholastic.

Sampson, A., Benson, S., Beck, A., Price, D., & Nimmer, C. (1999). Post-traumatic stress disorder in primary care. *Journal of Family Practice, 48*(3) 222–227.

Schubert, D., Yokley, J., Sloan, D., & Gottesman, H. (1995). Impact of the interaction of depression and physical illness on a psychiatric unit's length of stay. *General Hospital Psychiatry, 17,* 326–334.

Silverstone, P. (1996). Prevalence of psychiatric disorders in medical patients. *Journal of Nervous and Mental Diseases, 84*(1), 43–50.

Speckens, A. E. M., van Hemert, A. M., Bolk, J. H., Rooijmans, H. G. M., & Hengeveld, M. W. (1996). Unexplained physical symptoms: Outcome, utilization of medical care and associated factors. *Psychological Medicine, 26,* 745–752.

Steer, R., Cavalieri, T., Leonard, D., & Beck, A. (1999). Use of the Beck inventory for primary care to screen for major depression disorders. *General Hospital Psychiatry, 21,* 106–111.

Stern, T., Herman, J., & Slavin, J. (1998). *The Massachusetts General Hospital (MGH) guide to psychiatry in primary care.* New York: McGraw-Hill.

Stewart, W. F., Ricci, J. A., Chee, E., Hahn, S., Morganstein, D. (2003). Cost of lost productive work time among US workers with depression. *Journal of the American Medical Association, 289* (23), 3135-3144.

Surgeon General's call to action to prevent suicide [Online]. (1999). Available: http://www. surgeongeneral.gov/osg/call to action

Sussman, N. (1993). Treating anxiety while minimizing abuse and dependence. *Journal of Clinical Psychiatry, 54*(5), 57–64.

Weisman, A. (1998). The patient with acute grief. In T. Stern, J. Herman, & J. Slavin (Eds.), *The Massachusetts General Hospital (MGH) guide to psychiatry in primary care* (pp. 25–31). New York: McGraw-Hill.

Wozniak, J., Biederman, J., Kiely, K., Albon, S., Faraone, S., Mundy, E., & Mennin, D. (1995). Manic-like symptoms suggestive of childhood-onset bipolar disorder in clinically-referred children. *Journal of the American Academy of Child and Adolescent Psychiatry, 34*(7), 867–876.

Zimmerman, M., & Mattia, J. (1999). Is post-traumatic stress disorder underdiagnosed in routine clinical settings? *Journal of Nervous and Mental Disease, 187*(7), 420–428.

Zornber, G., & Pope, H. (1993). Treatment of depression in bipolar disorder: New directions for research. *Journal of Clinical Psychopharmacology, 13*(6), 397–406.

# 17

# *Destructive Behaviors*

Heather Pomeroy came into the infant follow-up clinic again today with Paul, who is now 4 months old. When he was born, he was small for gestational age, which is why we are monitoring him. He's not developing as quickly as expected, and his head is still floppy. The doctor says he has low muscle tone. Despite our help, his weight is not catching up, and neither are his milestones. The pediatrician referred him to a specialist, who looked at his face and asked if his mother drank during her pregnancy. Heather does have a long history of alcohol abuse, and during her prenatal visits, she was counseled about not drinking. She swore she had stopped and would do nothing that might hurt her baby. I wonder if she lied. How could someone do this to an innocent child?

—*From the journal of Larissa Montgomery, nursing student*

One of the motivators to enter a health profession is a desire to want to help people. Health care providers often assume that clients are equally motivated to follow their advice and work toward improvement. Therefore, it can be frustrating when clients fail to follow treatment plans and continue engaging in behaviors that hurt rather than help. Their self-destructive behaviors, especially those that cause severe negative consequences, may be puzzling to the health professionals who care for them. "Why don't they just stop doing those things that cause them so much harm?"

In this chapter, we describe several types of destructive behaviors, including substance use disorders, eating disorders, self-injurious behaviors, and suicide. Because many of these behaviors occur in clients who have been mistreated as children or adolescents, we first briefly discuss the effects of family violence and abuse. Our goal is for the reader to recognize the signs and consequences of these behaviors and to develop strategies to refer and support clients, enabling them to receive and benefit from appropriate care.

# Family Violence and Abuse

Family abuse can take many forms. Neglect, which is failing to adequately provide for an individual's physical, medical, financial, and/or psychological needs, can cause extreme emotional harm. Abuse is "the experience of highly stressful events inflicted by another person that is beyond the individual's capacity to cope and that impairs the individual's sense of well-being. Abused persons' effectiveness in living and the quality of their relationships are also impaired" (Evans & Sullivan, 1995, p. 31). Abuse can be physical, psychological, sexual, or a combination of these aspects. Even if physical damage is not inflicted, emotional harm can result. For instance, yelling, criticizing, name-calling, and making fun of children's weaknesses can severely damage their self-esteem and confidence.

Typically, a stronger, more powerful individual exerts this abuse or neglect on a weaker or more vulnerable person. Infants, children, adolescents, spouses or partners, people who are elderly, and those with disabilities are often easier targets for abuse. In a significant number of children with disabilities, the abuse may actually precipitate the disability (Groce, 1988). Many abusers have been abused themselves and have not learned appropriate nurturing skills. Others may have a psychiatric disorder and/or abuse alcohol or drugs. The vulnerable individual may place significant stress or demands on the abuser that are beyond his or her ability to meet. Consider Vanessa, a fussy and demanding baby, the youngest of four children all living in a small home with their parents. During the day, her father worked two jobs, and her mother cared for the children. In the evenings, her mother went to work. After a long workday, her father could not tolerate Vanessa's continual need to be held and comforted. He would yell and slap her. One night, he went too far, and Vanessa ended up in the emergency room with multiple fractures.

While it is tempting to look for an easy formula to identify potential abusers, there are few clear descriptors because abuse occurs across the spectrum of lifestyles and family situations. Poor education, particularly that of the mother, lack of access to health care, inadequate nutrition, and lack of day care and social supports all increase the risk of family violence (Birns, 1988). Social isolation is another significant factor. Families who live in remote, rural areas may not have family and friends nearby. Others may live in dense, urban communities but lack connections to schools, churches, family members, or neighbors who can provide support. Many abusers consciously isolate the family from others to be able to exert greater control. In addition, drug and alcohol abuse frequently contribute to all types of abuse and neglect (Birns, 1988).

It is difficult to obtain accurate statistics on the incidence of family violence. These events usually occur behind closed doors, and participants make great efforts to ensure that they remain private, due to shame and fear of social or legal consequences. Furthermore, there is no consensus of an exact description or definition of problem behaviors that constitute the various forms of abuse (Ammerman & Hersen, 1992). There is, however, a consensus that abuse is underreported and underidentified. One survey estimated that as many as one in four women and one in seven men has been sexually abused, with one in three women never revealing the abuse (Evans & Sullivan, 1995).

Abuse is harmful in many ways, and "the psychological effects can be devastating at all stages of development" (Strauss, 1988, p. 3). Survivors of abuse show an array of emotional, behavioral, and physical symptoms at the time of the abuse and across the lifespan (Evans & Sullivan, 1995). Imagine how it feels to be a child whose parents do not provide adequate food or clothing and medical care when you are sick or who constantly yell at you and call you stupid and lazy. Physical and sexual assaults can cause profound damage (Strauss, 1988). Abused adolescents may manifest "acting-out" behaviors that can be self-destructive, provocative, and harmful to others. They may become truant from school, abuse alcohol and/or drugs, run away, become sexually promiscuous, or get into trouble with the law (Strauss, 1988).

Childhood abuse and neglect have been linked to adult psychiatric disorders. Research indicates that 40 to 70 percent of clients in psychiatric hospitals have histories of abuse and/or neglect (Ammerman & Hersen, 1992). Anxiety, posttraumatic stress disorder, depression, fear, and anger can be sequelae of childhood abuse and sexual molestation, affecting the survivor for a lifetime (Kessler et al., 1995). Personality, eating, and attention-deficit disorders, as well as self-injurious behavior and substance abuse, have been linked to abuse and neglect (Evans & Sullivan, 1995). In addition, survivors often have difficulty developing intimate relationships built on mutual trust, especially if there has been sexual abuse.

Although there is no federal law mandating the reporting of domestic violence, most states mandate that all health care professionals report suspected abuse and neglect of vulnerable individuals. In some states, though, this is directed at children under the age of 18, while others include the elderly and people with disabilities. As caregivers, we need to be vigilant about observing bruises, burns, and other unexplained injuries in our clients. We must also be aware that clients who appear to be undernourished, dehydrated, dirty, or poorly groomed may not be receiving proper care and may be neglected by their caregivers. Failure to make and keep medical appointments, administer medication, provide wound care, or change the client's position often enough is considered medical neglect.

As health care professionals, it is our responsibility to assure the safety of all clients and thoroughly document what we observe. If we are concerned, we need to find a way to spend private time with clients to ask if they feel safe and are receiving adequate care. We can open a dialogue by saying something like, "I am aware that domestic violence is commonplace, so I ask all of my clients these questions: Do you feel safe? Is anyone hurting you at home or anywhere else? Are you receiving adequate care? Is there anything I can do to help you?"

Clients may be reluctant to divulge information and deny a problem exists. However, if we suspect abuse or neglect, we must make referrals to the appropriate professionals. Most agencies that employ health care providers have standard procedures for documenting and reporting abuse or neglect. In addition, if you feel the client is not receiving the prescribed medical care, you need to inform the appropriate medical provider. In most states, failure to report suspected abuse or neglect can result in legal penalties or fines.

For more detailed information, you may consult the following websites:

1. www.acf.hhs.gov/programs/cb/publications/cm02/cm02.pdf—Child Maltreatment 2002. Administration on Children, Youth and Families, Department of Health and Human Services.

2. www.cdc.gov/ncipc/factsheets/ipvfacts.htm—Intimate Partner Violence: Fact Sheet. National Center for Injury Prevention and Control, Centers for Disease Control and Prevention.

3. www.ojp.usdoj.gov/ovc/ncvrw/2001/statover7.htm—Elder Abuse and Neglect. Office of Victims of Crime, Office of Justice Programs, U.S. Department of Justice.

# Substance Use Disorders

In modern United States culture, the use of mind-altering substances is rampant. Alcohol-related advertising and its catchy slogans seem to be everywhere. The media even informed the public that a former president of the United States admitted to trying marijuana. Although some individuals appear to ingest mind-altering substances without obvious ill effects, many others have significant negative consequences. In the discussion of substance use disorders, we use the term "drug" to refer to alcohol and all other psychoactive substances. Use of psychoactive substances can be classified into three categories: substance use, substance abuse, and substance dependence or addiction. Refer to Table 17–1 for the key elements of each.

## Use

Substance use disorders constitute the most commonly reported psychiatric diagnosis (American Psychiatric Association, 2000a). The lifetime risk for a substance use disorder is 15 to 20 percent. Two out of every three Americans reported using alcohol, and 35.6 percent admitted using illicit drugs (Schuckit, 2000).

Anthropologic data tell us that alcohol has been used for 8,000 years. Marijuana, peyote, cocoa leaves, and tobacco have been used for over 1,000 years, most commonly in religious rituals and ceremonies (Betz, Mihalic, Pinto, & Raffa, 2000). However, occasional recreational or ceremonial use of psychoactive substances does not constitute abuse. Although drug use may impair thinking or motor skills while the user is intoxicated, he or she may still be able to fulfill major life roles and function competently. A person whose substance use is under control tends not to risk job, family, reputation, or financial security for the short-term pleasure of being intoxicated.

TABLE 17–1   Key Elements of Substance Use, Abuse, and Dependence or Addiction

| Substance Use | Substance Abuse | Substance Dependence or Addiction |
|---|---|---|
| • Occasional recreational use<br>• Creates no problems for the user | • Person engages in dangerous activities<br>• Drug use causes significant problems at home, work, or school that may be personal, financial, and/or legal | • Includes problems of substance abuse<br>• Activities revolve around acquiring, using, and recovering from drug use<br>• Person is unable to control or curtail use<br>• Issues of tolerance and withdrawal |

## Abuse

All substances that can be potentially abused are considered drugs and can be taken through many routes, including drinking, eating/swallowing, inhaling, or injecting. Although each drug causes unique physical and psychological effects, intoxication occurs when the substance changes mood, behavior, perception, or judgment (Schuckit, 2000). The *Diagnostic and Statistical Manual IV—Text Revision* lists several categories of substances of abuse, including alcohol, cocaine and amphetamines (speed), caffeine, cannabis (marijuana), opiates (i.e., morphine and heroin), hallucinogens (i.e., LSD), inhalants, nicotine, sedatives, hypnotics, and anti-anxiety drugs (American Psychiatric Association, 2000a). Alcohol is the most frequently abused substance, and marijuana is the most frequently abused illicit drug (Winger, Hofmann, & Woods, 1992). Many individuals abuse more than one drug, a situation known as polysubstance abuse.

Substance abuse is a maladaptive pattern of drug use that causes significant impairment and distress (American Psychiatric Association, 2000a). It leads to difficulty performing major life role expectations at home, work, or school. The person often partakes in potentially dangerous activities while intoxicated, such as driving, skiing, flying a plane, fighting, unsafe sexual practices, or stunts or pranks. Someone with a substance abuse disorder continues to use the drug(s) of choice, despite persistent personal, social, or legal difficulties. The individual may lose a job due to repeated mistakes and absences, have conflicts with family members, and get arrested by police for driving under the influence or for disorderly conduct.

## Addiction

To be considered a dependence or addiction, drug use is compulsive, even when it results in serious negative consequences (Betz et al., 2000). Life revolves around the drug use, which becomes increasingly more difficult to control. An individual who is addicted spends considerable time obtaining the substance, using the substance, and recovering from use. Social, recreational, or occupational activities are sacrificed, with devastating consequences for the individual and family. Although there are persistent physical or psychological problems that the person knows are caused by the substance abuse, he or she is unable to curtail its use (American Psychiatric Association, 2000a). Drug dependence results in expensive social problems, such as lost time from work and foster care, costing millions of dollars annually in the United States (McLellan, Lewis, O'Brien, & Kleber, 2000).

Two other criteria to determine dependence or addiction involve the issues of tolerance and withdrawal. Tolerance for a substance develops with habitual use. It is evident when a person ingests large quantities of the substance without showing visible effects. After prolonged use, when the substance leaves the body, withdrawal symptoms develop. However, the inclusion of tolerance and withdrawal as criteria for addiction is controversial. Some people who abuse substances but are not addicted need increasing quantities of their drug(s) of choice to provide the desired results, and withdrawal of the substance causes extremely unpleasant effects (Schuckit, 2000).

Although substance use can become abuse, there is no simple progression to addiction. The addicted brain is neurobiologically different from the nonaddicted brain (Ketchum & Asbury, 2000). Researchers believe that different drugs use multiple neurochemical pathways in the central nervous system (CNS), and there are common effects. All addictive substances affect dopamine receptors that regulate pleasure responses. Stimulating these pleasure responses positively reinforces a pattern of drug-seeking behavior and causes withdrawal symptoms when the drug is no longer present in the body (Betz et al., 2000). These CNS effects can cause permanent changes in synaptic function that make abstinence and treatment difficult. This may also explain the addictive properties of less harmful substances or activities, such as chocolate, caffeine, sex, excessive Internet use, and gambling.

The effects of substance abuse and addiction can be devastating. People cause injury to themselves and others while under the influence of a drug. Employees, including stockbrokers, lawyers, and even health care professionals, may come to work with impaired judgment, secondary to drug use, and be unable to perform their jobs competently. Consider Donald, an accountant who was responsible for managing his clients' money and reporting taxes. When he developed a cocaine addiction, he was unable to support his habit on his own income and embezzled money from client accounts. Discovered during a routine audit, his actions cost him his job, home, family, and, ultimately, his freedom. He was imprisoned.

## Alcoholism

I have been working with Tom for the last three months trying to find an appropriate wheelchair and seating system for him. He's 26 years old and has a spinal cord injury at the sixth cervical level as a result of an automobile accident he caused while driving drunk. When he was referred to us, he had a deep pressure sore in the area of his left buttock that kept him from getting out of bed and into his old chair. He had been in bed for months and was very depressed.

My supervisor and I identified a seating system that allowed him to be out of bed for up to 6 hours a day without any signs of redness. Since he's been home, he's having problems again. He swears he's using the equipment the right way and limiting his use to 6 hours a day. Last night, I saw him steering his wheelchair into a local tavern. I wonder if this has anything to do with his current problem.

*—From the journal of Zack McIntyre, physical therapist student*

Alcohol is the most frequently used and abused drug in the United States. While many individuals use it without harm, its negative consequences cannot be underestimated. Three criteria are necessary to establish a diagnosis of alcoholism (Ketchum & Asbury, 2000):

- A large quantity of alcohol must be consumed over a number of years.
- There must be a chronic loss of control over alcohol use, with an inability to decrease its use.
- There must be significant negative effects on physical health and social functioning.

It is beyond the scope of this chapter to provide a detailed list of problems that develop as a result of alcohol abuse. However, literally every organ and system of the body is affected. Chronic alcohol use affects the cardiovascular system, causing hypertension, arrhythmia, and increased risk of stroke. In the digestive system, the liver, kidneys, stomach, and pancreas are affected. Risk is significantly increased for pancreatitis, gastritis, ulcers, diabetes, cirrhosis, and cancer. The nervous system is affected by loss of nutrients, leading to brain damage, with memory loss and poor judgment. Chronic alcohol abuse can also cause peripheral neuropathies (Ketchum & Asbury, 2000).

It is no surprise that people with alcohol-related problems use more health care resources than others and utilize 10 to 50 percent of hospital beds (Epperly & Moore, 2000). Unfortunately, when they are ill or hospitalized for an alcohol-related disorder, many health care providers fail to recognize the antecedent problem and do not question them about substance use and abuse. This omission causes a missed opportunity for intervention.

Health-related effects of alcohol are not limited to the poor health of the person who uses the substances. There is a clear link between alcohol and all forms of trauma (Maull, Kinning, & Hickman, 1984). Even in moderate amounts, alcohol can have profound effects on a developing fetus, causing low birth weight, social and learning problems, and fetal alcohol syndrome (Olson et al., 1997). Alcohol abuse affects spouses, children, friends, emotional support and caretaking, employment, income, and leads to family violence and emotional abuse. The personal costs are enormous and may last a lifetime.

Accidents and violent crimes are also frequently associated with alcohol use. As a result of alcohol-impaired drivers, thousands of deaths annually occur in motor vehicle accidents, with millions of resulting injuries (Schuckit, 2000). For example, between 25 and 49 percent of clients with spinal cord injuries were intoxicated at the time of their injury. These clients are also more likely to have difficulty adhering to rehabilitation plans. Therefore, they have a higher incidence of medical complications, such as urinary tract infections and pressure sores (McKinley, Kolakowsky, & Kreutzer, 1999).

It is important for health care professionals to know the signs and medical consequences of alcohol abuse so it can be diagnosed and the appropriate treatment recommendations made. If alcohol abuse is suspected, there is a simple, cost-effective screening tool called CAGE. This acronym gets to the heart of the problems and involves asking the client four questions (Epperly & Moore, 2000):

- **C**ut—Have you ever tried unsuccessfully to **C**ut down your drinking?
- **A**ngry—Does it make you **A**ngry when people suggest that you stop drinking?
- **G**uilty—Do you feel **G**uilty when you drink?
- **E**ye-opener—Do you need an **E**ye-opener to get started in the morning?

This questionnaire is easy to administer. Two or more "yes" answers are a signal for the care provider to open a dialogue with the goal of encouraging treatment.

One possible source of intervention might be attendance at a meeting of a peer support group, such as Alcoholics Anonymous. In addition, Al-Anon helps families and friends who have been affected by someone else's drinking by providing understanding, hope, and strength. Alateen, a part of Al-Anon, is for young people who have been affected by the problem drinking of a friend or relative.

There is a complex relationship between substance use disorders and psychiatric disorders. It has been estimated that as many as 50 percent of people with psychiatric disorders abuse alcohol or other drugs (Marsden, Gossop, Stewart, Rolfe, & Farrell, 2000; Moore et al., 1989). In a study of clients seeking psychiatric care for personal difficulties, 60 percent were found to have both a substance abuse disorder and a personality disorder (Skodol, Oldham, & Gallagher, 1999). In the psychiatric population, polydrug use is common. Some clinicians have hypothesized that the use of psychoactive substances is a way of "self-medicating" to at least temporarily ameliorate distressing psychiatric symptoms. Unfortunately, psychoactive substances frequently exacerbate the psychiatric disorder. Clients who have dual diagnoses of psychiatric and substance use disorders are more difficult to treat and must receive care for both disorders (Najavits & Weiss, 1994). Conversely, substance use can cause psychiatric symptoms and disorders or trigger an escalation of symptom severity. For example, depression is frequently seen in clients who abuse alcohol and other drugs (American Psychiatric Association, 2000a; Ketchum & Asbury, 2000). Because substance use and withdrawal produce symptoms that mimic psychiatric diagnoses, a differential diagnosis may be difficult to establish when a client presents with behavior that is "out of control."

# Eating Disorders

Jayme is so thin! She came in for a nutritional assessment today because her family and her pediatrician are worried about all the weight that she has lost. When she was 13, she was a little chubby and was unhappy about it. Now, she has lost too much weight and is so frail, you can see all her bones and count her ribs. She still thinks that she's too heavy and worries about the little bit of fat that she carries on her hips. It makes her sick to think about food. To look at her, you'd think she's 12 instead of 15. Our measurements indicate she has only 4 percent body fat. I've heard about eating disorders, but I've never actually seen someone with one before.
—*From the journal of Christy Marks, nutrition student*

Eating disorders are a category of health challenges that include a broad range of behaviors, habits, and weight. At one end of the spectrum are individuals who are obese and at least 20 percent overweight (Greenberg, Chan, & Blackburn, 1999). At the other end of the spectrum are individuals with anorexia nervosa, who are at least 15 percent below ideal weight and may literally be starving to death (American Psychiatric Association, 2000b). Clients with bulimia nervosa are between the two ends of the spectrum. They tend to be in the normal weight range but have eating and weight control behaviors that are both physically and emotionally unhealthy. Because each of these disorders may have a different etiology, the treatment interventions differ.

Eating disorders, like other psychological and behavioral problems, are complex, and the cause is not clear. There are multiple factors that trigger the onset of the disordered eating or weight-maintenance behaviors, including brain chemistry, genetics, psychological issues, family factors, such as abuse and neglect, behavioral reinforcers, and activity/exercise level (American Psychiatric Association, 2000b). Stressful life events and attitudes about food and appearance are also factors. Persistent dieting is considered a risk factor for developing an eating disorder. Fifteen-year-old girls who diet are eight times more likely to develop an eating disorder than nondieters. Both dieting and fear of being fat have been documented in girls as young as 7 years of age (Ghaderi & Scott, 2000).

The brain, in particular the limbic system, is responsible for hunger, thirst, and feeling satisfied with the amount of food ingested. There is ongoing research related to brain mechanisms that control eating behaviors. For example, eating foods high in carbohydrates may flood the body with the amino acid tryptophan that in turn triggers the release of serotonin in the brain, causing a sensation of calmness and well-being, with appetite suppression (Wurtman & Wurtman, 1995). The neurotransmitters dopamine and norepinephrine have also been found to be involved in the control of food intake (Wolfe, 1998).

Currently, anorexia and bulimia are receiving a great deal of coverage in the press and popular literature. It is important to put these problems in perspective. Anorexia and bulimia occur in 1 to 4 percent of the population (American Psychiatric Association, 2000b). Obesity is a much more significant problem, occurring in 24 percent of men and 27 percent of women (Honig & Blackburn, 1994). All clients with disordered eating face health and quality-of-life problems that are a result of being over- or underweight or using unhealthy weight management behaviors.

## Anorexia

There is significant overlap between symptoms of anorexia and bulimia. "Weight preoccupation and excessive self-evaluation of size and shape are primary symptoms of anorexia and bulimia" (American Psychiatric Association, 2000b, p. 3). Fifty percent of clients with anorexia also exhibit symptoms of bulimia, and some clients may switch or alternate between different types of weight-restricting behaviors. In addition, clients with anorexia and bulimia often demonstrate symptoms of psychiatric disorders such as depression, which may occur in up to 55 percent of clients with eating disorders (Herzog, 1984).

Anorexia is an eating disorder that occurs when an individual refuses to maintain an appropriate body weight and is at least 15 percent below ideal weight for height and age. Refusal to gain weight is accompanied by an extreme fear of getting fat and a distorted perception of body size, weight, and appearance (American Psychiatric Association, 2000b). Anorexia does not cause a loss of appetite, but the loss of normal perception about appropriate body size and appearance causes the individual to severely reduce caloric intake.

Some people with anorexia control weight by stringently restricting the amount of food eaten. Others combine severe caloric restriction with binge eating, followed by purging through vomiting or use of laxatives and/or diuretics. Excessive exercising, to the point where it becomes obsessive, may also be used to burn "extra" calories that have been consumed (American Psychiatric Association, 2000b).

Anorexia typically begins in adolescence, when a young person, most often female, decides to diet to become more attractive. Many of today's role models, such as actresses and female rock stars, may be shockingly thin. They send a message that in order to be popular and successful, you need to be very thin (Wolfe, 1998). Furthermore, many popular activities encourage young people to have unrealistically thin bodies. Wrestlers, dancers, gymnasts, and ice skaters are all encouraged to keep their weight low, often without regard to health needs or risks.

Why do some adolescents progress from dieting to anorexia? Clients with anorexia often present with emotional and behavioral differences that may predispose them to developing this disorder. The young person with anorexia stands out not just for excessive thinness, but as an "isolated, self-absorbed, and otherwise wary, young woman" (Crisp, 1984, p. 210). Although there are boys with anorexia, it is a condition that is prevalent among girls. Family conflict or worries about reaching sexual maturity may also appear during adolescence and result in anxiety. Severe anxiety may trigger the client to begin abnormal eating behaviors because the client feels this provides some emotional control and can delay the onset of sexual maturity. Weight phobia is the cardinal symptom of anorexia and is at the core of the young person's avoidance of developing a mature body weight (Crisp, 1984).

Depression, anxiety, obsessions, perfectionism, and a rigid cognitive style, with lack of sexual interest, are frequently seen in clients with anorexia (American Psychiatric Association, 2000b). Some psychiatrists consider anorexia a form of self-destructive and suicidal behavior (American Psychiatric Association, 2000b). There are also numerous medical complications associated with anorexia, including loss of menstrual cycle (amenorrhea) in postpubescent women, hypotension, cardiac abnormalities and arrhythmia, dehydration, anemia, and osteoporosis. As many as 10 percent of people with anorexia die as a result of these medical problems, malnutrition, or starvation (Wolfe, 1998).

## Bulimia

Unlike the client with anorexia, a person with bulimia has a normal or near-normal body weight. However, eating behaviors are "chaotic," with extremely abnormal patterns of caloric intake and control. "The essential features of bulimia are binge eating and inappropriate methods to prevent weight gain" (American Psychiatric Association, 2000b, p. 589). Clients with bulimia may consume over 1,000 calories of food in less than 30 minutes (binging). Afterward, they may feel so distressed by this that they induce vomiting (purging). Between binges, clients with bulimia may restrict food or eat "normal" amounts. Excessive exercising, which can interfere with performing other life activities, is also common. Most clients are ashamed of their disordered eating patterns and hide this behavior from others (American Psychiatric Association, 2000a).

Clients with bulimia often manifest symptoms of depression, anxiety, poor impulse control, sexual conflicts, personality disorders, and have problems with intimacy. As many as 50 percent of clients with bulimia have reported being sexually abused, and approximately 30 percent have a substance use disorder (Wolfe, 1998). It has been suggested that during periods of food restriction, tryptophan intake is reduced, thereby lowering levels of serotonin in the brain. Perhaps because of the reduced amount of this neurotransmitter, which helps prevent depression, a majority of clients with bulimia show signs of depression (Wolfe, 1998).

Bulimia carries health risks that are less severe than those of anorexia and are usually not life-threatening. Because weight tends to be near normal, there are no severe weight fluctuations or starvation. However, bradycardia, hypotension, dehydration, hypoglycemia, and anemia can occur. Stomach acids from recurrent vomiting may affect the esophagus and oral area, including the teeth (Wolfe, 1998).

It may not be difficult to recognize an individual with anorexia, especially if the health provider asks the client to undress or checks the client's weight. There are often additional indicators of poor health, such as electrolyte imbalances, skin changes, cardiac abnormalities, or fatigue. In contrast, bulimia can be more difficult to identify, with the most visible signs on the hands or oral area as a result of self-induced vomiting. A careful health history, including questions about activity and exercise levels, may reveal unhealthy eating or weight maintenance behavior. "Psychiatric management forms the foundation of treatment for patients/clients with eating disorders and should be instituted for all patients/clients in combination with other specific treatment modalities" (American Psychiatric Association, 2000b, p. 1). Other treatments must be individualized to client needs and include nutritional counseling, individual or family psychotherapy, medication, behavioral therapy, and twelve-step programs.

## Obesity

Being thin is a desirable trait in contemporary U.S. society, and people may be well respected and admired by their peers for this attribute. However, the same does not hold true for those who are overweight. The social stigma and risks associated with obesity may be a greater disability than the physical health risks (Foster & Wadden, 1994).

There are strong cultural messages about the desirability of various physical traits. Although during the Renaissance Period, "Rubenesque" women were the height of fashion, they are considered obese by today's standards. There is often an inverse relationship between weight and social class in women. In developed countries, women of a higher socioeconomic status tend to have lower weight, and those of lower socioeconomic levels often weigh more. In contrast, the reverse is true in underdeveloped countries (Kumanyika, 1995). Discrimination against people who are overweight is omnipresent. It negatively affects social desirability and success in work, school, and life. Lessons are learned early. Children as young as 7 years old rated people who were overweight as lazy, stupid, and ugly (Foster & Wadden, 1994).

The health consequences of obesity affect morbidity and mortality. Multiple medical problems are caused or exacerbated by significant weight. Cardiac disease, hypertension, diabetes, gall bladder disease, metabolic and endocrine diseases, cancer, and strokes have all been linked to high weight. Excess weight loads put added stress on joints and increase the effects of arthritis and other joint dysfunctions. In addition, there are increased demands on the respiratory system, causing pulmonary problems, which can increase the risk of surgical procedures and anesthesia (Dwyer, 1994).

Why do people let themselves "get" so fat, and why can't they lose the weight once it is present? Obesity is affected by many factors, including genetics, culture, lifestyle and health behaviors, and socioeconomic and situational issues (Hayward et al., 2000). Women tend to gain weight during pregnancy, and it is difficult to return to previous patterns of eating and exercise. As people face increasing career and relationship responsibilities and demands on their time, they may become more sedentary, which can contribute to decreasing metabolism. Over the years, it is not unusual for people to gain weight. Because metabolic rates slow with age, weight becomes more difficult to lose. Endocrine imbalances and other diseases may play a role in achieving and maintaining an ideal weight. Finally, many medications, especially psychotropic drugs, can cause weight gains as a side effect of their therapeutic actions (Greenberg et al., 1999).

Although it is tempting to assume that individuals who are seriously overweight have psychological problems, research does not strongly support this premise. Psychological testing does not reveal any significant differences between obese and nonobese persons (Foster & Wadden, 1994). However, clients who are morbidly obese, more than 100 percent overweight, do have psychological difficulties. Black, Goldstein, and Mason (1992) found a significant incidence of mood and anxiety disorders, bulimia, and tobacco dependence. In addition, clients who are morbidly obese, a group that comprises only 1 percent of obese persons, may have extreme difficulty with mobility due to their weight and require the use of specialized beds and other equipment, such as specially fitted wheelchairs. Some people may be unable to leave their homes.

Once weight is gained, it can be extremely difficult to lose. Current literature supports a three-pronged approach to weight loss for clients with mild obesity, generally considered to be 20 to 40 percent overweight. This includes diet, exercise, and behavior-management techniques. For clients with moderate obesity, there is no clear indication of the "best" treatment, but for morbid obesity, surgical procedures, such as stomach stapling, appear to be most successful (Stunkard, 1992).

Clients often have an overly optimistic view of how much weight can be lost and how quickly the loss can occur. It is realistic to expect a 10 to 15 percent weight loss over a period of six months to a year. While clients may be disappointed by this "modest" loss, losing even 10 percent of body weight can significantly improve health and lower risk factors for diabetes, heart disease, and hypertension (Greenberg et al., 1992).

Most weight loss regimes include exercise or increased physical activity to promote weight loss. While this makes intuitive sense, the benefits of exercise are not always definitive. Although some studies clearly indicate a good outcome, others show little or no benefit (Fox, 1992; Greenberg et al., 1992; Whatley & Poehlman, 1994). Studying the effects of exercise on weight loss and maintenance of the loss is difficult because of many variables, including duration of activity, degree of energy expended, and type of exercise, such as aerobic or nonaerobic and high or low resistance activities. Many people who are overweight are unaccustomed to physical activity and may lack coordination and motor skills. Some consider exercise to be aversive, and it may be difficult to elicit and maintain adherence to programs. Research is working to identify biochemical triggers for appetite and eating. Finding a safe medication to promote weight loss is alluring for many people, but at this time, there is no "magic pill."

It is especially important for health care professionals who promote exercise and healthy lifestyles to be supportive and sensitive of clients who are overweight who come to them for care. Entering a gym amidst trim people who are comfortable exercising, and often wearing form-fitting attire, can be difficult for those who want to work on an obesity problem. They may need to exercise in a more private area, receive a modified exercise program, or individualized instructions. Providing extra praise for efforts to exercise and reinforcement for small successes may help sustain motivation and retention.

Health care professionals need to be alert to the signs, symptoms, and consequences of eating disorders. Many clients will present with health problems or diseases that are directly caused or amplified by disordered eating. They may also be suffering from emotional distress as a result of their eating habits, their weight, or a life event that triggered unhealthy patterns of eating and weight control. If we are aware of signs and symptoms of eating disorders, we can ask nonjudgmental questions that can help identify potential problems. Making appropriate referrals to mental health or medical professionals who specialize in eating disorders and weight management can help clients adjust to healthier eating patterns and weight and improve health and life satisfaction.

# Self-Injurious Behavior

All of the disorders we have discussed in this chapter can be considered self-injurious. Family violence does not physically harm the perpetrator but causes emotional harm by destroying relationships and putting the individual at risk for legal consequences. Substance abuse and eating disorders cause harm to the client but may not cause visible tissue damage or injury. The physical effects of disordered eating behavior may take many years to develop. However, there is a cluster of disturbing behaviors that result in immediate, direct, physical harm.

Self-injurious behaviors, also called self-mutilation or self-harm, are a complex group of behaviors that involve an individual causing direct physical harm to him- or herself, without intending to commit suicide. Seen more often in women, self-harm typically begins in adolescence. It has been reported in clients not only with a history of sexual abuse but also those with posttraumatic stress, borderline personality, and affective disorders. Many clients who harm themselves also have other self-destructive behaviors, such as eating and substance abuse disorders.

This behavior is a symptom, not a diagnosis, and is seen in heterogeneous groups of clients and settings, frequently in clients with psychiatric disorders, eating disorders, and prison populations (Favaro & Santonastaso, 1999, 2000; Favazza, 1998). Self-injurious behavior, or self-mutilation, is classified into three distinct types of behaviors—major self-mutilation, superficial or moderate self-mutilation, and stereotypical self-injurious behavior (Favazza, 1998). The range of behaviors is both lengthy and shocking. Cutting, burning, biting, head-banging, eye-gouging, skin-picking or scratching, and hair-pulling are classic behaviors. At the extreme end of the self-injurious behavior continuum are clients who cause enucleation, castration, or even amputation (Winchel & Stanley, 1991). It has been suggested that excessive body piercing and tattooing may also be forms of self-mutilation in mainstream U.S. culture. Why would someone do this to him- or herself?

Major self-mutilation is a particularly horrifying form of self-harm. It consists of extremely bloody acts that cause permanent or severe damage, such as removing one or both eyes or other body parts. These acts are most commonly committed by clients who are in a psychotic state and may be "hearing" commands or experiencing hallucinations. People who are extremely intoxicated may also cause severe self-harm. When the clients' minds clear, they are aghast at what they have done (Favazza, 1998).

Superficial or moderate self-mutilation describes behaviors that cause pain but do not inflict permanent injury, such as nail-biting, hair-pulling, scratching, cutting, or burning. This set of behaviors, particularly burning and cutting, are the most common. They have been reported in a diverse group of clients with various psychiatric disorders but are not psychotic (Favazza, 1998). Many clients who exhibit moderate self-harm have been sexually abused. Disorders of mood, personality, eating, and substance use are also reported (Dallarm, 1997; Favazza, 1998; Winchel & Stanley, 1991). These individuals are vulnerable and emotionally fragile.

Stereotypical self-injurious behavior refers to behaviors that are repetitive, rhythmic, and monotonous, as is sometimes seen in individuals with certain types of autism and mental retardation. Many of these actions are "mild," such as rocking, spinning, or twirling. However, head-banging, eye-poking, self-biting, and repetitive hitting are also common. One young man with autism repeatedly hit himself in the left eye, causing so much trauma he developed an infection. The eye needed to be surgically removed (Favazza, 1998).

These stereotypical self-injurious behaviors tend to occur most often in clients who have mental retardation or some types of autism. In the past, they were referred to as self-stimulating behaviors. Because autism and mental retardation are notable for producing abnormal sensory control and processing functions, clients respond atypically to normal levels of stimuli. They may be easily overwhelmed or feel understimulated. Self-injurious behaviors may represent a way of regulating or responding to abnormal sensory perceptions (Reisman, 1993).

Clients with psychiatric disorders who cause intentional self-harm often feel either significant emotional pain or numbing. Some clients report feelings of agitation or distress, and the physical act of the self-injurious behavior calms them. Other clients describe being in a dissociative state prior to cutting themselves, and seeing blood or feeling pain reconnects them to reality. The actual cutting is reported to be relatively painless, and seeing blood brings relief (Dallarm, 1997; Pies & Popli, 1994; Winchel & Stanley, 1991). "As I started to cut, the physical pain and blood became a welcome distraction. As I cut deeper, my mind began to feel relieved of the torment, my body eased of the tension, and I began to feel comforted" (Winchel & Stanley, 1991, p. 308). Inflicting self-harm causes pain that triggers the release of endorphins, the body's internal pain-reducing drugs, modulating the emotional pain. It provides a mechanism to regulate emotions or release tension (Dallarm, 1997).

Because there are multiple emotional and biological mechanisms causing self-injurious behavior, multiple approaches to treatment are needed. Behavioral therapy, especially applied behavior analysis, has been shown to be most effective with clients who have mental retardation, autism, or other biological disorders. For clients who cause severe self-harm while in an altered mental state due to psychosis, antipsychotic drugs are prescribed and can prevent further self-harm by stabilizing the underlying psychiatric disorder. For the majority of clients who self-injure using moderate or superficial means, treatment options are varied and need to be individualized to the client situation. Psychotherapy, various behavioral therapies, support groups, and medication can all be helpful (Favazza, 1998).

However, before therapy can begin, we need to identify clients who need assistance. Clients are generally ashamed of their self-injurious behavior and take great pains to conceal it or provide excuses for how they became injured. Health care providers need to be extremely sensitive and nonjudgmental to encourage open communication about these behaviors. We can provide physical and emotional support after an episode of injury to make the client comfortable and continue competent medical care. Making a referral to a mental health professional is an essential component of that care. Clients can be assisted in finding alternate, healthier means to deal with the tension or stress they may be feeling prior to self-injury. When we work with people who self-injure, we must take care "to be present and to listen to someone disclosing information that can be difficult for clients to articulate and clinicians to hear" (Connors, 1996, p. 207).

In the past, self-injury was frequently erroneously determined to be a suicide attempt. At first glance, all attempts to self-injure may appear to be suicidal gestures or suggest suicidal intent. In fact, most self-injurious behavior is not severe enough to be life-threatening and is characteristically an adaptive coping mechanism, intended to ameliorate emotional pain and obtain help (Connors, 1996).

## Suicide

The ultimate act of self-injury is suicide, a permanent solution to a temporary problem. Virtually all clients who attempt suicide have a psychiatric and/or substance abuse disorder. Suicide is more likely to occur if a psychiatric and substance abuse disorder are both present because impaired judgment may cause the clients to act impulsively, without regard to consequences (Surgeon General, 1999).

I have been taking an abnormal psych course this semester, and yesterday, the instructor discussed the symptoms of depression. When I was in high school, my best friend committed suicide, and none of us could figure out why. Her life seemed so perfect. She was smart, pretty, and a good athlete. Now, I see that she had all the symptoms of depression. Why didn't some adult notice? Why couldn't anyone have helped her? I feel so sad to know this could have been prevented.
—*From the journal of Susan Lockhart, speech-language pathology student*

Unfortunately, many clients send out distress signals that do not get heard. We are often quick to assume that "all teenagers act like this," or "of course, he's acting withdrawn; his wife recently died." Most people are not trained to recognize symptoms of psychiatric disorders, and many who seek care are not appropriately diagnosed. Half of all people who attempt or complete suicide have visited a health care provider in the month prior to their attempt, and the provider failed to recognize the risk or offer supportive treatment (Surgeon General, 1999).

The Surgeon General's *Call to Action to Prevent Suicide* (1999) identifies several characteristics of individuals who successfully complete suicide. The "successful suicide" is most likely to be a white male at either end of the age spectrum—adolescent or elderly. While females make more attempts than men, males are four times more likely to be successful. Males also tend to use more violent methods. For both genders, access to a gun is a major risk factor for completing suicide.

There are several situational factors that make an individual a greater suicide risk. As noted above, mental illness, especially depression, and substance abuse are known risk factors. Individuals who live alone or are socially isolated are at particularly high risk. Poor health, lack of social supports, and stressful life events may also trigger a suicide attempt (Glod, 1998).

Clients who verbalize feeling helpless, hopeless, and worthless or have excessive guilt are a concern, especially if they are socially withdrawn or isolated. Other examples of critical cues of suicide risk are giving away beloved items, voicing a plan, or becoming suddenly brighter in affect. Some clients state that they wish they were dead or want to die. In this case, health professionals need to ask the clients if they have a suicide plan. If they answer yes, the professional needs to determine if the clients have the means to carry out the plan. When a client has the intent, the plan, and the means to attempt suicide, the provider must summon immediate mental health intervention and keep the client under observation until help arrives.

This is an area where all health care providers can intervene and literally save someone's life. As with substance abuse, all clients can be screened during regular health care visits for symptoms of emotional distress or disorders by asking a few simple questions, such as those in the BATHE questionnaire (Lieberman, 1997, p. 5):

- **B**ackground—"What's going on in your life?"
- **A**ffect—"How do you feel about that?"
- **T**rouble—"What about the situation troubles you the most?"
- **H**andling—"How are you handling that?"
- **E**mpathy—"That must be very difficult."

We can ask how things are in their personal lives and if anything is bothering them. If problems are identified, we can ask clients if they have the resources to handle the situation and offer assistance finding appropriate supports. Once again, sensitive, nonjudgmental questioning and listening are essential to allow clients to feel sufficiently safe to talk about their feelings and discuss problems that may threaten their health or well-being. It can be difficult knowing what to say or how to recommend mental health care. Letting clients know that you care and are worried about them and that you want to make sure they are safe is a good place to start.

## SUMMARY

In this chapter, we have discussed destructive behaviors that put the clients' well-being at risk, including family violence, substance abuse, eating disorders, and other self-injurious behaviors. It can be difficult to broach these subjects during a client interview and find ways to effectively discuss them. Sometimes it seems easier to remain silent or pretend that these situations do not exist. However, the competent health care provider is concerned about all aspects of the client's health and welfare and needs to develop screening and referral strategies.

## REFLECTIVE QUESTIONS

1. Working with clients and families can be very challenging. This is especially true when you suspect that the family may be neglecting to provide adequate care or may be abusive.
   a. What are your feelings about families who are abusive or neglectful?
   b. What strategies could you use to help put your feelings aside and work effectively with families where abuse or neglect is present?
   c. What can you do to protect the vulnerable family member?
2. Alcohol and other drugs are readily available and frequently used. You or someone you know may have used them.
   a. How do you feel about drug and alcohol use? Under what circumstances might they be used?
   b. Based on your experiences, what behaviors or problems would indicate that someone has moved from substance use to abuse? What behaviors or problems would indicate that someone has moved from substance abuse to addiction?
   c. As a health care practitioner, you may need to suggest interventions for people with drug or alcohol problems. How will your personal experiences affect your judgment in making these decisions? What strategies do you think you could use to offer help?
3. Appearance and weight are important concerns in our culture.
   a. How will you be able to recognize a client with an inappropriate weight or with an eating disorder?
   b. How do you feel about people who are too overweight and those who are too underweight?
   c. Would these feelings affect your ability to work with a client?
   d. What strategies could you use to offer clients help with their weight or eating patterns?
   e. Think about your own values, beliefs, and behaviors around food. Would you be a good role model for your clients? Why or why not?

4. Clients sometimes intentionally harm themselves or attempt suicide. It can be shocking to discover these situations.
   a. How do you think you might feel about a client who you discover has been harming him- or herself?
   b. How do you think you might feel about a client who reveals that he or she wants to commit suicide?
   c. How might you respond to the client?
5. All the problem behaviors described in this chapter can trigger powerful emotions for us, particularly if we have had personal experiences with these problems.
   a. Are there any groups of clients with whom you think you might have difficulty working?
   b. How might you be able to manage your emotional responses to your clients and their behaviors and develop a therapeutic relationship?

## CASE STUDY

Samantha Davis is a junior in high school who excels academically and athletically. She is being admitted to an ambulatory surgicenter for day surgery. While taking the history and recording vital signs prior to the procedure, the nurse notes that Samantha's weight is well below the standard for someone her age and height, although she comments that she needs to lose a few more pounds. After the client disrobes, the nurse notices several scars that appear to be burnmarks on the inner thighs. The nurse is concerned and tells Samantha that there are things she will need to discuss with Samantha's parents. Samantha begins to sob and begs the nurse not to tell them anything because they will "kill" her if they find out she has any problems.

1. What could be possible explanations for all of the physical findings?
2. For a licensed health care provider, what is the role and the legal and ethical obligations to document and share this information?
3. If a student were the examining clinician, how would the role and legal and ethical obligations differ from those of a licensed health care provider?
4. Identify resources that could provide optimal care for Samantha.

## REFERENCES

American Psychiatric Association. (2000a). *Diagnostic and statistical manual IV—text revision* (4th ed.). Washington, DC: Author.

American Psychiatric Association (2000b). Practice guidelines for the treatment of patients with eating disorders (rev. ed.). *American Journal of Psychiatry, 157* (Suppl. 1), 1–23.

Ammerman, R., & Hersen, M. (1992). Current issues in the assessment of family violence. In R. Ammerman & M. Hersen (Eds.), *Assessment of family violence* (pp. 3–26). Canada: Wiley.

Betz, C., Mihalic, D., Pinto, M. E., & Raffa, R. B. (2000). Could a common biochemical mechanism underlie addictions? *Journal of Clinical Pharmacy and Therapeutics, 25,* 11–20.

Birns, B. (1988). The mother–infant tie: Of bonding and abuse. In M. Strauss (Ed.), *Abuse and victimization across the lifespan* (pp. 9–31). Baltimore: Johns Hopkins University Press.

Black, D. W., Goldstein, R. B., & Mason, E. E. (1992). Prevalence of mental disorder in 88 morbidly obese bariatric clinic patients. *American Journal of Psychiatry, 149,* 227–234.

Connors, R. (1996). Self-injury in trauma survivors. *American Journal of Orthopsychiatry, 66*(2), 207–216.

Crisp, A. H. (1984). The psychopathology of anorexia nervosa: Getting the "heat" out of the system. In A. J. Stunkard & E. Stellar (Eds.), *Eating and its disorders* (pp. 209–234). New York: Raven Press.

Dallarm, S. J. (1997). The identification and management of self-mutilating patients in primary care. *The Nurse Practitioner, 22*(5), 151–170.

Dwyer, J. T. (1994). Medical evaluation and classification of obesity. In G. L. Blackburn & B. S. Kanders (Eds.), *Obesity pathophysiology, psychology, and treatment* (pp. 9–39). New York: Plenum Press.

Epperly, T., & Moore, K. (2000). Health issues in men: Part II. *American Family Physician, 62*(1), 117–124.

Evans, K., & Sullivan, J. M., (1995). *Treating addicted survivors of trauma.* New York: Guilford Press.

Favaro, A., & Santonastaso, P. (1999). Different types of self-injurious behavior in bulimia nervosa. *Comprehensive Psychiatry, 40*(1), 57–60.

Favaro, A., & Santonastaso, P. (2000). Self-injurious behavior in anorexia nervosa. *Journal of Nervous and Mental Disorders, 188*(8), 537–542.

Favazza, A. R. (1998). The coming of age of self-mutilation. *Journal of Mental and Nervous Disorders, 185*(5), 259–268.

Foster, G. D., & Wadden, T. A. (1994). The psychology of obesity, weight loss, and weight regain: Research and clinical findings. In G. Blackburn & B. Kanders (Eds.), *Obesity pathophysiology, psychology, and treatment* (pp. 140–162). New York: Chapman and Hall.

Fox, K. R. (1992). A clinical approach to exercise in the markedly obese. In T. A. Wadden & T. B. Vanitallie (Eds.), *Treatment of the seriously obese patient* (pp. 354–382). New York: Guilford Press.

Ghaderi, A., & Scott, B. (2000). Coping in dieting and eating disorders. *Journal of Nervous and Mental Disease, 188*(5), 273–279.

Glod, C. (1998). Mood disorders. In C. Glod (Ed.), *Contemporary psychiatric-mental health nursing* (pp. 343–376). Philadelphia: F. A. Davis.

Greenberg, I., Chan, S., & Blackburn, G. L. (1999). Non-pharmacologic and pharmacologic management of weight gain. *Journal of Clinical Psychiatry, 60*(21), 31–36.

Groce, N. (1988). Special groups at risk of abuse: The disabled. In M. Straus (Ed.), *Abuse and victimization across the lifespan* (pp. 223–239). Baltimore: Johns Hopkins University Press.

Hayward, L. M., Nixon, C., Jasper, M. P., Murphy, K. M., Harlan, V., Swirda, L., & Hayward, K. (2000). The process of restructuring and the treatment of obesity. *Health Care for Women International, 21,* 615–630.

Herzog, D. B. (1984). Are anorexic and bulimic patients depressed? *American Journal of Psychiatry, 141,* 1594–1597.

Honig, J., & Blackburn, G. (1994). The problem of obesity: An overview. In G. Blackburn & G. Kanders (Eds.), *Obesity pathophysiology, psychology, and treatment* (pp. 1–8). New York: Chapman and Hall.

Kessler, R., Sonnega, A., Bromet, E., Hughes, M., & Nelson, C. (1995). Post-traumatic stress disorder in the national co-morbidity survey. *Archives of General Psychiatry, 22,* 1048–1060.

Ketchum, K., & Asbury, W. (2000). *Beyond the influence.* New York: Bantam Books.

Kumanyika, S. (1995). Cultural factors in desirable body shapes and their impact on weight loss and maintenance. In D. B. Allison & R. X. Pi-Sunyer (Eds.), *Obesity treatment* (pp. 79–83). New York: Plenum Press.

Lieberman, J. A. (1997). BATHE: An approach to the interview process in the primary care setting. *Journal of Clinical Psychiatry, 58*(Suppl. 3), 3–6.

Marsden, J., Gossop, M., Stewart, D., Rolfe, A., & Farrell, M. (2000). Psychiatric symptoms among clients seeking treatment for drug dependence. *British Journal of Psychiatry, 176,* 285–289.

Maull, K. I., Kinning, L. S., & Hickman, J. K. (1984). Culpability and accountability of hospitalized injured alcohol-impaired drivers. *Journal of the American Medical Association, 252*(14), 1880–1883.

McKinley, W. O., Kolakowsky, S. A., & Kreutzer, J. S. (1999). Substance abuse, violence, and outcome after traumatic spinal cord injury. *American Journal of Medical Rehabilitation, 78,* 306–312.

McLellan, A. T., Lewis, D. C., O'Brien, C. P., & Kleber, H. D. (2000). Drug dependence: A chronic medical illness. *Journal of the American Medical Association, 284* (13), 1689–1695.

Moore, R., Bone, L. R., Geller, G., Mamon, J., Stokes, E. J., & Levine, D. (1989). Prevalence, detection and treatment of alcoholism in hospitalized patients. *Journal of the American Medical Association, 262*(30), 403–407.

Najavits, L. M., & Weiss, R. D. (1994). The role of psychotherapy in the treatment of substance-use disorders. *Harvard Review of Psychiatry, 1994*(2), 84–96.

Olson, H. C., Streissguth, A. P., Sampson, P. D., Barr, H. M., Bookstein, F. L., & Thiede, K. (1997). Association of prenatal alcohol exposure with behavioral and learning problems in early adolescence. *Journal of the American Academy of Child and Adolescent Psychiatry, 36*(9), 1187–1194.

Pies, R. W., & Popli, A. P. (1994). Self-injurious behavior: Pathophysiology and implications for treatment. *Journal of Clinical Psychiatry, 56,* 580–588.

Reisman, J. (1993). Using a sensory integrative approach to treat self-injurious behavior in profound mental retardation. *American Journal of Occupational Therapy, 47*(5), 403–411.

Schuckit, M. (2000). *Drug and alcohol abuse.* New York: Kluwer Academic/Plenum Press.

Skodol, A. E., Oldham, J. M., & Gallagher, P. E. (1999). Axis II comorbidity of substance use disorders among patients referred for treatment of personality disorders. *American Journal of Psychiatry, 156,* 734–738.

Strauss, M. (1988). Family violence across the lifespan. In M. Strauss (Ed.), *Abuse and victimization across the lifespan* (pp. 1–8). Baltimore: Johns Hopkins University Press.

Stunkard, A. J. (1992). An overview of current treatments for obesity. In T. A. Wadden & T. B. Vanitallie (Eds.), *Treatment of the seriously obese patient* (pp. 33–44). New York: Guilford Press.

Surgeon General. (1999). *Call to action to prevent suicide* [Online]. Available: .surgeongeneral.gov/osg/calltoaction. Date accessed: 1/2/02.

Whatley, J. E., & Poehlman, E. T. (1994). Obesity and exercise. In G. L. Blackburn & B. S. Kanders (Eds.), *Obesity pathophysiology, psychology, and treatment* (pp. 123–140). New York: Chapman and Hall.

Winchel, R. M., & Stanley, M. (1991). Self-injurious behavior: A review of the behavior and biology of self-mutilation. *American Journal of Psychiatry, 148,* 306–317.

Winger, G., Hofmann, F., & Woods, G. (1992). A handbook on drug and alcohol abuse. New York: Oxford University Press.

Wolfe, B. (1998). *Eating disorders.* In C. Glod (Ed.), *Contemporary psychiatric-mental health nursing* (pp. 461–478). New York: F. A. Davis.

Wurtman, R. J., & Wurtman, J. J. (1995). Brain serotonin, carbohydrate-craving, obesity and depression: Nutrients, neurotransmitter synthesis, and the control of food intake. *Obesity Research, 3* (Suppl. 4), 477S–480S.

# ADDITIONAL READINGS FOR PART V

Armstrong, L., & Jenkins, S. (2000). *It's not about the bike.* New York: Berkley Books.

Bauby, J. D. (1999). *The diving bell and the butterfly.* New York: Random House.

Dorris, M. (1989). *The broken cord.* New York: Harper & Row.

Dubus, A. (1991). *Broken vessels.* Boston: David Godine.

Dubus, A. (1997). *Meditations from a moveable chair.* New York: Vintage Press.

Frank, A. (1992). *At the will of the body.* Boston: Houghton Mifflin.

Jamison, K. (1995). *An unquiet mind.* New York: Alfred A. Knopf.

Karp, D. (1996). *Speaking of sadness.* New York: Oxford Press.

Karp, D. (2000). *Burden of sympathy.* New York: Oxford Press.

Lydon, J. (1997). *Daughter of the Queen of Sheba.* Boston: Houghton Mifflin.

Manning, M. (1996). *Undercurrents: A life beneath the surface.* San Francisco: Harper Perenial.

Osborn, C. (2000). *Over my head: A doctor's own story of head injury from the inside looking out.* Kansas City, MO: Andrews McMeel.

Rose, L. (1995). *Show me the way to go home.* New York: Elder Books.

Sacks, O. (1990). *Awakenings.* New York: Harper Perenial.

Simon, C. (1997). *Madhouse.* New York: Penguin.

Slater, L. (1996). *Welcome to my country.* New York: Random House.

Slater, L. (1998). *Prozac diary.* New York: Random House.

Solomon, A. (2001). *The noonday demon.* New York: Scribner.

# Index

## A

Abuse
  caregiver, 95
  childhood, 337
  defined, 336
  elderly, 95
  family, 336–37
  sexual, 95, 347
  substance, 339, 340–41
Acceptance
  of change in body image, 189–91
  stage of grieving, 253
  of sudden-onset disability, 202
Accommodation, 49
Acculturation, 60–61
Acquired immune deficiency syndrome (AIDS), 13,
    169, 233
  healing process, spirituality as, 170
  loss associated with, 233
Active listening, 32–33
Activities of daily living (ADLs), 84, 116, 137, 280
Activity orientation, 63–64
Acupuncture, 63
Acute grief, 245, 246, 247
Acute loss, 235, 258
Acute or rapidly progressive diseases, 203–5
Acute pain, 300
  progressing to chronic pain, 300–301
Adaptation strategies, 269–79
  bereavement services, 277–78
  cognitive reframing, 270–71
  counseling, 273–76
  emotional and practical support, 272–73
  hope, 278–79
  meaning of life, 271–72
  support groups, 276–77
Adapting
  to changes in body image, 189–91
  to illness, 157
Addiction, substance, 339–40
Adherence. *See* Motivation and adherence
A dimension characteristics, 60
Adjustment, 203
  coping behavior, 264–69
  health care providers' role in, 269–79
  psychosocial adaptation strategies, 269–79
Adolescents
  with bipolar disorder, 322

caring for a parent, 91, 92
  depression among, 321
  eating disorders among, 343
  self-mutilation among, 347
  sexual abuse of, 337
  sexual development among, 216–17
  with spinal cord injuries, 185
  spirituality, benefits of, 165
  suicide among, 349
Adults
  with developmental disabilities, 198–200
  with facial disfiguration, 188
  home care for, 151
  with posttraumatic stress disorder (PTSD), 327
Advanced directives, 124
Advocacy
  by caregivers, 87–88
  client-provider, 121
Ageism, 9–11
Age of Autonomy, 110
Age of Bureaucracy, 110–12
Age of Justice, 112–13
Age of Paternalism, 108, 110
Age-related disability, 206–7
Alcohol, 338
  abuse of, 218
Alcoholics Anonymous, 341
Alcoholism, 340–42
  establishing diagnosis of, 340
  health-related effects of, 341
Altruism, 163
Alzheimer's disease, 85, 207, 236
American Medical Association, 113
American Nursing Association, 113
American Occupational Therapy Association, 113
American Physical Therapy Association, 113
American Speech-Language-Hearing Association,
    113
Americans with Disabilities Act (ADA), 303
Amyotrophic lateral sclerosis (ALS), 269, 270
*Anatomy of Melancholy* (Burton), 37
Anger
  associated with chronic pain, 300
  change in body image and, 188
  childhood abuse and, 337
  stage of grieving, 249–50, 253
Angina, 8
Anorexia, 244, 343–44
Anticipatory grief, 244, 245

Insomnia, 244
associated with chronic pain, 300
Institutionalized racism, 12
Instrumental activities of daily living (IADLs), 116
Integrative theory of bereavement, 254–55
Intelligence, interpersonal/intrapersonal, 4
Intergroup conflict, 45–46
Internalized racism, 12
International Center for the Integration of Health and Spirituality (ICIHS), 162, 163
International Classification of Impairments, Disabilities, and Handicaps (ICIDH), 117
Internet, 36, 139
Interpersonal
communication, 27
conflict, 44
intelligence, 4
Intervention programs, 150
Intimate zone, 64
Intragroup conflict, 45
Intrapersonal
communication, 27
intelligence, 4

## J

Justice, 5, 125–26

## K

Kant, Immanuel, 37
Kleinman, Arthur, 299
Kübler-Ross, Elisabeth, 253
Kurtzke's Status Disability Scale, 180

## L

Language
barriers, 41–42, 65–66
client-sensitive, 29
cultural differences, 65–66
Laryngectomy, 187
Latino/Hispanic cultures
activity orientation/environmental control and, 63
cross-cultural differences, 62t
health beliefs and practices, 70–71
poverty and, 67, 68
treatment of, bias affecting, 11, 12
Learning disabilities, 196
Learning styles, 138–39
Legal and ethical principles, 122–26
Legislation, disability rights, 148, 149t
Life's activities, 191
Limbic system, function of, 166–68
Listening
active, 32–33
selective, 42
Literature, adults with developmental disabilities, 198
Living will, 124
Locus of control, 132

Loss, 231–39
acute, 235, 258
age-related, 233
associated with chronic conditions, 234–35
current, 182
and grief, 186
for the health care professional, 237–39
of intimacy, 236
for the personal caregiver, 236–37
primary internal and secondary external, 233
prior, 182
response to, 231
types of, 232–34
Lou Gehrig's disease, 232, 269; *see also* Amyotrophic lateral sclerosis (ALS)

## M

Magnetic resonance imaging (MRI), 120
Major depressive disorder (MDD), 319
Malingering, 306–7
defined, 306
symptoms of, 306
worker's compensation and, 307
Mania, 323, 324
Manic episode, defined, 322
Maslow's hierarchy of needs, 197
Mastectomy, 187
Material culture, 58, 59
McGill Quality of Life Questionnaire, 205
Meals on Wheels, 88
Meaning of life, 271–72
Media, 36
Mediation, 51
Medicaid, 122, 305
Medical examination, 119
Medical Outcomes Study (MOS) Short From, SF-36, 115
Medical records, confidentiality of, 111
Medicare, 85, 112, 122
Medicine, culture of, 71–72
Meditation, 163, 164, 169
Men. *See* Gender differences
Menopause, 220
Mental illness, 316
and chronic health conditions, 297
clients with, bias affecting treatment of, 14–15
defined, 315–16
etiology of, 316
screening for, 317
spirituality as healing process, use of, 170
suicide associated with, 349
Mental retardation, 196
self-injurious behaviors associated with, 347
Mind/Body Institute at the Beth Israel Deaconess Medical Center, 164
Mind-body-spirit connection, 161–71
ancient insights and modern practices, 163–65
holism, 162–63
limbic system, function of, 166–68
pain and, 302
spirituality and, 163